PROFESSIONAL PARAMEDIC

MEDICAL EMERGENCIES, MATERNAL HEALTH & PEDIATRICS

STUDY GUIDE

VOLUME II

RICHARD BEEBE

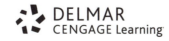

DELMAR
CENGAGE Learning

Australia • Brazil • Japan • Korea • Mexico • Singapore • Spain • United Kingdom • United States

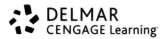

Professional Paramedic: Medical Emergencies, Maternal Health & Pediatrics Study Guide
Richard Beebe

Vice President, Career and Professional Editorial: Dave Garza

Director of Learning Solutions: Sandy Clark

Product Development Manager: Janet Maker

Managing Editor: Larry Main

Senior Product Manager: Jennifer A. Starr

Editorial Assistant: Amy Wetsel

Vice President, Career and Professional Marketing: Jennifer Baker

Executive Marketing Manager: Deborah S. Yarnell

Senior Marketing Manager: Erin Coffin

Associate Marketing Manager: Shanna Gibbs

Production Director: Wendy Troeger

Production Manager: Mark Bernard

Senior Content Project Manager: Jennifer Hanley

Art Director: Benj Gleeksman

For product information and technology assistance, contact us at
Cengage Learning Customer & Sales Support, 1-800-354-9706

For permission to use material from this text or product, submit all requests online at **www.cengage.com/permissions.** Further permissions questions can be e-mailed to
permissionrequest@cengage.com.

ISBN-13: 978-1-4283-2352-0
ISBN-10: 1-4283-2352-X

Delmar
5 Maxwell Drive
Clifton Park, NY 12065-2919
USA

Cengage Learning is a leading provider of customized learning solutions with office locations around the globe, including Singapore, the United Kingdom, Australia, Mexico, Brazil and Japan. Locate your local office at: **international.cengage.com/region**

Cengage Learning products are represented in Canada by Nelson Education, Ltd.

To learn more about Delmar, visit **www.cengage.com/delmar**

Purchase any of our products at your local college store or at our preferred online store **www.cengagebrain.com**

NOTICE TO THE READER
Publisher does not warrant or guarantee any of the products described herein or perform any independent analysis in connection with any of the product information contained herein. Publisher does not assume, and expressly disclaims, any obligation to obtain and include information other than that provided to it by the manufacturer. The reader is expressly warned to consider and adopt all safety precautions that might be indicated by the activities described herein and to avoid all potential hazards. By following the instructions contained herein, the reader willingly assumes all risks in connection with such instructions. The publisher makes no representations or warranties of any kind, including but not limited to, the warranties of fitness for particular purpose or merchantability, nor are any such representations implied with respect to the material set forth herein, and the publisher takes no responsibility with respect to such material. The publisher shall not be liable for any special, consequential, or exemplary damages resulting, in whole or part, from the readers' use of, or reliance upon, this material.

Printed in the United States of America
1 2 3 4 5 6 7 14 13 12 11 10

CONTENTS

PREFACE

We are pleased to offer a *Study Guide* to accompany *Professional Paramedic, Volume II: Medical Emergencies, Maternal Health, and Pediatrics*. Inside these pages you will find tools to help you practice and prepare for success in your Paramedic program, on the certification exam, and beyond.

Features

This Study Guide contains the following features.

Section I: Case Studies & Practice Questions

Divided by chapters, these features review the terms and concepts that are discussed in the corresponding chapter in the textbook.

- *Case studies* present a new scenario intended to reinforce content contained within each chapter. Like the case studies in the textbook, each of the cases includes critical thinking questions that prompt you to test your knowledge of the concepts presented in the case, and likewise the corresponding chapter. These activities help you develop and fine tune the decision-making skills that ultimately relate to treating patients in the field.
- *25 practice questions* per chapter allow you to practice your knowledge of the content presented in the textbook. Questions are asked in a variety of styles—multiple choice, short answer, and fill in the blank—to ensure that you master the content.

Section II: NREMT Skills for Paramedic Certification

This section contains the Paramedic skills that you will be tested on as part of the National Registry exam. You will want to practice the steps in the skills and ensure that you are confident you can successfully complete each skill prior to the exam.

Visit **http://www.nremt.org** for up-to-date information on the National Registry and certification exams.

Section III: Answers to Questions

The answers to the questions provided in this *Study Guide* offer you an opportunity to evaluate your knowledge of the terms and concepts presented in the textbook, *Professional Paramedic, Volume II: Medical Emergencies, Maternal Health, and Pediatrics*.

About The Technical Writer/Series Co-Authors

Richard Beebe, MS, BSN, NREMT-P

Richard Beebe is a Chief Training Officer for MedicThink, LLC. with over two decades of experience teaching Paramedics, over three decades of field experience, and continues to be a practicing field Paramedic with the Guilderland Police Department.

Dr. Jeff Myers, DO, EdM, NREMT-P, FAAEM

Dr. Myers is board certified in Emergency Medicine. He is currently on faculty at the State University of New York, University at Buffalo; and serves as the Associate System EMS Medical Director and EMS Fellowship Director at the Erie County Medical Center, where he is an active member of the physician response team. Dr. Myers is also the director of the Behling Simulation Center at the University at Buffalo.

Also Available

- *Professional Paramedic, Volume I: Foundations of Paramedic Care*/Order#: 978-1-4283-2345-2
- *Study Guide to accompany Professional Paramedic, Volume I: Foundations of Paramedic Care*/Order#: 978-1-4283-2346-9
- *Professional Paramedic, Volume III: Trauma Care and EMS Operations*/Order#: 978-1-4283-2348-3
- *Study Guide to accompany Professional Paramedic, Volume III: Trauma Care and EMS Operations*/Order#: 978-1-4283-2349-0

Please visit us at our *Online Companion* site for more learning tools for the *Professional Paramedic* series, as well as to view other EMS titles: **http://www.cengage.com/community/ems**

ACING THE CERTIFICATION EXAM: AN INTRODUCTION TO TEST-TAKING STRATEGIES

Introduction

Test time. Whether you are preparing for a certification test or a hiring test, the thought of an examination strikes fear in many people's hearts. The fear is so common that psychologists even have a diagnosis called test anxiety. However, testing does not have to be that way. Evaluations are simply an instrument to determine if you were effectively taught the information intended, or if you have the knowledge base necessary to do the job. That's all! If the purpose of testing is so simple, then why do so many people become so anxious when test time comes? Several factors play into test anxiety and why so many people have such fears of testing. However, these can be overcome. With the assistance of this guide, you too can be better prepared and calmer on examination day.

Test Obstacles

Test obstacles are issues that complicate test taking. If we view test taking as simply an avenue to determine the individual's comprehension of the material, then test obstacles are barriers to the process. There are many issues that may create test obstacles. We will discuss a few.

Mental

Mental test obstacles can sometimes be the greatest hurdles to overcome. Mental preparation for a test can be as important as intellectual preparation. So often, many people have failed an exam before they even begin. Issues that arise out of mental obstacles are:

- feeling unprepared
- feeling incompetent
- fear of taking tests
- fear of failure

Overcoming these obstacles can be your greatest asset when testing. Not allowing yourself to be beaten before entering the testing area can make the difference between success and failure on the exam.

Physical

Improper rest, poor eating habits, and lack of exercise can be some of the physical obstacles to overcome. When preparing for tests, always ensure that you get plenty of rest the night before, have a well-balanced meal before the test, and ensure you have a regiment of proper exercise. Physical obstacles are typically the easiest to overcome; however, they are the most overlooked.

Emotional

The emotional obstacles are often the most vague with which to deal. Much like mental obstacles, emotional obstacles can cause a person to do poorly on an exam well before they enter the room. Stress related issues that can interfere with test taking are:

- family concerns
- work-related concerns
- financial concerns

Emotional issues can cause a person to lose focus, cloud decision-making skills, and become distracted. Overcoming these obstacles requires a conscious effort to ensure that emotions do not interfere with the test.

Preparing to Take a Test

Before the Test

1. Start preparing for the examination. For certification exams, start the first day of class. You can do this by reading your syllabus carefully to find out when your exams will be, how many there will be, and how much they are weighed into your grade.
2. For certification classes, plan reviews as part of your regular weekly study schedule; a significant amount of time should be used to review the entire material for the class.
3. Reviews are much more than reading and reviewing class assignments. You need to read over your class notes and ask yourself questions on the material you don't know well. (If your notes are relatively complete and well organized, you may find that very little rereading of the textbook for detail is needed.) You may want to create a study group for these reviews to reinforce your learning.
4. Review for several short periods rather than one long period. You will find that you are able to retain information better and get less fatigued.
5. Turn the main points of each topic or heading into questions and check to see if the answers come to you quickly and correctly. Do not try to guess the types of questions; instead, concentrate on understanding the material.

During the Test

1. Preview the test before you answer anything. This gets you thinking about the material. Make sure to note the point value of each question. This will give you some ideas on how best to allocate your time.
2. Quickly calculate how much time you should allow for each question. A general rule of thumb is that you should be able to answer 50 questions per hour. This averages out to one question every 1.2 seconds. However, make sure you clearly understand the amount of time you have to complete the test.
3. Read the directions CAREFULLY. (Can more than one answer be correct? Are you penalized for guessing?) Never assume that you know what the directions say.
4. Answer the easy questions first. This will give you confidence and a feel for the flow of the test. Only answer the ones for which you are sure of the correct answer.
5. Go back to the difficult questions. The questions you have answered so far may provide some indication of the answers.
6. Answer all questions (unless you are penalized for wrong answers).
7. Generally, once the test begins, the proctor can ONLY reread the question. He/she cannot provide any further information.
8. Circle key words in difficult questions. This will force you to focus on the central point.
9. Narrow your options on the question to two answers. Many times, a question will be worded with two answers that are obviously inaccurate, and two answers that are close. However, only one is correct. If you can narrow your options to two, guessing may be easier. For example, if you have four options on a question, then you have a 25% chance of getting the question correct when guessing. If you can narrow the options to two answers, then you increase to a 50% chance of selecting the correct choice.
10. Use all of the time allotted for the test. If you have extra time, review your answers for accuracy. However, be careful of making changes on questions of which you are not sure. People often change the answers to questions of which they were not sure, when their first guess was correct.

After the Test

Relax. The test has been turned in. You can spend hours second-guessing what you could have done, but the test is complete. For certification tests, follow up to see if you can find out what objectives you did well and what areas you could improve. Review your test if you can; otherwise, try to remap the areas of question and refocus your studying.

Summary

Test taking does not have to be overwhelming. The obstacles to testing can be overcome and conquered through solid strategies and preparation. Initiating an effective plan, following it, and mentally preparing for a test can be your greatest tools to test success.

CASE STUDIES & PRACTICE QUESTIONS

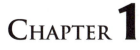

CHAPTER 1

DIAGNOSTIC ECG—THE 12-LEAD

Case Study

Chief Concern

Rocky's New Year's resolution was to lose weight, stop smoking, and go to the gym. At age 50, he knows that he can't live forever and has to start taking care of his health. After finishing his run at the gym, Rocky starts to head to the showers but stops along the way due to a wave of crushing substernal chest pain. Staffers at the gym call 9-1-1 and retrieve the AED before the Paramedics arrive.

Rocky is seated in the lobby, with a clenched fist on his chest, looking very pale and diaphoretic. The Paramedic recognizes the clenched fist as Levine's sign. Moving quickly, the Paramedic places the electrodes on Rocky for a quick rhythm check while the EMT checks his vital signs. Rocky is dismissing the pain as a "pulled muscle," and even though the monitor shows a normal sinus rhythm the Paramedic knows enough to get a 12-lead ECG.

Critical Thinking Questions

1. What indicators prompted the Paramedic to obtain a 12-lead ECG?

_____

_____

2. Based on the patient presentation, what type of myocardial infarction should be suspected and where would the ECG changes be seen?

_____

_____

Case Study Conclusion

The Paramedic properly prepares Rocky for the electrode placement and then asks him to lie down, arms to his side. The 12-lead ECG does not show any ST segment elevations but does show other ECG changes that concern the Paramedic.

Starting the standard medication regime, with oxygen first, Rocky is packaged for transport to the cardiac center. While en route, the Paramedic gives a full report including electronic transmission of the 12-lead ECG.

Critical Thinking Questions

1. Why would the 12-lead ECG not show ST elevations if the patient is experiencing a myocardial infarction in evolution?

_____

_____

2. What other ECG changes may have alerted the Paramedic to the potential for a myocardial infarction in evolution?

_____

_____

Practice Questions
Multiple Choice

Select the best answer for each of the following questions.

1. The mnemonic for treating a suspected MI is MONA. Which treatment comes first?
   a. morphine
   b. oxygen
   c. nitrates
   d. aspirin

2. Which of the following is NOT a typical presentation of a post-menopausal woman experiencing a myocardial infarction?
   a. chest pain
   b. unexplained weakness
   c. sudden diaphoresis
   d. shortness of breath

3. Which of the following leads is considered bipolar?
   a. Lead I
   b. aVL
   c. V1
   d. V4R

4. Which of the following leads does NOT look at the lateral wall of the left ventricle?
   a. Lead I
   b. aVL
   c. V1
   d. V6

5. Who originated the central terminal theory?
   a. Einthoven
   b. Wilson
   c. Goldberger
   d. Waller

6. What is the frequency range for a diagnostic ECG?
   a. 0.05 to 150 Hz
   b. 0.5 to 100 Hz
   c. 0.5 to 50 Hz
   d. 0.5 to 5 Hz

7. Which of the following will NOT create 60-cycle electromagnetic interference (EMI)?
   a. pulse oximeter
   b. malfunctioning ballast
   c. fluorescent lights
   d. poorly shielded ambulance convertor

8. Which of the following is NOT used to prepare a patient for an ECG?
    a. place patient in position of comfort
    b. clip the patient's chest hair as needed
    c. debride the patient's skin
    d. use antiperspirant

9. Which preparation for electrode placement reduces the skin's resistance the most?
    a. de-fatting the skin with an alcohol prep pad
    b. shaving the skin with a commercially prepared razor
    c. wiping the surface with a gauze pad to remove dirt
    d. debriding the skin with sandpaper

10. Which of the following is NOT shown on a standard 12-lead ECG?
    a. inferior wall
    b. right ventricle
    c. anterolateral wall
    d. common septum

11. What would ST segment changes in leads V1/V2/V3/V4 be called?
    a. pure changes
    b. mixed changes
    c. global changes
    d. diverse changes

12. Which coronary artery provides blood to the AV node in some 90% of the population?
    a. anterior coronary artery
    b. septal perforators
    c. right coronary artery
    d. circumflex coronary artery

13. Three changes in the ECG represent changes in the myocardium from coronary occlusion. What does ST elevation represent?
    a. insult
    b. injury
    c. infarction
    d. ischemia

14. Which of the following ECG changes is NOT consistent with ischemia?
    a. lengthening QT interval
    b. hyperacute T waves
    c. inverted T waves
    d. ST segment depression

15. Which of the following ECG changes is most suggestive of an anterior wall myocardial infarction?
    a. reverse R wave progression
    b. new onset left bundle branch block
    c. reciprocal changes
    d. widened QRS

Short Answer

Write a brief answer to each of the following questions.

16. Who standardized electrode placement?

_____

_____

17. What common mistake causes V1 and V2 to be placed too high?

_____

_____

18. Which electrode is placed "out of order"?

_____

_____

19. What does it mean to be "left dominate"?

_____

_____

20. What are reciprocal changes, which are most commonly seen in inferior wall myocardial infarctions?

_____

_____

Fill in the Blank

Complete each sentence by adding the appropriate word in the provided blanks.

21. Traditionally limb electrodes are placed at the _____ and _____; however, the Mason–Likar modification permits the electrodes to be placed on the _____ and _____.

22. The printout at the bottom of a four-channel ECG is called a _____ _____, emphasizing dysrhythmia analysis as first priority.

23. A positive deflection, followed by a negative deflection, then another positive deflection of the QRS is a _____ complex.

24. "Tombstone" ST elevations are seen in the _____ wall myocardial infarction.

25. Pathologic Q waves are _____ deeper than the R wave and _____.

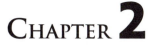
ACUTE CORONARY SYNDROME

Case Study

Chief Concern

"Jeez, Sam. You look terrible!" comments Bonnie, Sam's secretary. Sam—a middle-aged, overweight chain smoker—is pale, diaphoretic, and looks like he just ran a marathon, yet he has been sitting at his desk all morning. Not more than a couple seconds after the words are out of Bonnie's mouth, Sam starts to vomit into the garbage can next to his desk.

Bonnie, concerned that something serious is happening, says she is going to call emergency services. Sam waves her off, "It's only some food poisoning, I'll get over it," then he vomits some more. "Baloney," Bonnie replies, knowing he hadn't eaten all morning. "I am calling 9-1-1."

Paramedics Reba and Roger arrive to find Sam lying on the floor next to a garbage can. Though the report came in as "man vomiting," Reba is surprised by the scant amount of vomitus. Roger, while introducing himself, takes Sam's pulse and shoots a look at Reba. "I have no more than a beat a second."

Critical Thinking Questions

1. What are some of the possible causes of Sam's symptoms?

   _____

   _____

2. How can the bradycardia be related?

   _____

   _____

History

While Roger obtains a set of vital signs, Reba starts a medical history. Sam's symptoms started suddenly and without explanation. Although Sam continues to suggest food poisoning, he admits that he has not eaten anything that day, "just my usual, black coffee and a cigarette in the morning." He denies having any abdominal distress and states he does not have diarrhea. Changing course away from the abdominal etiology, Reba asks Sam about chest pain or shortness of breath. Sam denies both but offers a history including elevated cholesterol levels, treated with a "statin"; hypertension, treated with an ACE inhibitor; and a 40-plus year history of smoking that started in his early teens.

Critical Thinking Questions

1. What are the important elements of the history that a Paramedic should obtain?

   _____

   _____

2. What are the risk factors associated with coronary artery disease?

_____

_____

Examination

Roger's vital signs reveal a heart rate of 40 and a blood pressure of 120/98. The blood pressure puzzles Roger. Even though the patient stated he was on an ACE inhibitor for his blood pressure, he is hypertensive. Continuing with his examination, Roger notes no jugular venous distention; clear lung sounds apices to bases, and no hint of a murmur or ventricular gallop. However, Sam's abdomen is tender at the epigastrium, perhaps secondary to the vomiting, but is otherwise noncontributory. The patient does not have a hepatic jugular reflex and no peripheral edema is noted at the ankles.

Roger proceeds to place Sam on the ECG monitor, which immediately displays the bradycardia and an ST elevation in Lead II. Roger knows not to trust the monitor and elects to perform a diagnostic 12-lead ECG. While waiting for the 12-lead readout, Reba prepares for intravenous access. "What's that for?" Sam protests. Roger hands the 12-lead ECG to Reba and says, "The IV is for this." The 12-lead shows ST elevations in Leads II, III, and aVF.

Critical Thinking Questions

1. What are the elements of the physical examination of a patient with suspected acute coronary syndrome?

_____

_____

2. Why is a 12-lead ECG a critical element in this examination?

_____

_____

Assessment

Sam starts to get up, stating empathetically that he does not need to go to the hospital. As he sits up, he gets dizzy and lies back down. "Hmmm, Sam, maybe you should go to the hospital," Reba states. "It's not natural to get dizzy when you stand like that. Plus, your heart rate is questionable."

Critical Thinking Questions

1. Hemodynamically speaking, what is the significance of dizziness and the bradydysrhythmia?

_____

_____

2. What diagnosis did the Paramedic announce to the patient?

_____

_____

Treatment

Roger consults the pulse oximeter, which reads 95%. According to protocol, he administers oxygen 2 liters by nasal cannula. After ascertaining that the patient does not have an allergy to aspirin, Roger administers four 81 mg baby aspirin. Reba recognizes the treatment regime as MONA and cautions Roger that she wants to get venous access before giving any nitrates.

Critical Thinking Questions

1. What is the standard of care of patients with suspected inferior wall myocardial infarction?

_____

_____

2. Why did Reba want venous access prior to Roger's administration of nitrates?

_____

_____

Evaluation

While Reba obtains venous access, Sam complains of dizziness. Roger immediately leans over to grasp a radial pulse. It is gone. Roger is stunned. It seems as if Reba is clairvoyant. Moving to the carotid, where there is a pulse, Reba asks Roger to place an electrode in V4R while she does another primary assessment. While the patient is hypotensive, the lungs have rales (crackles) apices to base and the only notable finding is a loud machinery murmur appreciated in the left axilla.

Critical Thinking Questions

1. What are some of the predictable complications associated with an inferior wall myocardial infarction?

_____

_____

2. Why did Reba request V4R?

_____

_____

Disposition

Roger calls out to the driver to "light it up" as they proceed to the hospital. Over the din of the ambulance siren, Roger asks Reba what to do next. She asks for a second venous access and says, "Keep one eye on his breathing and his saturations."

Reba is already on the radio talking to the base hospital when Roger looks up after starting the venous access. Following her hand signal, Roger opens the second intravenous solution wide open as well and then reassesses the patient's blood pressure.

Critical Thinking Questions

1. What is the most appropriate transport decision that will get the patient to definitive care?

_____

_____

2. While en route, what treatments should be instituted?

_____

_____

Practice Questions
Multiple Choice

Select the best answer for each of the following questions.

1. Which of the following complaints is NOT associated with myocardial infarction?
    a. jaw pain
    b. headache
    c. shortness of breath
    d. nausea

2. What is the most common cause of myocardial infarction?
    a. embolus
    b. vasospasm
    c. aneurysm
    d. thrombus

3. Which mechanism will create a myocardial infarction in atrial fibrillation?
   a. embolus
   b. vasospasm
   c. aneurysm
   d. thrombus

4. Which mechanism will create a myocardial infarction in a patient with cocaine intoxication?
   a. embolus
   b. vasospasm
   c. aneurysm
   d. thrombus

5. A non-ST elevation myocardial infarction is diagnosed with all of the following EXCEPT _____.
   a. reciprocal changes
   b. troponin levels
   c. history
   d. ST elevation

6. Which condition can cause an almost instantaneous pericardial tamponade, which occurs in less than 1 minute?
   a. renal failure
   b. thoracic aneurysm
   c. malignancy
   d. pericarditis

7. Which of the following is NOT part of Beck's triad?
   a. hypotension
   b. jugular venous distention
   c. aortic murmur
   d. diminished heart sounds

8. What causes the vast majority of myocarditis cases?
   a. dental surgery
   b. intravenous drug abuse
   c. environmental poisons
   d. viral infections

9. Which of the following is NOT included in the classic symptom pattern for aortic stenosis?
   a. dyspnea
   b. ST elevations
   c. chest pain
   d. syncope

10. Stenosis of the pulmonary valve results in all of the following EXCEPT _____.
    a. pulmonary edema
    b. jugular venous distention
    c. hepatic distention
    d. peripheral edema

11. Patients with obstructive sleep apnea can develop what condition?
    a. chronic pulmonary embolism
    b. chronic obstructive pulmonary disease
    c. collagen vascular disease
    d. pulmonary hypertension

12. Which myocardial infarction is likely to present with atypical symptoms?
    a. inferior
    b. lateral
    c. septal
    d. anterior

13. Which of the following may NOT experience a silent myocardial infarction?
    a. diabetics
    b. obese
    c. women
    d. elderly

14. Which of the following is NOT a presentation sign for cresendo angina?
    a. increasing frequency
    b. relief with nitroglycerine only
    c. longer duration
    d. increasing intensity

15. Peripheral edema and jugular venous distention, with clear lung sounds, is most likely to be seen with which condition?
    a. anterior MI
    b. inferior MI
    c. posterior MI
    d. right ventricular MI

Short Answer

Write a brief answer to each of the following questions.

16. In simple terms, what is the mechanism that will create a myocardial infarction during hyperventilation?

    _____

    _____

17. What are the three ways that the coronary arteries can be revascularized?

    _____

    _____

18. Why would a myocardial infarction not show ST changes on the ECG?

    _____

    _____

19. Define unstable angina.

    _____

    _____

20. Name three of the six listed causes of pericarditis.

    _____

    _____

Fill in the Blank

Complete each sentence by adding the appropriate word in the provided blanks.

21. The coronary arteries fill during _____ when the _____ valve closes.

22. The other name for unstable angina is _____ angina.

23. Pulmonary edema occurs with _____ valve failure and not with _____ valve failure (hint: both are in the left ventricle).

24. The harsh murmur of aortic stenosis is best heard at the _____.

25. _____ or _____ is commonly used to deny myocardial infarction.

CHAPTER **3**

HEART FAILURE

Case Study

Chief Concern

As the alarm lights flash and the room lights come on, Nick looks over at the clock, which reads 2 a.m. As he slips on his pants and shoes, the squawk box bellows, "65-year-old male, sudden shortness of breath, history of cardiac disease, address 345 Old Irvine Manor, time out 0200 hours."

After sliding down the pole and leaping into the jump seat, Nick buckles up as the Q winds up and the engine goes screaming down the street. During the trip, Nick spends his time trying to figure out what could cause shortness of breath at 2 a.m. The engine's sudden lurch as they arrive at the house shakes Nick out of his mental fog. Jumping out of the engine, Nick approaches the front steps of the house and is greeted by an elderly woman who leads him to the second-floor bedroom. The patient is sitting next to an open window in a straight-back kitchen chair. Nick is struck by the sight and thinks, "It must be freezing outside."

Critical Thinking Questions

1. What are some of the possible causes of sudden shortness of breath?

_____

_____

2. How can a history of cardiac disease be related to shortness of breath?

_____

_____

History

The woman explains that her husband, Kareem, woke up from a sound sleep, which was not unusual as he normally woke up during the night to go to the bathroom. Tonight, though, he rushed to the window, opened it, and stuck his head outside. The rush of cold air woke her, and when she asked what was wrong all he could say was, "Get . . . help."

She notes that Kareem had been watching the late show, as he often did, but then decided to go to bed early, around midnight, because of a nagging nonproductive cough and fatigue. He admits that many nights he sleeps upright in a lounge chair because he has trouble walking up the stairs. Tonight, however, he was sound asleep in his bed when he suddenly awoke and couldn't catch his breath.

Kareem has an extensive past medical history that includes a lifetime of cigarette smoking (>40 pack/years), hypertension controlled by diuretics and ACE inhibitors, as well as being status post-coronary artery bypass graft (CABG). He suffered a heart attack five years ago, after which his doctor said he was lucky to be alive. Kareem denies syncope but admits to some chest heaviness that he attributes to his heavy breathing.

Critical Thinking Questions

1. What are the important elements of the history that a Paramedic should obtain?

_____

_____

2. What is the symptom pattern associated with a backward failure?

_____

_____

Examination

While the engine crew finishes taking the vital signs, Nick sets up the ECG monitor and obtains a quick 12-lead ECG. While scanning the 12-lead ECG, Nick's concentration is interrupted when the EMT whispers, "His pulse is funny." Following the lead, Nick reaches down and grasps the patient's pulse at the radial. Every time Kareem takes a deep breath, the pulse weakens.

"Heart rate 120, blood pressure 118/98, respiratory rate 28 and labored, pulse ox reads 90% on room air" the EMT calls out while Nick starts performing his head-to-toe examination. Kareem is open mouth breathing, a sign of air hunger or pain; his jugular veins are markedly distended; and there are diffuse wheezes as well as fine rales (crackles) at the base of the lungs. Nick remembers the department's training officer saying, "Not all that wheezes is asthma" during the last in-service. Straining to hear over the wheezes, Nick can definitely hear the ventricular gallop but does not appreciate any murmurs that would signify valve damage.

Moving to the abdomen, Nick palpates the left upper quadrant to try to elicit a hepatic jugular reflex. After he does, he assesses for abdominal tenderness, which Kareem does not have. Finally, Nick ends with an assessment of Kareem's ankles, noting there is no pedal edema.

Critical Thinking Questions

1. What are the elements of the physical examination of a patient with suspected heart failure?

_____

_____

2. Why is a 12-lead ECG a critical element in this examination?

_____

_____

Assessment

Although the EMT placed Kareem on high-flow, high-concentration oxygen, his respiratory distress does not seem to be appreciably improving. Nick calls for the crew to get the patient ready for transport, as the ambulance has just arrived.

Kareem reaches his hand out to Nick and says, "I feel like I am dying." Nick puts a reassuring hand on Kareem's shoulder and replies, "You've got a touch of heart failure but we can fix you right up, don't you worry." Nick marvels at how much more relaxed the patient seems with just a few encouraging words, a hand on the shoulder, and a hearty smile.

Critical Thinking Questions

1. What were the symptoms, in the symptom complex, that led the Paramedic to the diagnosis?

_____

_____

2. What diagnosis did the Paramedic announce to the patient?

_____

_____

Treatment

First things first, Nick thought. Although the patient's oxygen saturation remains above 90%, it is still cause for concern. That, coupled with the increasing dyspnea, convinces Nick to give the patient a trial of continuous positive airway pressure (CPAP). Nick had previously seen CPAP resolve mild cases of heart failure without any other interventions. Following that, Nick considered nitroglycerine.

Although Kareem's blood pressure is borderline, Nick remembers what the doctor had told the assembled Paramedics at the last CME: "Give nitroglycerine until your thumbs cramp and as long as the patient's pressure holds up."

Ever the cautious medic, Nick elects to start venous access first, just in case a bolus is needed. As he starts the venous access, the EMT gives the patient four baby aspirin, after inquiring if the patient has any allergies. With an IV in place, Nick administers the first nitro, asking the EMT to note the time of administration and reminding her that she needs to take vital signs every five minutes.

Critical Thinking Questions

1. What is the standard of care of patients with suspected heart failure?

_____

_____

2. Why was aspirin administered?

_____

_____

Evaluation

Despite the careful titration of the nitroglycerine (a total of three doses were administered), Kareem continues to deteriorate. Even with CPAP, his lungs continue to fill and his breathing becomes more labored. Nick elects to intubate Kareem using conscious sedation and provide positive pressure ventilation, coupled with PEEP. By intubating Kareem he can closely trend the end-tidal carbon dioxide levels.

Soon, the patient's pressure drops and Kareem starts losing consciousness. His MAP is less than 60 mmHg, and Kareem cannot afford any more fluids. While waiting for the last nitrate to wear off, to ensure the hypotension is not caused by the nitro, Nick starts a second venous access and hangs a dopamine drip. He decides to start the drip at the lower beta range and titrates carefully, every five minutes, to a mean blood pressure of 60 mmHg.

Critical Thinking Questions

1. What are some of the predictable complications associated with heart failure?

_____

_____

2. What are some of the predictable complications associated with the treatments for heart failure?

_____

_____

Disposition

Understanding the nature of the patient's condition, Nick elects to prioritize calling the hospital above providing other urgent treatments. Nick understands that he is just the first step in what is likely going to be a prolonged process of critical care.

Donning the headset, Nick describes the patient's condition, briefly explaining the reason for EMS, and asks for further instructions. The voice on the other end says, "Keep doing what you are doing. You are doing a great job and we will see you in ten."

Critical Thinking Questions

1. What is the most appropriate transport decision that will get the patient to definitive care?

   _____

   _____

2. What are some of the transportation considerations?

   _____

   _____

Practice Questions
Multiple Choice

Select the best answer for each of the following questions.

1. Which of the following conditions results in heart failure?
   a. volume overload
   b. increased vascular resistance
   c. ventricular dysfunction
   d. all of the above

2. What is the first effect of the sympathetic nervous system to hypotension?
   a. increased heart rate (chronotropy)
   b. increased force of contraction (inotropy)
   c. increased speed of contraction (dromotropy)
   d. increased ventricular tension (isotropy)

3. As part of the renin–angiotensin–aldosterone mechanism, aldosterone effects on the kidneys can lead to _____, thereby worsening heart failure.
   a. hyponatremia
   b. hypernatremia
   c. hyperkalemia
   d. hypokalemia

4. Which hormone is most likely to cause fluid overload in heart failure?
   a. vasopressin
   b. aldosterone
   c. renin
   d. angiotensin

5. What is the leading intrinsic cause of heart failure?
   a. myocarditis
   b. cardiomyopathy
   c. coronary artery disease
   d. toxicity from substance abuse

6. Increased volume load, leading to heart failure, can be due to all of the following EXCEPT _____.
   a. excessive sodium consumption
   b. renal failure
   c. acute hypertension
   d. cardiomyopathy

7. High output failure can be the result of all of the following EXCEPT _____.
   a. hyperthyroidism
   b. chronic anemia
   c. high fever
   d. renal failure

8. Which of the following restrictive diseases does NOT lead to heart failure?
   a. pericarditis
   b. pericardial tamponade
   c. cardiomyopathy
   d. tension pneumothorax

9. Which of the following is NOT a common patient complaint related to heart failure?
   a. headache
   b. shortness of breath
   c. syncope
   d. chest pain

10. Which of the following medications are NOT used to treat both heart failure and hypertension?
    a. nitrates
    b. digoxin
    c. angiotensin converting enzyme inhibitors
    d. beta blockers

11. Which of the following is NOT a leading cause of heart failure?
    a. sleep apnea
    b. diabetes
    c. hypertension
    d. myocardial infarction

12. Which of the following ECG rhythms can lead to heart failure?
    a. sustained ventricular tachycardia
    b. atrial fibrillation with rapid ventricular response
    c. Type I, third-degree heart block with junctional escape rhythm
    d. all of the above

13. Which form of edema is associated with heart failure?
    a. pitting
    b. nonpitting
    c. hard
    d. shiny

14. Which of the following is ECG evidence of left ventricular hypertrophy?
    a. absence of ST segment elevation during ischemia
    b. presence of elevated T waves
    c. exaggerated R waves in the precordial leads
    d. notched P wave

15. Which of the following is NOT a sign of right-sided heart failure?
    a. pulmonary edema
    b. nocturia
    c. jugular venous distention
    d. abdominal tenderness and ascites

Short Answer

Write a brief answer to each of the following questions.

16. What is the pathological progression of heart failure?

_____

_____

17. What is the progression of pulmonary changes in backward failure?

_____

_____

18. What is the pathological process of paroxysmal nocturnal dyspnea?

_____

_____

19. What are the six signs of heart failure?

_____

_____

20. What three abdominal signs are suggestive of heart failure?

_____

_____

Fill in the Blank

Complete each sentence by adding the appropriate word in the provided blanks.

21. A patient with a complaint of shortness of breath despite clear lung sounds and an adequate oxygen saturation may have _____ _____ _____.

22. The therapeutic goal of management of heart failure is to maintain _____ _____ _____.

23. When the ventricle chambers are reshaped, secondary to hypertrophy, this leads to decreased ventricular filling and _____ _____.

24. Patients with heart failure often have a pulse that is _____ and _____.

25. The sign of impending respiratory failure, secondary to heart failure, is _____.

CHAPTER **4**

ERRORS OF AUTOMATICITY

Case Study
Chief Concern

Sofia is the life of the unit at the nursing home. Since she was admitted some six months ago, the staff has become accustomed to her witty, good-hearted tweaks of the staff. Although Sofia is not a complainer, she asks to go back to bed right after breakfast one morning. As the nurse gets her back in bed she quickly grabs a pulse and finds it irregularly irregular. The nurse calls her attending physician and tells him that Sofia just doesn't seem right. The attending physician knows better than to question her, as she has a curious ability to divine problems intuitively, so he orders the transport.

Critical Thinking Questions

1. What are some of the possible causes of Sofia's weakness?

   _____

   _____

2. What is the implication of an irregularly irregular pulse?

   _____

   _____

History

The nurse explains that Sofia is an 87-year-old client who has been admitted for rehabilitation following a hip fracture. Her medical history is relatively scant considering her advanced age but does include osteoporosis and some renal failure.

Sofia is indeed very pleasant, preferring to sit up to greet her guests but feeling too weak to do so without assistance. Sofia says she felt fine yesterday but when she awoke this morning she felt "out of sorts" and dismisses her concerns with, "Oh I probably have a cold or something." She denies any chest pressure or shortness of breath. Although she admits to feeling dizzy when standing, she denies having passed out. Sofia does express some anxiety about the "fluttering" in her chest and admits to being a little frightened.

Critical Thinking Questions

1. What are the important elements of the history that a Paramedic should obtain?

   _____

   _____

2. What is the cause of the "fluttering" and why would it invoke anxiety?

   _____

   _____

Examination

With Sofia's permission, the Paramedic proceeds with a physical examination. Starting from the top, the Paramedic elects to do a baseline neurological examination, even though Sofia has no indications of neurological deficits, rather than a cardiopulmonary examination.

Sofia has mild JVD to the angle of her jaw and some fine rales (crackles) at the base of the lungs that clear with deep inspiration. Otherwise, her cardiac examination is noncontributory. The ECG monitor shows an irregularly irregular narrow complex tachycardia with a variable ventricular response between 120 and 140 beats per minute. The initial assessment of peripheral pulses, taken with the pulse oximeter, and the rate on the ECG monitor show a 30 to 40 beat per minute pulse deficit, which is a significant finding.

Critical Thinking Questions

1. What are the elements of the physical examination of a patient with suspected new onset atrial fibrillation?

_____

_____

2. Why is a 12-lead ECG a critical element in this examination?

_____

_____

Assessment

At first Sofia resists the idea of going to the hospital, though her protest is not vigorous. After the Paramedic explains that her heart is beating unnaturally and this could be the cause of her problem, she agrees to go get her heart "checked out."

Critical Thinking Questions

1. What were the symptoms, in the symptom complex, that led the Paramedic to the diagnosis?

_____

_____

2. What diagnosis did the Paramedic announce to the patient?

_____

_____

Treatment

While en route to the hospital, the Paramedic continues to monitor Sofia's heart rhythm as well as her pulse rate, noting the pulse deficit in the process. The Paramedic performs all of the routine procedures (i.e., O_2, IV, and ECG administration). After obtaining venous access, the Paramedic pulls the diltiazem from the drug box and places it next to the monitor, telling Sofia the drug is there "just in case."

Critical Thinking Questions

1. What is the standard of care of patients with suspected errors of automaticity?

_____

_____

2. What are some of the patient-specific concerns and considerations that the Paramedic should consider when applying this plan of care that is intended to treat a broad patient population presenting with atrial fibrillation?

_____

_____

Evaluation

As they continue en route, Sofia complains that she feels lightheaded. The Paramedic immediately reassesses Sofia and finds that she is neurologically intact, although her blood pressure has taken a nosedive. Although treatment with a calcium channel blocker would effectively lower the heart rate without converting the rhythm, effectively avoiding the risk of a thromboembolic event leading to stroke, the Paramedic decides that is a "big hammer" for a small nail. Instead, the Paramedic elects to use a small fluid bolus that would take advantage of Starling's law. Sofia's lungs are essentially clear and her pulse oximeter reading is greater than 95% on 4 lpm by nasal cannula, so it is a safe bet.

Patiently waiting for the fluid bolus to take its effect, and hoping Sofia is a brisk responder, the Paramedic reassesses Sofia's lungs every time vital signs are obtained.

Critical Thinking Questions

1. What are some of the predictable complications associated with atrial fibrillation with rapid ventricular response?

   _____

   _____

2. What are some of the predictable complications associated with the treatments for sustained wide complex tachycardia?

   _____

   _____

Disposition

Sofia responds to a small 250 cc fluid bolus, increasing both her blood pressure and her mentation. She exclaims she is "right as rain," and wants to go back to her friends at the nursing home. The Paramedic convinces her to at least say hello to the doctor. After all, he has already been introduced by radio and is expecting her. Always the lady, Sofia agrees.

Critical Thinking Questions

1. What is the most appropriate transport decision that will get the patient to definitive care?

   _____

   _____

2. What are some of the transportation considerations?

   _____

   _____

Practice Questions
Multiple Choice

Select the best answer for each of the following questions.

1. Which of the following will NOT accelerate automaticity?
   a. atropine
   b. hypoxia
   c. pain
   d. beta-agonists

2. Which of the following does NOT lead to a narrow complex tachycardia?
   a. cocaine
   b. methamphetamine
   c. digitalis
   d. epinephrine

3. Which of the following pathologic "hypo's" does NOT lead to increased automaticity in the sinus node?
   a. hypokalemia
   b. hypoglycemia
   c. hypoxia
   d. hypovolemia

4. Which syndrome of dysautonomia is seen in young women?
   a. syndrome of inappropriate sinus tachycardia
   b. syndrome of reflexive tachycardia
   c. autonomic dysfunction syndrome
   d. postural orthostatic tachycardia syndrome

5. What ECG finding distinguishes focal atrial tachycardia from sinus tachycardia?
   a. QT interval
   b. ST segment depression
   c. PR interval
   d. QRS width

6. A wandering atrial pacemaker is akin to a(n) _____.
   a. sinus tachycardia
   b. atrial fibrillation
   c. atrial flutter
   d. multifocal atrial tachycardia

7. Xanthine compounds have been implicated in wandering atrial pacemakers. Which of the following does NOT contain xanthine compounds?
   a. adenosine
   b. coffee
   c. chocolate
   d. theophylline

8. Which of the following can cause junctional ectopic tachycardia?
   a. AV node ischemia
   b. digitalis toxicity
   c. hypoxia
   d. cocaine

9. What is the most common dysrhythmia?
   a. atrial fibrillation
   b. ventricular fibrillation
   c. bundle branch block
   d. sinus arrest

10. Which of the following is NOT included in the three classifications of atrial fibrillation?
    a. uncontrolled atrial fibrillation
    b. multifocal atrial fibrillation
    c. paroxysmal atrial fibrillation
    d. persistent atrial fibrillation

11. Which of the following does NOT lead to digitalis toxicity?
    a. depression
    b. diarrhea
    c. diuretics
    d. drugs (i.e., Vaughn–Williams class I)

12. Which symptom of digitalis toxicity should alert the Paramedic to potential cardiotoxic effects and dysrhythmia?
    a. yellow-green halos around lights
    b. nausea and vomiting
    c. diarrhea
    d. lethargy

13. Which term describes an ectopic complex every other complex?
    a. bigeminy
    b. trigeminy
    c. quadrageminy
    d. quatrogeminy

14. A premature atrial complex may be the precursor for which of the following?
    a. multifocal atrial tachycardia
    b. sinus tachycardia
    c. atrial fibrillation
    d. accelerated atrial tachycardia

15. According to Lown's criteria, what are the most dangerous premature ventricular complexes?
    a. couplets
    b. multifocal PVC
    c. frequent PVC
    d. R on T PVC

Short Answer

Write a brief answer to each of the following questions.

16. What are the two origins of dysrhythmia and what is the importance of knowing these origins?

    _____

    _____

17. What are the three chemical factors most likely to influence errors of automaticity?

    _____

    _____

18. Name three suspected causes of atrial fibrillation.

    _____

    _____

19. What is the remarkable pharmacological property of digitalis?

    _____

    _____

20. What is the "cycle" of digitalis toxicity?

    _____

    _____

Fill in the Blank

Complete each sentence by adding the appropriate word in the provided blanks.

21. Understanding the concept of _____ is key to understanding errors of automaticity.

22. _____ _____ _____ is the result of enhanced automaticity of the bundle of His.

23. The key feature of an ectopic beat is _____.

24. The relationship between the premature complex and the preceding complex is called the _____ _____.

25. A Stokes–Adams attack is characterized by _____.

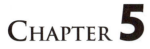

CHAPTER **5**

ERRORS OF CONDUCTION: TACHYCARDIA

Case Study

Chief Concern

The Paramedics receive a call regarding a middle-aged woman with syncope who is now complaining of feeling weak and dizzy and that her heart is racing. While en route, Jesse mulls over the potential causes of the patient's weakness and dizziness. Problems from hypoxia to hypoglycemia cross his mind, and he makes a mental note to check those out early on. However, it could also be a problem of hypotension. Remembering how his ACLS instructor had broken it down for him, it could be a problem of the pipes, pump, or fluids. Upon arrival, Jesse calls out, "Mrs. Beckerman!" She replies, "In here!"

Critical Thinking Questions

1. What are some of the possible cardiac causes of Mrs. Beckerman's weakness?

    _____

    _____

2. How can the dizziness be related?

    _____

    _____

History

Mrs. Beckerman is lying on the floor of her studio apartment, legs elevated, and is being attended to by a concerned friend. It seems that Mrs. Beckerman has been working long hours and is, as her friend put it, "just exhausted." In addition, Mrs. Beckerman had a fourth cup of coffee that morning and had even forgotten to eat.

She explains she was bending down to pick up a book from off the floor. When she sat up, she suddenly felt her heart start to race, causing a fluttering in her chest, and she "nearly passed out." She was gently assisted to the floor while her friend called emergency services.

At present, she is resting comfortably but feels dizzy whenever she sits up, which Jesse discourages her from doing. She denies any chest discomfort, shortness of breath, or even nausea, yet she appears pale and diaphoretic as she remains on the floor.

Critical Thinking Questions

1. What are the important elements of the history that a Paramedic should obtain?

    _____

    _____

2. What history would explain the diaphoresis?

_____

_____

Examination

While Mrs. Beckerman is talking, Jesse takes a routine set of vital signs and places her on the monitor. Her pulse oximeter reading is good. Although she is not a diabetic, Jesse checks her blood sugar anyway. Her heart rate at the radial pulse is faster than two beats a second and almost too fast to count, which the pulse oximeter confirms. A glance at the ECG monitor gives Jesse pause. The heart rate counter says 200 and a wide complex tachycardia of unknown origin appears on the monitor. Yet Mrs. Beckerman is awake and alert without complaints of shortness of breath or chest pain.

Critical Thinking Questions

1. What are the elements of the physical examination of a patient with suspected tachydysrhythmia?

_____

_____

2. Why is a 12-lead ECG a critical element in this examination?

_____

_____

Assessment

The ECG monitor shows a wide complex tachycardia of unknown origin. Because Mrs. Beckerman is stable, and therefore does not need immediate cardioversion, Jesse feels it prudent to obtain a 12-lead ECG so that the most effective treatment can be used. The 12-lead ECG shows an extreme left axis deviation as well as concordance, although he cannot discern P waves to make a statement about A/V dissociation. Nevertheless, he feels confident that he is dealing with a monomorphic ventricular tachycardia.

With the obvious implications of ventricular tachycardia, Jesse feels it is wisest to stay on-scene and provide supportive care, including gaining venous access and treating Mrs. Beckerman prior to transport. Mrs. Beckerman, sensing the anxiety in the room, asks why they aren't on their way to the hospital.

Critical Thinking Questions

1. What were the symptoms, in the symptom complex, that led the Paramedic to the diagnosis?

_____

_____

2. What diagnosis did the Paramedic announce to the patient?

_____

_____

Treatment

After obtaining venous access, Jesse hangs the amiodarone drip, 150 mg in 100 mL to run over 10 minutes, while continuously monitoring the patient for signs of hypotension, such as loss of consciousness and bradycardia. In this case, these signs would be a blessed relief.

Once the drip is established, as well as a secondary line, Mrs. Beckerman is strapped to the stretcher and moved to the ambulance. Jesse, anxious to see the results of his treatment, walks next to Mrs. Beckerman, making small talk while keeping a constant eye on the monitor for signs of change.

Critical Thinking Questions

1. What is the standard of care of stable patients with suspected ventricular tachycardia?

2. What are some of the patient-specific concerns and considerations that the Paramedic should consider when applying this plan of care that is intended to treat a broad patient population presenting with stable ventricular tachycardia?

Evaluation

Mrs. Beckerman is not responding to the amiodarone infusion as Jesse had hoped. Her monomorphic ventricular tachycardia remains. For a moment, Jesse considers overdrive pacing, and then remembers that is for polymorphic ventricular tachycardia. Mrs. Beckerman's level of consciousness is declining along with her blood pressure. Biting the bullet, Jesse elects to perform synchronized cardioversion.

Critical Thinking Questions

1. What are some of the predictable complications associated with a synchronized elective cardioversion?

2. What is the greatest risk in applying this plan of care?

Disposition

The elective synchronized cardioversion does the trick. Mrs. Beckerman converts into a normal sinus rhythm and within moments she awakens. Her first comment is, "Why does my chest hurt?" to which Jesse smiles and tells her he had to do something "dramatic," but that she is all right. Resting back on the stretcher, with Jesse's encouragement, Mrs. Beckerman closes her eyes as the ambulance pulls onto the ramp at the hospital.

Critical Thinking Questions

1. What is the most appropriate transport decision that will get the patient to definitive care?

2. What other concerns should the Paramedic have for this patient?

Practice Questions

Multiple Choice

Select the best answer for each of the following questions.

1. Which of the following dysrhythmias is NOT created by macrocircuits?
   a. atrial flutter
   b. atrial fibrillation
   c. atrial tachycardia
   d. AV nodal re-entrant tachycardia

2. Which of the following characteristics is NOT characteristic of Type I atrial flutter?
   a. flutter waves between 250 and 350 beats per minute
   b. regular block (i.e., 2:1 or 3:1 or 4:1)
   c. irregular ventricular response
   d. originate in the atria

3. Patients with a history of which condition are prone to atrial flutter?
   a. heart failure
   b. tricuspid regurgitation
   c. chronic obstructive pulmonary disease
   d. all of the above

4. What is the most common supraventricular tachycardia?
   a. atrial flutter
   b. atrial fibrillation
   c. A/V nodal re-entry tachycardia
   d. multifocal atrial tachycardia

5. Which of the following does NOT cause heart rates above 350 beats a minute?
   a. Type II atrial fibrillation
   b. Wolfe–Parkinson–White syndrome
   c. Long–Ganong–Levine syndrome
   d. A/V nodal re-entry tachycardia

6. Which of the following does NOT have congenital accessory pathways?
   a. A/V re-entry tachycardia
   b. A/V nodal re-entry tachycardia
   c. Wolfe–Parkinson–White syndrome
   d. Long–Ganong–Levine syndrome

7. What is the usual origin of ventricular tachycardia?
   a. ischemia
   b. prolonged QT
   c. sympathomimetics, such as cocaine
   d. mitral valve prolapse

8. Hypomagnesemia can lead to polymorphic ventricular tachycardia. Which of the following can lead to hypomagnesemia?
   a. alcoholism
   b. diuretics
   c. certain antibiotics
   d. all of the above

9. Polymorphic ventricular tachycardia is usually preceded by an ECG with which reading?
   a. elevated ST segment
   b. prolonged QT interval
   c. prolonged PR interval
   d. widened QRS

10. Which congenital cardiac conduction condition can lead to polymorphic ventricular tachycardia?
   a. Wolfe–Parkinson–White syndrome
   b. Romano–Ward syndrome
   c. Long–Ganong–Levine syndrome
   d. Cushing's syndrome

11. What is the most common symptom of tachydysrhythmia?
   a. palpitations
   b. chest pressure
   c. dyspnea
   d. dizziness

12. Which of the following vagal maneuvers should be avoided in the field?
   a. ice water immersion of the face
   b. Valsalva maneuver
   c. bearing down
   d. carotid sinus massage

13. What is the key ECG feature of a pre-excitation syndrome?
   a. shortened PR interval
   b. delta wave
   c. widened QRS
   d. prolonged QT interval

14. What ectopy is often a precursor to torsades de pointes?
   a. PAC
   b. atrial bigeminy
   c. PVC
   d. ventricular bigeminy

15. What is the first responsibility of a Paramedic when faced with a patient with a wide complex tachycardia of unknown origin?
   a. obtain a 12-lead ECG
   b. determine the origin
   c. determine if the patient is stable
   d. cardiovert

Short Answer

Write a brief answer to each of the following questions.

16. What are the two types of errors of conduction?

_____

_____

17. What is the underlying problem with tachycardias?

_____

_____

18. Explain how to perform the vagal maneuver called Valsalva and how it works.

_____

_____

19. Define a "rate related bundle branch."

_____

_____

20. What are the three steps to differentiate ventricular tachycardia from supraventricular tachycardia with aberrancy?

_____

_____

Fill in the Blank

Complete each sentence by adding the appropriate word in the provided blanks.

21. Typically a sustained sinus tachycardia cannot be maintained above 120 beats per minute, except for _____ _____ _____ _____.

22. Conduction down a pathway (anterograde) and up a pathway (retrograde) is called _____ conduction.

23. Both Wolfe–Parkinson–White and Long–Ganong–Levine syndromes are examples of _____ _____ _____.

24. Supraventricular tachycardias tend to stop and re-start _____ following vagal maneuvers whereas sinus tachycardia tends to stop and re-start _____.

25. When faced with a sustained tachycardia above 150 bpm, whether ventricular or atrial in origin, _____ is always an acceptable treatment.

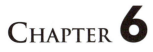

CHAPTER 6

ERRORS OF CONDUCTION: BRADYCARDIA

Case Study

Chief Concern

"I've fallen and I can't get up," Andre quips in a high-pitched voice. His partner Aimee looks at him quizzically. "It was a funny commercial for a life alert system in the 80s" Andre explains. Again, Aimee, a twentysomething-year-old Paramedic in her first year, gives him a sideways glance. "Forget it," Andre mumbles. "So, what was the nature of the call?" Their call is for an elderly female who has fallen. Security footage reveals that that she did not trip and witnesses say she was unconscious. As the field training officer, Andre's job is to put Aimee through her paces. "So, what do you think could be the cause of the syncope?" Andre asks as they arrive at the scene.

Critical Thinking Questions

1. What are some of the possible causes of cardiac-related syncope?

   _____

   _____

2. Why is the cause of the fall more important than the fall?

   _____

   _____

History

Mall security officers are already on-scene. The patient is laid down with an emergency blanket folded under her neck. Aimee winces as she looks at the folded blanket. If she has a cervical spine injury, the blanket can compromise the cervical spine. However, the lady's companion tells them that he was walking next to her, arm-in-arm, when she said she felt lightheaded. Before they could get to the bench, he felt her go limp and lowered her to the ground. He is sure that she didn't hit her head and there was not any seizure activity. He explains that he already told that to the officers. Aimee sighs in relief.

The patient, Mrs. Granger, has an extensive past medical history and an equally impressive list of medications that she keeps on a list in her purse. While fishing through her purse for the list, she explains that she suddenly became lightheaded. She denies chest pain, shortness of breath, or abdominal pain.

Reviewing the list quickly, Aimee notes a potpourri of medications from numerous doctors, from atropine-like eye drops to beta blockers and a host of vitamin supplements. From her study of pharmacology, she knows there is no way to figure out which medication—or combination of medications—may have caused or contributed to Mrs. Granger's syncope. Aimee resolves to treat the patient where she is.

Critical Thinking Questions

1. What are the important elements of the history that a Paramedic should obtain?

_____

_____

2. What is the symptom pattern associated with a bradydysrhythmia?

_____

_____

Examination

The first responders have already obtained a set of vital signs, which are all within normal limits. Mrs. Granger insists she is all right and wants to go on her way with her companion. However, Aimee is not satisfied. She wonders why Mrs. Granger isn't more tachycardiac with all this excitement? Are her medications stopping her heart from racing, or is there another issue?

Putting on a smile, Aimee asks Mrs. Granger if she can just place her on the monitor and give her a "quick checkup." Although both the gross neurological examination and the cardiac examination are noncontributory, the ECG is different as it shows the patient is dropping beats. Aimee reminds herself to get back to the first responders and remind them that regularity and strength of pulse is as important as the number.

Critical Thinking Questions

1. What are the elements of the physical examination of a patient with suspected bradydysrhythmia?

_____

_____

2. What is the advantage of a 12-lead ECG in this case?

_____

_____

Assessment

Closely examining the ECG, Aimee notes dropped beats, not even a P wave, and that the P-to-P interval changes the rhythm. That finding helps Aimee to suspect sick sinus syndrome. She decides she needs a 12-lead ECG and that the patient needs to go to the hospital, despite her protestations, for a possible pacemaker insertion.

Critical Thinking Questions

1. What diagnosis did the Paramedic announce to the patient?

_____

_____

2. Why is a 12-lead ECG a critical element in this examination?

_____

_____

Treatment

As the patient is not grossly symptomatic, and despite the high-degree heart block, Aimee elects to perform supportive care, including venous access, oxygen as needed, and an ECG monitor. Andre concurs, and Mrs. Granger is packaged for transport with a pulse oximeter, noninvasive blood pressure cuff, and ECG monitor in place.

Critical Thinking Questions

1. What is the standard of care of patients with suspected bradydysrhythmia?

   _____

   _____

2. What are some of the patient-specific concerns that the Paramedic should consider when applying this plan of care that is intended to treat a broad patient population presenting with bradycardia?

   _____

   _____

Evaluation

"Oh dear," Mrs. Granger exclaims, " I don't feel good." Simultaneously, Aimee grabs Mrs. Granger's radial pulse and looks at the monitor. The pulse is gone and the heart rate counter reads 30.

Mrs. Granger is still conscious, barely, and her blood pressure is "in the toilet." Andre suggests transcutaneous pacing. However, Aimee prefers a trial of atropine to see if that will hold her until she reaches the hospital. However, Andre knows that sooner or later Mrs. Granger will need the pacemaker.

The atropine appears to do the trick. Mrs. Granger's heart rate is climbing, so Aimee grabs a quick 12-lead ECG. This ECG shows ST elevations in the lateral leads. Aimee quickly surmises that Mrs. Granger is probably having a lateral wall myocardial infarction that originated in the circumflex and impacts the SA node.

Critical Thinking Questions

1. What are some of the predictable complications associated with an SA node infarction?

   _____

   _____

2. What are some of the predictable complications associated with the treatments for sustained wide complex tachycardia?

   _____

   _____

Disposition

As predicted, the atropine works for about 5 minutes. However, a repeat dose of 0.5 mg of atropine is ineffective. Mrs. Granger slips into a junctional escape rhythm but maintains a minimal perfusion pressure as evidenced by her mental status. Fortunately, the ambulance arrives at the hospital and Mrs. Granger is transported immediately to the interventional cardiology center, bypassing the emergency department, to an awaiting cardiologist. As she says goodbye to Mrs. Granger, she is thankful that they have bluetooth technology and are capable of transmitting the 12-lead ECG to the cardiologists.

Critical Thinking Questions

1. What is the most appropriate transport decision that will get the patient to definitive care?

   _____

   _____

2. Why would an interventional cardiology center be helpful?

   _____

   _____

Practice Questions

Multiple Choice

Select the best answer for each of the following questions.

1. Which of the following is NOT considered a diastolic disorder?
   a. tension pneumothorax
   b. cardiomyopathy
   c. pericardial tamponade
   d. dysrhythmia

2. Which of the following does NOT precede orthostatic hypotension?
   a. aura
   b. lightheadedness
   c. dizziness
   d. blurred vision

3. Which of the following is NOT considered an outflow obstruction?
   a. dysrhythmia
   b. aortic stenosis
   c. intracardiac tumor
   d. pulmonary embolism

4. Which of the following medications has NOT been implicated in sick sinus syndrome?
   a. metoprolol beta blockers
   b. diltiazem–calcium channel blockers
   c. procainamide–sodium channel blockers
   d. amiodarone–potassium channel blockers

5. What is the first sign of A/V ischemia?
   a. lengthening PR interval
   b. ST segment elevation
   c. bradycardia
   d. axis deviation

6. What is another name for Wenckebach's phenomena?
   a. Mobitz I
   b. classic heart block
   c. Mobitz II
   d. Type II second degree A/V heart block

7. What does dropped beats without a change in the PR interval of preceding beats suggest?
   a. Mobitz I
   b. classic heart block
   c. Wenckebach's phenomena
   d. Type I second degree A/V heart block

8. Which of the following is NOT a noncardiac cause of bradycardia?
   a. small bowel obstruction
   b. traumatic brain injury
   c. calcium channel blockers overdose
   d. hypothermia

9. Transcutaneous pacing has an American Heart Association class I indication for _____.
   a. prolonged asystole
   b. witnessed Type I first degree heart block
   c. witnessed asystole
   d. symptomatic bradycardia

10. What is another name for asynchronous mode pacing?
    a. demand pacing
    b. fixed mode
    c. sensing option
    d. permanent

11. Which of the following is NOT a sign of mechanical capture?
    a. spike followed by QRS on ECG
    b. improvement in patient mentation
    c. return of spontaneous circulation
    d. palpable blood pressure

12. Which of the following is NOT a circuit in the pacemaker's microprocessor?
    a. reed switch
    b. sensing
    c. pulse maker
    d. fail-safe

13. In the future _____ batteries will be used in pacemakers.
    a. nuclear
    b. biological
    c. lithium
    d. mercury–zinc

14. What is the code for a trancutaneous pacemaker?
    a. VVI
    b. DDD
    c. VOO
    d. DVO

15. What is the most common cause of pacemaker malfunction?
    a. failure to discharge
    b. depleted batteries
    c. failure to sense
    d. broken lead wire

Short Answer

Write a brief answer to each of the following questions.

16. Explain how bradydysrhythmias cause cerebral hypoperfusion.

   _____

   _____

17. Explain vasovagal syncope.

   _____

   _____

18. What is the distinguishing characteristic of a third degree heart block?

_____

_____

19. What are the two pacemaker pad placements?

_____

_____

20. What triad of symptoms is associated with pacemaker failure?

_____

_____

Fill in the Blank

Complete each sentence by adding the appropriate word in the provided blanks.

21. An infranodal block is also called a _____ _____ block.

22. A Stokes–Adams attack is the result of a _____ _____, as opposed to a sinus block.

23. The old name for a Type I second degree heart block is _____ phenomena.

24. The other name for overdrive pacing is _____ _____.

25. Elderly patients who accidentally disconnect their leads from the pacemaker by physically manipulating the pacemaker have _____ syndrome.

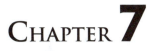

CHAPTER 7

CARDIAC RESUSCITATION

Case Study

Chief Concern

The din of the siren's wail almost drained out Dwayne's thoughts. The dispatcher's report had stated: "30ish-year-old male down at the YMCA with CPR in progress." Although there are many possible reasons for a cardiac arrest, Dwayne knows that younger people are less prone to have one. The ambulance pulled up on-scene.

Upon entering the Y, the crew is ushered into the center court. Looking around as he enters the room, Dwayne sees concerned teammates standing on the sidelines and a row of people crowding the rail on the indoor running track over his head. Dwayne groans, as he is not a fan of audiences at resuscitations. Looking forward toward the patient, Dwayne sees the bright orange AED next to the patient's head, someone doing compressions, and another person at the head of the patient with what appears to be a pocket mask. Dwayne quickly finds out the person doing compressions is a cardiologist.

Critical Thinking Questions

1. What is the importance of early bystander CPR?

   _____

   _____

2. What is the importance of early citizen defibrillation?

   _____

   _____

History

The story starts to come together. Fellow team members tell Dwayne how the patient was suddenly short of breath and went to one knee center court, clutching his chest as he suddenly collapsed. He was cyanotic and unresponsive. Dr. Putnam, the cardiologist, started doing compressions and a fellow ballplayer called for someone to get an AED and call 9-1-1.

Critical Thinking Questions

1. What is the importance of having an AED on-scene?

   _____

   _____

2. What is the implication of a "do not shock" warning from the AED?

   _____

   _____

Examination

Hurrying to the patient's side, Dwayne reaches down and confirms the adequacy of the CPR. CPR was started immediately upon the patient's collapse and has been continuous. Since it took the ambulance at least four minutes to get to the scene, the total elapsed time is between six to eight minutes. Dwayne is relieved the patient is still in the window of opportunity. The EMT on crew takes over compressions from an obviously exhausted bystander who leans over the EMT's shoulder and reminds him to compress often and deep.

While this is going on, Dwayne disconnects the AED and plugs the AED pads into his ECG monitor. One of the staffers from the YMCA says, "I think the AED might be broke. It said no shock advised and we got to him as soon as we could. It couldn't have been more than two or three minutes." Dwayne looks at the monitor and finds the answer to the question. The patient has an organized rhythm that is fast with a narrow complex. That's good news, Dwayne thought. He calls for an interruption in CPR to check the patient's pulse. After what seems like forever, Dwayne announces there is no pulse, and asks them to please continue the CPR.

Critical Thinking Questions

1. What are the causes of pulseless electrical activity?

   _____

   _____

2. Which of the causes of pulseless electrical activity can a Paramedic have an impact on while in the field?

   _____

   _____

Assessment

As Dwayne starts an intraosseous access in the patient's tibia, his partner prepares to intubate. While administering the first round of epinephrine and preparing a fluid bolus, Dwayne goes over the causes of PEA in his head, using the mnemonic ITCH PAD. The patient's color is still poor despite being ventilated and the EMT states it is getting harder and harder to bag the patient. Before the words escape the EMT's lips, Dwayne places his stethoscope on the patient's chest. Bingo! Dwayne thought, as he notes diminished breath sounds on the right side. Pulling a decompression needle from the venous access kit, Dwayne "darts" the chest. Almost instantly, the patient's color improves, as does his bag–mask compliance.

With hesitation and hope, Dwayne reaches for a carotid pulse. "We got one," Dwayne proudly announces. Dwayne knows it is time to change from resuscitation mode to post-resuscitation mode.

Critical Thinking Questions

1. What are the next priorities for the patient with a return of spontaneous circulation (ROSC)?

   _____

   _____

2. What is "reverse CPR"?

   _____

   _____

Treatment

Dwayne calls to the EMT, "Grab some ice packs and the stretcher and let's get this guy loaded up." Although therapeutic hypothermia is new to the crew, they have already seen one successful case: a 50-year-old cardiac arrest survivor who was a "suitcase carrier" (i.e., discharged neurologically intact). Dwayne is hopeful in this case. Even though the patient remains unconscious, he had a quick reversal so the brain damage should be minimal.

Critical Thinking Questions

1. What are the indications for therapeutic hypothermia?

_____

_____

2. What is the standard of care for therapeutic hypothermia status post-return of spontaneous circulation?

_____

_____

Evaluation

Although the patient's blood pressure stabilizes, Dwayne remains worried about rebound hypertension, a phenomena he saw in a previous ROSC. The antidysrhythmic ordered, amiodarone, is infusing and a 12-lead ECG is obtained and transmitted with a confirmation. Although the 12-lead ECG is negative for ST elevation, it does show a prolonged QT interval, which may be an effect of the amiodarone or may be the cause of the arrest. Dwayne doesn't know which. His therapeutic goal is to maintain the patient's blood pressure with a mean arterial pressure (MAP) greater than 65 mmHg, per his protocols, and an end-tidal between 35 and 45 mmHg.

Critical Thinking Questions

1. What are the hemodynamic parameters that the Paramedic should maintain?

_____

_____

2. How does the Paramedic maintain these hemodynamic parameters?

_____

_____

Disposition

The locals affectionately called the hospital "St. Elsewhere." Dwayne just knows that it is a cardiac center capable of accepting patients treated with therapeutic hypothermia in the field. They are met at the door by the cardiologist who started compressions. Still dressed in his sweat pants, he directs Dwayne and the crew to take the patient into the resuscitation room where a team is standing by.

Critical Thinking Questions

1. What is the most appropriate transport decision that will get the patient to definitive care?

_____

_____

2. Why was a 12-lead ECG indicated following the return of spontaneous circulation?

_____

_____

Practice Questions

Multiple Choice

Select the best answer for each of the following questions.

1. Which of the following is NOT a relative blood volume loss?
   a. gastrointestinal bleeding
   b. anaphylaxis
   c. systemic inflammatory response syndrome
   d. septic shock

2. Errors of automaticity can be caused by hyperkalemia. Which of the following is NOT a cause of hyperkalemia?
   a. acute renal failure
   b. Addison's disease
   c. hyperthyroidism
   d. diabetic ketoacidosis

3. What is the drug of choice for a beta blocker overdose?
   a. magnesium sulfate
   b. sodium bicarbonate
   c. high-dose intravenous glucagon
   d. atropine

4. What does the T in the mnemonic ITCH PAD stand for?
   a. tension pneumothorax
   b. thrombosis
   c. trauma
   d. tamponade

5. Purpura can be mistaken for all of the following EXCEPT _____.
   a. livor mortis
   b. dependent lividity
   c. petechiae
   d. rigor mortis

6. Which of the following is NOT included in the classic triad of death?
   a. unresponsiveness
   b. apnea
   c. pulselessness
   d. asystole

7. Which of the following will NOT increase the likelihood of success with defibrillation?
   a. inhalation of oxygen
   b. administration of epinephrine
   c. exhalation of carbon dioxide
   d. administration of sodium bicarbonate

8. What components make up a duty cycle?
   a. ventilation and compression
   b. compression and decompression
   c. adequate depth of compression
   d. two minutes of compression

9. In which situation is a precordial thump acceptable?
   a. witnessed asystole
   b. prior to CPR in unwitnessed arrest
   c. witnessed ventricular fibrillation
   d. pulsed ventricular tachycardia

10. What is the initial drug of choice in cardiac arrest?
    a. amiodarone
    b. lidocaine
    c. procainamide
    d. epinephrine

11. What is the first action when confronted with asystole?
    a. administer epinephrine
    b. endotracheal intubation
    c. confirm in two perpendicular leads
    d. establish venous access

12. What is the first action when confronted with pulseless electrical activity?
    a. fluid bolus
    b. epinephrine bolus
    c. atropine bolus
    d. amiodarone bolus

13. Which of the following antidysrhythmics should be administered following return of spontaneous circulation (ROSC)?
    a. amiodarone
    b. last effective antidysrhythmic
    c. beta blocker
    d. all of the above

14. Which of the following is an indication for termination of resuscitation?
    a. refractory ventricular fibrillation
    b. asystole despite standard medical treatment
    c. end-tidal carbon dioxide ($EtCO_2$) less than 10 mmHg
    d. all of the above

15. Which of the following does NOT need to precede a decision to terminate a resuscitation?
    a. confirmed asystole
    b. inclusion criteria for termination
    c. family wishes
    d. grief counseling

Short Answer

Write a brief answer to each of the following questions.

16. What are the four identifiable causes of cardiac arrest, from a mechanistic perspective?

_____

_____

17. What is the treatment regime for a tricyclic overdose?

_____

_____

18. What is the advantage of ventilating a patient with room air over ventilating a patient with exhaled air?

_____

_____

19. What are the immediate therapeutic goals of resuscitation during pulseless electrical activity?

_____

_____

20. What is the danger of hyperventilation and "air stacking"?

_____

_____

Fill in the Blank

Complete each sentence by adding the appropriate word in the provided blanks.

21. The goal of defibrillation is _____.

22. The danger of hyperventilation is _____ and a shift of the oxyhemoglobin curve.

23. To prevent gastric distention, _____ _____ (i.e., Sellick's maneuver) should be applied.

24. Both the CPR vest and the circumferential chest band depend on _____ _____ theory.

25. Biphasic defibrillation is intended to mimic the _____ _____.

CHAPTER **8**

DISORDERS OF OXYGENATION

Case Study

Chief Concern

"3 a.m. The only people up at this hour are truckers and cops," Adriana sighs as the ambulance pulls into the rest area next to the interstate. Although the throaty rumble of the trucks drowns out the ambulance siren, the flashing lights catch the eye of a trucker who waves them down. "He's in here!" he calls, pointing to the cab of a tractor–trailer. "We went to get him up for breakfast and he told us he couldn't breathe."

While perched on the step, Adriana peers into the cab. Sure enough, the fifty-something trucker sitting in the cab is a peculiar shade of blue. The color may be due to the lights, Adriana considers. She decides to get him out of the cab to make sure. Several other truckers climb into the cab and drag the patient, named Darin, out to the waiting stretcher.

Critical Thinking Questions

1. What are some of the possible causes of shortness of breath for a trucker?

_____

_____

2. Which of the possible causes of shortness of breath could be directly related to the patient being a truck driver?

_____

_____

History

Darin has been a long-haul trucker for the last 20 years. When he isn't trucking he hangs out with his fellow truckers late into the night. His eating habits are bad enough to make a cardiologist recoil. In addition, he smokes at least two packs of cigarettes a day, and thinks taking medicine for his hypertension is hogwash. Since he hurt his back helping to unload cargo, he has stopped doing any form of exercise and has subsequently gained 70 pounds, most of which is found on his midsection.

Lately, he has been having trouble with his sugar. Darin's doctor revealed he was a diabetic, and he recently had unexplained swelling in his legs that made it difficult for him to get into and out of the cab.

Darin says his trouble breathing came on all of a sudden as he got up to get out of the cab and that he is having chest pain that worsens with every breath. Darin has trouble completing his sentences because he keeps coughing.

Critical Thinking Questions

1. What are the important elements of the history that a Paramedic should obtain?

_____

_____

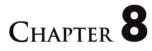

2. What is the symptom pattern associated with pulmonary embolism?

_____

_____

Examination

Adriana's primary assessment of Darin shows that he is stable for the moment. His lungs are clear apices to base, helping to eliminate the possibility of backward heart failure. Of greater concern to Adriana is Darin's borderline oxygen saturation, even though he is on high-flow, high-concentration oxygen. Admittedly, though, his cyanosis has cleared up, and his blood pressure is low for a man claiming to have a history of hypertension.

Turning to his legs, Adriana splits Darin's pant leg up the seam with her scissors. The left leg is visibly larger and a beefy red, suggesting that it is inflamed. Grasping his toes, she pushes upward, announcing "toes to the nose," to which Darin lets out a yelp and grabs his knee.

Critical Thinking Questions

1. What are the elements of the physical examination of a patient with suspected deep vein thrombus?

_____

_____

2. Why is a Homans' sign a critical element in this examination?

_____

_____

Assessment

Adriana lets Darin know that they are going to use the lights and siren. Without uttering a word, Darin waves Adriana off. He really didn't care. "I know that you are having trouble breathing and we are going to try to get you some help. Hang in there," Adriana says in an effort to comfort Darin. However, she isn't sure if her words are simply falling on deaf ears. Darin seems focused on his increasing difficulty breathing.

Critical Thinking Questions

1. What diagnosis did the Paramedic announce to the patient?

_____

_____

2. Why is a 12-lead ECG a critical element in this examination?

_____

_____

Treatment

Adriana sits Darin upright while adjusting his oxygen mask. He is obviously working hard to breathe. She considers using a nebulizer treatment and then realizes it will not really help the problem, which is on the circulatory side. She makes herself content with starting intravenous access and monitoring Darin while they are en route to the hospital.

Critical Thinking Questions

1. What is the standard of care of patients with suspected pulmonary embolism?

_____

_____

2. What additional treatment might be considered in this case?

_____

_____

Evaluation

Suddenly Darin passes out. Adriana finds a carotid pulse but not a radial one. Looking toward the ECG monitor, she notices Darin's oxygen saturation has plummeted, obviously meeting the downward slope of the oxyhemoglobin curve. He has slid into hypoxia that will be unresolved despite the administration of oxygen. Adriana prepares to intubate Darin, which is a daunting task considering Darin's size.

Critical Thinking Questions

1. What are some of the predictable complications associated with a pulmonary embolism?

_____

_____

2. What are some of the predictable complications associated with a saddle embolism?

_____

_____

Disposition

When they leave the scene Darin is awake and speaking to the Paramedics. However, en route he becomes unconscious. Darin's blue color also starts to return. Adriana intubates and ventilates him, then starts performing compressions. As the ambulance arrives at the hospital, Adriana continues with her "One–two–three" cadence as the ambulance driver opens the back doors. Quickly they wheel Darin into the hospital.

Critical Thinking Questions

1. What is the most appropriate transport decision that will get the patient to definitive care?

_____

_____

2. What are some of the transportation considerations?

_____

_____

Practice Questions
Multiple Choice

Select the best answer for each of the following questions.

1. Which respiratory disease is the result of structural damage to the alveoli?
   a. emphysema
   b. pulmonary edema
   c. asthma
   d. pulmonary embolism

2. What is the cause of the Bohr effect?
   a. lowered pH
   b. increased temperature
   c. oxyhemoglobin shift left
   d. increased carbon dioxide

3. Which of the following would NOT be considered an oxygen-poor environment (i.e., <21%)?
   a. grain silo
   b. ship hold
   c. sewer manhole
   d. high altitude

4. Which of the following is an oxygen gas that is "heavier than air"?
   a. ammonia
   b. natural gas
   c. carbon monoxide
   d. none of the above

5. Which of the following would be an extrapulmonary cause of alveolar hypoventilation leading to hypoxia?
   a. hyperthyroidism
   b. opiate overdose
   c. shock
   d. asthma

6. Which alveolar–capillary impairment would have clear lung sounds?
   a. pneumonia
   b. pulmonary edema
   c. pulmonary embolism
   d. asthma

7. Which of the following often leads to pulmonary embolism during childbirth?
   a. fat embolism
   b. air embolism
   c. thrombus formation
   d. amniotic fluid embolism

8. Which factors put a woman at risk for a pulmonary embolism?
   a. oral contraceptives
   b. obesity
   c. smoking
   d. all of the above

9. Which of the following is NOT part of Virchow's triad?
   a. infection
   b. venous stasis
   c. hypercoagulability
   d. inflammation

10. Which of the following will NOT cause a V–Q mismatch?
    a. pneumonia
    b. pulmonary embolism
    c. pulmonary edema
    d. asthma

11. Which of the following is NOT included in the classic triad of symptoms of pneumonia?
    a. fever
    b. night sweats
    c. cough
    d. shortness of breath

12. Patients with which of the following conditions are at risk for pneumonia?
    a. poliomyelitis
    b. myasthenia gravis
    c. muscular dystrophy
    d. all of the above

13. What is a collection of pus in the pleural space called?
    a. pneumonia
    b. consolidation
    c. empyema
    d. pneumocyst

14. False low oxygen saturations can occur with which substance?
    a. carboxyhemoglobin
    b. carbon monoxide
    c. methemoglobin
    d. methylene blue

15. Which of the following should NOT be used to treat patients with ARDS?
    a. higher concentrations of oxygen
    b. higher ventilation pressures
    c. lower ventilation volumes
    d. lower ventilation rates

Short Answer

Write a brief answer to each of the following questions.

16. Define Type I respiratory failure.

_____

_____

17. What is the traditional symptom complex for pulmonary embolism?

_____

_____

18. What are the ECG changes associated with pulmonary embolism?

_____

_____

19. What is the Fick equation?

_____

_____

20. How does CPAP/PEEP work?

_____

_____

Fill in the Blank

Complete each sentence by adding the appropriate word in the provided blanks.

21. The most common source of pulmonary embolism is _____ _____ _____.

22. Pain in the back of the knee with dorsiflexion is called _____ sign.

23. Hypoxia in the face of high-flow, high-concentration oxygen and clear lungs suggests _____ _____.

24. Pneumocystis jirovecii, formerly known as Pneumocystis carinii, pneumonia is most likely to be found in _____ patients.

25. The other name for shaking chills associated with pneumonia is _____.

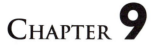

CHAPTER **9**

DISORDERS OF VENTILATION

Case Study
Chief Concern

As they wake up from their deep slumber, the crew can hear a cigarette smoker's hack from the front room. The experienced crew members knew that was a clear sign the boss was into work early again. Terrance, known as Terry by the crew, slowly rises to his feet. He has some questions to ask the boss and he knows from experience that the boss is most approachable in the morning.

Walking into the front office from the ambulance bay, he sees the boss leaning over. Stepping through the doorway, he notices that something is wrong. His boss isn't leaning over. Instead, he is tripod and his color is gray, not the deep tan Terry is used to seeing from all those vacations his boss took to the Cape. He really appears to have trouble breathing.

Critical Thinking Questions

1. What are some of the possible respiratory-related causes of shortness of breath?

   _____

   _____

2. How is the patient's shortness of breath possibly related to the early morning?

   _____

   _____

History

The boss has a smoking history that extends for over 40 years. He started smoking in the U.S. Army during World War II, when soldiers were encouraged to smoke during breaks; after all, cigarettes were part of the rations. He has matured his smoking habit to two and a half packs a day, and despite the rising costs of cigarettes always manages to find his "butts."

Critical Thinking Questions

1. What are the important elements of the history that a Paramedic should obtain?

   _____

   _____

2. What is the symptom pattern for Type II respiratory failure?

   _____

   _____

Examination

By now the duty crew has assembled and brought a stretcher into the room. Using the pulse oximeter, Terry notices that the reading is low despite the administration of high-flow, high-concentration oxygen by partial nonrebreather mask. This is an ominous sign.

Auscultation of the barrel chest reveals some faint wheezes over distant breath sounds. The boss is using all of his accessory muscles to breathe—strap muscles, intercostals, and even the diaphragm—as evidenced by the seesaw motion. All the while he looks like he is trying to whistle.

Critical Thinking Questions

1. What are the elements of the physical examination of a patient with suspected Type II respiratory failure?

_____

_____

2. What assessment tools are critical elements in this examination?

_____

_____

Assessment

The boss is not answering questions very quickly, and when he does the answers are monosyllabic. He also seems "out of it," as he keeps bobbing his head. In addition, the end-tidal CO_2 reading is high, very high. "Let's get him moving." Terry orders.

As the crew picks up the boss to put him on the stretcher, an inhaler falls out of his pants pocket. Picking it up, Terry shakes it and notices that it is empty even though the prescription is brand new.

Critical Thinking Questions

1. What is the significance of the elevated end-tidal carbon dioxide level?

_____

_____

2. What does the use of a rescue inhaler suggest?

_____

_____

Treatment

Fearing imminent respiratory arrest, Terry orders that his boss be ventilated, slowly and carefully, with a bag–mask assembly. While preparing his intubation kit for what seems like an inevitable intubation, Terry considers the boss's early morning statement made several months back. "Kid," he said, "I don't want to be intubated and I don't want to be placed on no damn respirator." It seems he had seen one of his childhood buddies die in an iron lung.

"Let's set up a neb treatment and please try to keep his end-tidal ($EtCO_2$) around 50," Terry instructs his teammates. "I would like to try to avoid intubating if I can."

Critical Thinking Questions

1. What is the standard of care of patients with suspected Type II respiratory failure?

_____

_____

2. What are some of the patient-specific concerns and considerations that the Paramedic should consider when applying this plan of care that is intended to treat a broad patient population presenting with acute respiratory failure?

_____

_____

Evaluation

"Terry, it's getting harder to bag him!" his colleagues note. It wasn't easy to bag him in the first place, as increased airway resistance has decreased compliance. However, they are using two hands to bag him now. "Stop bagging," Terry orders as he checks his boss's lung sounds. Glancing at the monitor, he sees the heart rate skyrocket, the blood pressure plummet, and the end-tidal go through the roof.

Critical Thinking Questions

1. What are some of the predictable complications associated with ventilation of the emphysemic patient in Type II respiratory failure?

_____

_____

2. What are some of the predictable complications associated with the treatments for acute respiratory distress?

_____

_____

Disposition

The ambulance "on the red" is followed by a parade of ambulances from the company. Quickly unloading the boss, Terry is met by the ED attending, who states, "Give me the short version." Terry's booming voice can be heard trailing off as the boss enters the emergency department.

Critical Thinking Questions

1. What is the most appropriate transport decision that will get the patient to definitive care?

_____

_____

2. Why choose this hospital even if it means bypassing other hospitals?

_____

_____

Practice Questions
Multiple Choice

Select the best answer for each of the following questions.

1. Neuromuscular disease can lead to hypoventilation. Which of the following is NOT a neuromuscular disease?
   a. stroke
   b. myasthenia gravis
   c. Guillain–Barré
   d. amyotrophic lateral sclerosis

2. Which of the following chest wall deformities, that leads to hypoventilation, is NOT congenital?
   a. pectus excavatum
   b. pectus carinatum
   c. scoliosis
   d. kyphosis

3. Which of the following is NOT a primary disease?
   a. asthma
   b. chronic obstructive pulmonary disease
   c. emphysema
   d. chronic bronchitis

4. Emphysema is primarily characterized by which of the following?
   a. reduced effort to breath
   b. increased resistance to airflow
   c. decreased lung surface area
   d. increased secretions

5. What is a primary characteristic of asthma?
   a. reduced effort to breath
   b. increased resistance to airflow
   c. decreased lung surface area
   d. increased secretions

6. What is a primary characteristic of chronic bronchitis?
   a. reduced effort to breath
   b. increased resistance to airflow
   c. decreased lung surface area
   d. increased secretions

7. Hemoptysis is NOT seen in which of the following conditions?
   a. pneumonia
   b. pulmonary embolism
   c. cor pulmonale
   d. tuberculosis

8. What is another name for asbestosis?
   a. black lung
   b. farmer's lung
   c. white lung
   d. popcorn packer's lung

9. What classification is given to an asthmatic who is symptomatic twice a week, with less than two nocturnal episodes a month?
   a. mild intermittent asthma
   b. mild persistent asthma
   c. moderate persistent asthma
   d. severe asthma

10. Which of the following is NOT related to intrinsic asthma?
    a. drug allergies
    b. dust–mold allergies
    c. nasal polyps
    d. sinusitis

11. Asthma should be suspected in patients presenting with all of the following EXCEPT _____.
    a. persistent cough
    b. headache
    c. chest tightness
    d. awakened with a cough

12. Which of the following is NOT a color of mucoid sputum?
    a. clear
    b. red
    c. white
    d. grey

13. A patient with a peak flow meter reading less than 50% is in the _____ zone.
    a. white
    b. yellow
    c. green
    d. red

14. Permissive hypercarbia is useful in patients with which condition?
    a. reduced effort to breath
    b. increased resistance to airflow
    c. decreased lung surface area
    d. increased secretions

15. Which of the following is NOT a side effect of sympathomimetic medications, such as beta agonist inhalers?
    a. tachycardia
    b. tremors
    c. hyperkalemia
    d. muscle cramps

Short Answer

Write a brief answer to each of the following questions.

16. Define Type II respiratory failure.

_____

_____

17. List the causes of wheezing.

_____

_____

18. What two cardiac medications may induce asthma?

_____

_____

19. What is the downward spiral of asthma?

_____

_____

20. Describe hypoxic drive.

_____

_____

Fill in the Blank

Complete each sentence by adding the appropriate word in the provided blanks.

21. _____ pack/years or greater is considered significant.

22. Patients allergic to epinephrine are actually allergic to the _____ _____ preservative.

23. Cross allergy to _____ can induce an asthma attack in aspirin-sensitive asthmatics.

24. Pursed lip breathing is an attempt at _____.

25. Severe respiratory failure is manifest by an end-tidal carbon dioxide level of _____ mmHg.

CHAPTER **10**

DISORDERS OF BRAIN FUNCTION

Case Study

Chief Concern

The call comes in for a 1-year-old infant seizing. Fortunately, the ambulance is just around the corner from the address, standing by "at post" in the mid-zone. Total time from dispatch to arrival is less than three minutes.

"It's my baby!" the woman cries as she clutches the infant tightly to her chest. Jolin, the Paramedic, moves to assist her, asking, "May we please take a look at your baby?"

"What took you so long? What's wrong with my baby? Why did this happen?" the mother asks. The barrage of questions continues.

"First, we are going to take care of your baby," Jolin assures her. "Now, can I ask you a few questions?"

Critical Thinking Questions

1. What are some of the possible causes of convulsions in an infant?

_____

_____

2. What immediate actions should the Paramedics take to safeguard this patient?

_____

_____

History

The mother explains to Jolin that the infant has never had a seizure. She was an on-time vaginal delivery without any birth trauma or anoxia that the mother knew about. The baby had been to the pediatrician earlier that morning for her "first ear infection" and her mother was on her way to the pharmacy to pick up a prescription for amoxicillin.

Although the infant's fever is relatively mild, less than 101°F rectal, the mother relates that the fever "spiked" about half an hour ago. Since she wasn't at home, she couldn't give the baby any acetaminophen for the fever.

Critical Thinking Questions

1. What are the important elements of the history that a Paramedic should obtain?

_____

_____

2. What is the symptom pattern associated with a seizure?

_____

_____

Examination

The infant is listless but breathing. Jolin makes a quick visual inspection of the infant's mouth, finding that it is clear. The infant's breathing is slightly rapid and is punctuated by yawns, but remains within acceptable limits according to the Broselow tape. Placing the pulse oximeter stripe on the infant's forehead confirms both heart rate (tachycardia within normal range) and oxygen saturations. While assessing the infant, Jolin notes that the skin is hot and dry to the touch. Since her ambulance does not have a thermometer, she estimates the infant's temperature as greater than 101°F. She plans to verify her guess at the hospital.

Critical Thinking Questions

1. What are the elements of the physical examination of a patient with suspected seizure disorder?

_____

_____

2. Why is an examination for meningeal signs a critical element in the neurological examination?

_____

_____

Assessment

"Ma'am," Jolin explains, "we think your baby had an infant's seizure but we can't be entirely sure here. We would like to go to the hospital." The mother, at first, insists that the crew take the patient to the pediatrician. However, after a short discussion emphasizing the special resources at the emergency department, the mother agrees to go to the hospital as long as the crew speaks to the doctor.

Critical Thinking Questions

1. What diagnosis did the Paramedic announce to the patient's mother?

_____

_____

2. Why should the Paramedic insist that the child be seen in the emergency department?

_____

_____

Treatment

"Yes, doctor, understood," Jolin acknowledges over the phone. "You will call into the emergency department with the baby's history. Hmm, yes, the baby appears post-ictal but it's only been 10 minutes since the seizure stopped. Yes, thank you, doctor." Jolin places the telephone back in her holster and explains what will happen to her baby while en route to the hospital.

Critical Thinking Questions

1. What is the standard of care of patients with suspected febrile seizure?

_____

_____

2. Why is the use of an oropharyngeal airway discouraged?

_____

_____

Evaluation

"Will my baby be epileptic?" the mother asks with a concerned look on her face. Jolin replies, "The chances of your baby having epilepsy, statistically speaking, is extremely low." As fate would have it, as if mocking Jolin's words, the infant begins having another seizure as soon as the words leave her mouth.

Critical Thinking Questions

1. What are some of the predictable complications associated with a seizure?

_____

_____

2. What are the treatments if this complication occurs?

_____

_____

Disposition

Turning the infant on its side, to let the airway drain naturally, Jolin starts to mull over the options. She can try to obtain venous access, which is tough on a kid, and give valium. She also considers giving versed intranasal, even though valium works faster IV than versed IN. Alternatively, she can give the valium per rectum. Owing to the immediacy of the situation, Jolin opts to give the versed intranasally and then call ahead to the emergency department to describe the situation.

Critical Thinking Questions

1. What is the most appropriate transport decision that will get the patient to definitive care?

_____

_____

2. Why should the Paramedic choose to go to a hospital with an available operating room?

_____

_____

Practice Questions
Multiple Choice

Select the best answer for each of the following questions.

1. At which level of consciousness can someone be aroused with a verbal stimulus?
   a. lethargy
   b. stupor
   c. obtunded
   d. coma

2. Which of the following is NOT suggestive of a psychogenic non-epileptic seizure?
   a. thrusting pelvic movements
   b. side-to-side head movements
   c. incontinence
   d. dystonic posturing

3. Which of the following is NOT an example of focal seizures?
   a. automatisms
   b. tonic–clonic movement
   c. narcolepsy
   d. unconscious repetitious actions

4. Which of the following is NOT an example of generalized seizures?
   a. atonic
   b. absence
   c. focal motor
   d. tonic–clonic

5. The "epileptic cry" is heard during the _____ phase of a convulsion.
   a. aura
   b. tonic
   c. clonic
   d. post-ictal

6. Breath-holding and cyanosis are seen during the _____ phase of a convulsion.
   a. aura
   b. tonic
   c. clonic
   d. post-ictal

7. What does a pediatric convulsion associated with projectile vomiting suggest?
   a. febrile seizure
   b. meningitis-induced seizure
   c. epilepsy
   d. traumatic brain injury

8. Which of the following is NOT a seizure disorder?
   a. epilepsy
   b. febrile seizure
   c. Tourette syndrome
   d. petit mal

9. What is the most common cause of new-onset seizures?
   a. unknown
   b. alcohol related
   c. brain tumor
   d. medication noncompliance

10. Which antidysrhythmic is known to induce seizures?
    a. amiodarone
    b. procainamide
    c. lidocaine
    d. magnesium

11. Which of the following anticonvulsants does NOT affect the GABA neuroreceptors?
    a. hydantoins such as phenytoin
    b. barbiturates such as phenobarbital
    c. benzodiazepines such as clonazepam
    d. carboxylic acids such as valproic acid

12. Which of the following would suggest a pontine hemorrhage of the brainstem as the origin for a seizure?
    a. unilateral dilated pupil
    b. bilateral dilated pupil
    c. doll's eyes
    d. pinpoint pupils

13. Which of the following would NOT be normal following an epileptic seizure?
    a. hypertension
    b. irregular respirations such as yawning
    c. bradycardia
    d. hypoglycemia

14. Which of the following is NOT a definition of status epilepticus?
    a. prolonged twilight
    b. continuous seizure lasting five minutes
    c. two or more seizures without intervening period of lucidity
    d. prolonged unconsciousness with automatisms

15. Which of the following does NOT represent unstable epilepsy?
    a. increasing frequency of seizures
    b. decreasing length of post-ictal period
    c. increasing duration of seizures
    d. decreasing medication requirements

Short Answer

Write a brief answer to each of the following questions.

16. Why should naxolone be avoided in treating an addicted mother's newborn?

_____

_____

17. What is an "electrical storm?" What is an analogy?

_____

_____

18. What is a Jacksonian march?

_____

_____

19. What is Brudzinski's sign? What is Kernig's sign?

_____

_____

20. What is the pathophysiology of status epilepticus?

_____

_____

Fill in the Blank

Complete each sentence by adding the appropriate word in the provided blanks.

21. Wakefulness is a function of the _____ _____ _____.

22. _____ is the key characteristic of a generalized seizure.

23. A(n) _____ seizure was formerly called a "drop attack."

24. _____ is a clue for a(n) _____ seizure, formerly called a petit mal.

25. Déjà vu is another name for the _____ phase of a generalized seizure.

Chapter 11

DISORDERS OF CEREBRAL CIRCULATION

Case Study
Chief Concern

Martin has been a faithful employee of the U.S. Postal Service for the past five years. His supervisors have always commented on how hard working Martin is; therefore, his coworkers are surprised one day when they see Martin in the break room.

"What's wrong?" Cecelia asks.

Martin replies, "This is the worst headache of my life! I tried aspirin, I tried ibuprofen, and nothing seems to work."

"Here," Cecelia offers, "let me put this ice pack on the back of your neck. You tell me if it helps. I'm going to get the plant nurse."

Jennifer, the occupational nurse on duty, is called to the break room. She knows at once that something is seriously wrong. The lights have been turned off, and when she tries to turn them on Martin cries out, "Turn the lights off!" Martin is seated at the table, cradling his head in his arms. Pressing her radio microphone, Jennifer requests EMS to the scene immediately.

Critical Thinking Questions

1. What are some of the possible causes of sudden headache?

   _____

   _____

2. How could the sudden headache be related to the patient's photophobia?

   _____

   _____

History

Aimee is the first arriving Paramedic and finds Martin, as Jennifer had described, sitting in the break room, cradling his head in his hands. He explains again that this is the worst headache of his life. It started at the back of his head and it came "out of the blue." Martin does not have a history of headaches, migraine or otherwise. In fact, in reviewing Martin's medical records, Jennifer declares him to be in perfect health. He has no hypertension, takes no medications, and has not even had so much as a broken fingernail in the past five years of working for the postal service.

Martin admits that he had a similar headache about two weeks ago, associated with some nausea and vomiting that he attributed to the flu. Since it was short-lived, he did not seek medical attention for it.

Aimee notices that Martin is rubbing his neck, so she asks him if his neck hurts as well. He responds by vomiting, unannounced, onto the tabletop.

Critical Thinking Questions

1. What are the important elements of the history that a Paramedic should obtain?

_____

_____

2. What is the importance of the previous headache?

_____

_____

Examination

Aimee checks Martin and finds that he has no fever. She sighs in relief, as that helps reduce the chance that the headache is due to meningitis. Nonetheless, Aimee elects to keep her mask on. Since flashing a penlight in Martin's eyes does not seem sensible, Aimee elects to perform the rest of examination.

Aimee stands on Martin's right side to ask him questions while she gets equipment out of her bag. She notices that he turns his head and scans the room, as if he is looking for her. "That's odd," she says to herself, "I better check his visual fields." Facing him, she tells Martin what she is going to do and she smiles at him, hoping to comfort him. Reflexively, he smiles back. However, it is a twisted grimace. Turning to Jennifer, Aimee asks if the facial droop is new.

Critical Thinking Questions

1. What are the elements of the physical examination of a patient with suspected disorder of cerebral circulation?

_____

_____

2. Why is a blood glucose test a critical element in this examination?

_____

_____

Assessment

Aimee suspects that Martin has a subarachnoid hemorrhage. She appreciates the severity of the situation and asks all present to help move Martin to the ambulance. Martin says he would like to go to Community Hospital but Aimee advises otherwise. "Martin," she says as she is picking up equipment, "you need Regional."

Critical Thinking Questions

1. What diagnosis did the Paramedic announce to the patient?

_____

_____

2. What symptoms led the Paramedic to the diagnosis?

_____

_____

Treatment

As Martin is loaded into the ambulance; Aimee thanks Jennifer for all of her help and climbs in. Concerned about Martin's dropping heart rate and rising blood pressure, she instructs the driver to use the lights and sirens judiciously.

While on the way to the hospital, Aimee places Martin on the monitor, establishes venous access, keeps the valium nearby in case it is needed, and uses all of the monitoring tools at her disposal, including pulse oximeter, automatic noninvasive blood pressure cuff, and end-tidal capnography.

Critical Thinking Questions

1. What is the standard of care of patients with suspected subarachnoid hemorrhage?

   _____

   _____

2. What are some of the patient-specific concerns that the Paramedic should consider when administering mannitol?

   _____

   _____

Evaluation

Suddenly Martin has a seizure and becomes unconscious and unresponsive. Aimee performs another primary assessment. His airway is clear, and Aimee knows an oral airway, along with a head-tilt, chin-lift, will help maintain its patency. Aimee plans to intubate Martin shortly, but wants to administer lidocaine prior to doing so. Martin's vital signs demonstrate Cushing's triad and a quick check of his pupils shows that they are midposition and unresponsive to light.

Aimee knows the situation is bad as she administers the diazepam prophylactically to prevent further seizures. Watching the end-tidal capnography, she elects to lower the $EtCO_2$. However, first she gives Martin lidocaine, ventilates him for a few minutes to let it work, and then intubates him before trying hypocarbia.

Critical Thinking Questions

1. What are some of the predictable complications associated with a subarachnoid hemorrhage?

   _____

   _____

2. What is the problem with rebleeding?

   _____

   _____

Disposition

Martin is wheeled straight into trauma one, where all the serious cases go, and is surrounded by a team of doctors and nurses led by a neurologist, Dr. Peters. "First things first," exclaims Dr. Peters. "Let's get some of that pressure off of his brain!"

Critical Thinking Questions

1. What is the most appropriate transport decision that will get the patient to definitive care?

   _____

   _____

2. What are some of the transportation considerations?

   _____

   _____

Practice Questions

Multiple Choice

Select the best answer for each of the following questions.

1. Which of the following conditions is the Paramedic unable to mitigate in the field?
   a. hypoxia
   b. hypoglycemia
   c. hypotension
   d. hyperglycemia

2. Which of the following is NOT an ischemic stroke?
   a. thrombotic stroke
   b. hemorrhagic stroke
   c. embolic stroke
   d. vasospastic stroke

3. Which cardiac dysrhythmia can cause a stroke?
   a. atrial fibrillation
   b. ventricular tachycardia
   c. supraventricular tachycardia
   d. heart block

4. A brainstem stroke can be caused by the occlusion of which of the following?
   a. middle cerebral artery
   b. internal carotid artery
   c. basilar artery
   d. circle of Willis

5. Which strokes are attributed to senility?
   a. basilar
   b. frontal
   c. subarachnoid
   d. lacunars

6. Which of the following does NOT result in a watershed stroke?
   a. hypoxia
   b. hypoglycemia
   c. hypotension
   d. hyponatremia

7. What distinguishes a subarachnoid hemorrhage from meningitis?
   a. nuchal rigidity
   b. fever
   c. headache
   d. photophobia

8. Which pathology can mimic a stroke?
   a. Bell's palsy
   b. Todd's paralysis
   c. thoracic outlet syndrome
   d. all of the above

9. Which of the following symptoms is NOT associated with right-sided strokes?
   a. contralateral paralysis
   b. difficulty speaking
   c. excessive speaking
   d. loss of left lateral gaze

10. Which of the following symptoms is NOT associated with left-sided strokes?
    a. contralateral paralysis
    b. difficulty speaking
    c. inability to read or write
    d. slurred monotone speech

11. Which of the following symptoms is NOT associated with brainstem strokes?
    a. double vision
    b. difficulty speaking
    c. difficulty swallowing
    d. loss of fine motor control

12. Which of the following symptoms is NOT associated with cerebellar strokes?
    a. double vision
    b. nystagmus
    c. ataxia
    d. slurred speech

13. Which of the following is NOT a way cranial nerves are tested in the Miami Emergency Neurologic Deficit (MEND) exam?
    a. smile
    b. Romberg
    c. cardinal gazes
    d. nystagmus

14. Which of the following visual disorders is NOT suggestive of stroke?
    a. agnosia
    b. homonymous hemianopia
    c. nystagmus
    d. diplopia

15. Which of the following terms is NOT used to describe a patient's inability to understand the spoken word?
    a. Broca's aphasia
    b. receptive aphasia
    c. Wernicke's aphasia
    d. fluent aphasia

Short Answer

Write a brief answer to each of the following questions.

16. Describe the Cincinnati Stroke Scale.

_____

_____

17. Describe loss of a visual field.

_____

_____

18. Describe monoparesis versus quadriparesis versus hemiparesis.

_____

_____

19. What stroke mimics drunkenness?

_____

_____

20. Describe the Romberg test.

_____

_____

Fill in the Blank

Complete each sentence by adding the appropriate word in the provided blanks.

21. A _____ bleed is a warning symptom of a future cerebral aneurysm rupture.

22. The _____ headache is a classic sign for a subarachnoid hemorrhage.

23. Brainstem strokes are the result of occlusion of the _____ artery.

24. Prior to a brainstem stroke the patient may complain of _____ in her ears.

25. The Los Angeles Prehospital Stroke Scale has the added advantage of time of onset and _____ _____ .

CHAPTER 12

DISORDERS OF THE PERIPHERAL NERVOUS SYSTEM

Case Study

Chief Concern

Mrs. Forness is a pleasant middle-aged woman who does not complain much. However, when her son finds her walking with crutches, he decides to call 9-1-1.

Upon arriving at the residence, Taine reviews with his partner, Alena, some of the atraumatic reasons for weakness. As they ring the doorbell, Mrs. Forness greets them at the door.

She explains that she has just started to have trouble walking, and does not want to be a bother. Therefore, she's using her son's crutches, left over from when he broke his leg in football during high school, to help her get around. "I planned to see the doctor next week," she explains. While talking to Mrs. Forness, Taine notes that she is having difficulty breathing and is speaking in word clusters.

Critical Thinking Questions

1. What are some of the possible causes of unexplained weakness?

   _____

   _____

2. How is trouble breathing related to the weakness?

   _____

   _____

History

Mrs. Forness denies any recent trauma including falls or motor vehicle collisions, explaining that her son does most of her shopping so she doesn't have to own a car.

She tells them the weakness started in her legs and she has noticed that she seems to be getting weaker "by the day." She is also experiencing those "pins and needles" in her legs, which is new.

Mrs. Forness's past medical history is unremarkable. This gives both Alena and Taine pause. There is no explanation for her shortness of breath.

Critical Thinking Questions

1. What are the elements of the physical examination of a patient with suspected neuromuscular disease?

_____

_____

2. What are the symptoms associated with peripheral nervous systems disorders?

_____

_____

Examination

Starting at her feet, Taine notes that Mrs. Forness has weakness in her legs. It seems remarkable that she can even walk, although truthfully she is dragging her legs around and using her arms and those crutches for locomotion.

Although Mrs. Forness's respiratory examination is unremarkable (i.e., lungs clear apices to base as well as a satisfactory SpO_2), she is still having trouble breathing.

Critical Thinking Questions

1. What are the elements of the physical examination of a patient with suspected peripheral nervous system disorder?

_____

_____

2. Why perform the physical examination by starting distal and working proximal?

_____

_____

Assessment

Taine's first thought is that maybe Mrs. Forness is having a stroke. However, his partner reminds him that the weakness is bilateral, which is not an indication of a cervical injury. Without further testing, they cannot be sure. However, for the moment, the diagnosis is peripheral nervous system disorder of unknown etiology.

Critical Thinking Questions

1. What diagnosis did the Paramedic announce to the patient?

_____

_____

2. Is it possible to have unilateral weakness from a spinal cord injury?

_____

_____

Treatment

Mrs. Forness is provided supplemental oxygen and positioned sitting upright on the stretcher for comfort. While venous access is obtained, Alena obtains a set of vital signs. "Hmmm," she mutters under her breath, "Mrs. Forness is bradycardiac. I think I will get a 12-lead ECG while I am at it."

Critical Thinking Questions

1. What is the standard of care of patients with suspected peripheral nervous system disorder?

_____

_____

2. Would it be inappropriate to stabilize the patient's spinal column?

_____

_____

Evaluation

The transport time is well over 30 minutes, so there is time to obtain blood samples (the blood sugar is normal) and a 12-lead ECG (which does not show any signs of ischemia yet was bradycardiac), as well as an end-tidal carbon dioxide reading.

The $EtCO_2$ is troubling. It reads a low CO_2 level, which is suggestive of either hypothermia or hypoventilation. Taine prepares the intubation tray, just in case.

Critical Thinking Questions

1. What are some of the predictable complications associated with peripheral nervous system disorders?

_____

_____

2. What is the greatest danger in Guillain–Barré syndrome?

_____

_____

Disposition

As the ambulance arrives at the regional medical center, Mrs. Forness is turned over to the nurses. Later, when returning with another patient, the emergency department attending physician approaches Taine and Alena. "Remember Mrs. Forness? Well, she is intubated and in the ICU." Both Paramedics look shocked. "She has Guillain–Barré, and if she had waited much longer you may have found her in respiratory arrest or worse."

Critical Thinking Questions

1. What is the most appropriate transport decision that will get the patient to definitive care?

_____

_____

2. Is it acceptable to transport the patient to a community hospital?

_____

_____

Practice Questions

Multiple Choice

Select the best answer for each of the following questions.

1. What is pain that is out of proportion to the stimulus called?
    a. allodynia
    b. hyperesthesia
    c. hyperalgesia
    d. analgesia

2. Which of the following causes an ascending paralysis?
    a. Guillain–Barré
    b. multiple sclerosis
    c. poliomyelitis
    d. amyotrophic lateral sclerosis

3. Which of the following peripheral nerve disorders will NOT cause respiratory paralysis?
   a. Guillain–Barré
   b. multiple sclerosis
   c. poliomyelitis
   d. amyotrophic lateral sclerosis

4. Which of the following peripheral nerve disorder symptoms fluctuate from week to week?
   a. Guillain–Barré
   b. multiple sclerosis
   c. poliomyelitis
   d. amyotrophic lateral sclerosis

5. Which of the following disorders is cured by vaccination?
   a. Guillain–Barré
   b. multiple sclerosis
   c. poliomyelitis
   d. amyotrophic lateral sclerosis

6. Which of the following disorders does NOT affect the neuromuscular junction?
   a. Guillain–Barré
   b. myasthenia gravis
   c. poliomyelitis
   d. amyotrophic lateral sclerosis

7. Which peripheral nerve disorder can be worsened by medications such as lidocaine, haloperidol, and beta blockers?
   a. Guillain–Barré
   b. myasthenia gravis
   c. poliomyelitis
   d. amyotrophic lateral sclerosis

8. Which of the following does NOT cause movement disorder?
   a. amyotrophic lateral sclerosis
   b. Parkinson's disease
   c. Huntington's disease
   d. myasthenia gravis

9. Which disease is genetic?
   a. amyotrophic lateral sclerosis
   b. Parkinson's disease
   c. Huntington's disease
   d. myasthenia gravis

10. Which peripheral nerve disease can be mistaken as a psychiatric disorder?
    a. amyotrophic lateral sclerosis
    b. Parkinson's disease
    c. Huntington's disease
    d. myasthenia gravis

11. Choking is NOT a hazard for which of the following peripheral nerve disorders?
    a. amyotrophic lateral sclerosis
    b. Parkinson's disease
    c. Huntington's disease
    d. myasthenia gravis

12. Which of the following peripheral nerve disorders does NOT mimic a stroke?
    a. Guillain–Barré
    b. myasthenia gravis
    c. Parkinson's disease
    d. multiple sclerosis

13. Which condition is worse in the afternoon than in the morning?
    a. amyotrophic lateral sclerosis
    b. Parkinson's disease
    c. Huntington's disease
    d. myasthenia gravis

14. Which disease causes the patient to have a shuffling gait when walking?
    a. amyotrophic lateral sclerosis
    b. Parkinson's disease
    c. Huntington's disease
    d. myasthenia gravis

15. Which disease causes the patient to develop an abnormal dancing gait?
    a. amyotrophic lateral sclerosis
    b. Parkinson's disease
    c. Huntington's disease
    d. myasthenia gravis

Short Answer

Write a brief answer to each of the following questions.

16. Describe post-polio syndrome.

_____

_____

17. What are several diseases that can cause peripheral nerve disorders?

_____

_____

18. What is complex regional pain syndrome?

_____

_____

19. What is the physical examination of the patient with a suspected peripheral nerve disorder?

_____

_____

20. How can myasthenia gravis mimic a stroke?

_____

_____

Fill in the Blank

Complete each sentence by adding the appropriate word in the provided blanks.

21. The most common peripheral neuropathy that affects the limbs symmetrically is _____-_____ syndrome.

22. _____ _____ _____ is also called Lou Gehrig's disease.

23. Cogwheeling is a side effect of haloperidol and _____ _____.

24. The Sabin and Salk vaccines are the cure for _____.

25. Peripheral nerve disorders generally produce _____ paresthesia in the hands and _____ paresthesia in the feet.

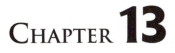

CHAPTER **13**

DISORDERS OF GLUCOSE METABOLISM

Case Study
Chief Concern

"Hope on the hill" laughs Roman, after the radio call stops. The local emergency services staff gave that affectionate name to Our Lady of Hope nursing home, which is incidentally located on an elevation of land. The call is for a routine transfer to Memorial Hospital for a diabetic patient with altered mental status.

Roman knows there is nothing routine about the transfer of a diabetic patient with altered mental status. "Let's step up our response," Roman says to Natalie as he leans over to flip on the lights, "Altered mental status could mean anything."

Critical Thinking Questions

1. What are some of the possible diabetic-related emergencies?

_____

_____

2. What are other conditions that could mimic a diabetic-related emergency?

_____

_____

History

The nurse meets Roman and Natalie at the nursing station. Wheeling the gurney toward the patient's room, he explains that the patient has a urinary tract infection and that he has finished his course of antibiotics. The patient's urine appears clear and his temperature has been near normal over the weekend, yet his mental status has not improved. Concerned about this development, he calls the attending physician, who orders the patient, Mr. O'Connor, to be transported to Memorial Hospital for further workup.

Mr. O'Connor has a history of type 2 diabetes that is controlled by a combination of oral hypoglycemic agents and diet. Mr. O'Connor's medication list includes heart failure medications such as furosemide and a beta blocker. However, conspicuously missing is a potassium supplement that almost always seems to accompany the furosemide. The nurse explains that Mr. O'Connor has some renal failure as a result of his diabetes and that, after several episodes of hyperkalemia, the medication was removed from his list.

Critical Thinking Questions

1. What are the important elements of the history that a Paramedic should obtain?

_____

_____

2. What is the symptom pattern associated with hyperosmolar nonketonic syndrome (HONKS)?

_____

_____

Examination

While Roman is getting the medical history from the nurse, Natalie proceeds to perform the primary assessment. Although Mr. O'Connor is obtunded, his airway is patent, his pulse oximeter reading is within normal limits, and his vital signs show he is tachycardiac.

Of course, Natalie feels the blood glucose reading is "too high." Their particular glucometer can accurately read up to 800 mg/dL. She wonders if Mr. O'Connor's blood sugar might be over 800 mg/dL?

She continues her assessment. She cannot smell acetone on his breath, which suggests ketoacidosis, nor does he have the rapid and deep, almost sighing, Kussmaul respirations. Looking down, she notes the almost full urine bag, to which the nurse replies, "We emptied that this morning. Let me get that before you leave."

Critical Thinking Questions

1. What are the elements of the physical examination of a patient with suspected hyperglycemia?

_____

_____

2. What is one key that helps differentiate HONKS and DKA?

_____

_____

Assessment

As the nurse leaves the room to get a urinal, Roman leans over Mr. O'Connor, as they are transferring him from the bed to the gurney, and whispers to Natalie, "HONKS."

"What?" Natalie whispers back.

"Hyperosmolar, nonketonic syndrome," Roman explains. "You know, HONKS!" Natalie looks down at Mr. O'Connor on the stretcher and the light bulb comes on.

Critical Thinking Questions

1. What diagnosis did the Paramedic announce to his partner?

_____

_____

2. How does the Paramedic differentiate between HONKS and DKA?

_____

_____

Treatment

Loading the patient into the ambulance, Natalie announces her treatment plan to Roman. "I think I will try to start tow lines and get a fluid bolus going, but only after I get him hooked up to our monitors." Roman nods in agreement and closes the ambulance doors.

Settling in for the ride, Natalie applies the ECG monitor, noninvasive blood pressure cuff, the pulse oximeter, and the end-tidal capnography to the patient following intubation.

Critical Thinking Questions

1. What is the standard of care of patients with suspected hyperglycemia?

_____

_____

2. What are some of the patient-specific concerns and considerations that the Paramedic should consider when applying this plan of care that is intended to treat a broad patient population presenting with hyperglycemia?

_____

_____

Evaluation

Almost as soon as Natalie establishes venous access, Mr. O'Connor seizes. Natalie quickly administers diazepam, which luckily was nearby. The seizure activity stops almost immediately and Natalie turns her attention to reassessing the patient's oxygenation and ventilation.

Critical Thinking Questions

1. What are some of the predictable complications associated with hyperglycemia?

_____

_____

2. What are some of the predictable complications associated with the treatments for seizures secondary to cerebral edema?

_____

_____

Disposition

Pulling into the emergency bay at Memorial Hospital, Roman helps Natalie unload Mr. O'Connor. Mr. O'Connor is intubated and on a transport ventilator. He has two saline solutions running wide up and is hooked up to the monitor. "So much for a routine transfer," Roman says to Natalie.

Critical Thinking Questions

1. What is the most appropriate transport decision that will get the patient to definitive care?

_____

_____

2. What is key to report when turning the patient over to the emergency department staff?

_____

_____

Practice Questions
Multiple Choice

Select the best answer for each of the following questions.

1. What is used to store glucose for immediate use?
    a. glycogen
    b. lipogenesis
    c. glycogenolysis
    d. gluconeogenesis

2. What process causes the creation of triglycerides from fatty acids?
   a. glycogen
   b. lipogenesis
   c. glycogenolysis
   d. gluconeogenesis

3. Which hormone lowers blood glucose levels?
   a. glucagon
   b. insulin
   c. epinephrine
   d. atropine

4. What stimulates the ketogenic pathway?
   a. glucagon
   b. lipogenesis
   c. glycogenolysis
   d. gluconeogenesis

5. Lack of insulin production results in _____ diabetes.
   a. adult onset
   b. type 1
   c. gestational
   d. type 2

6. Humulin R insulin, a regular insulin, is _____.
   a. rapid acting
   b. short acting
   c. intermediate acting
   d. long acting

7. Which type of insulin is most likely given immediately following a large meal?
   a. rapid acting
   b. short acting
   c. intermediate acting
   d. long acting

8. Insulin resistance is the hallmark of which type of diabetes?
   a. adult onset
   b. type 1
   c. gestational
   d. type 2

9. One form of diabetes has a cure. Which one?
   a. adult onset
   b. type 1
   c. gestational
   d. type 2

10. Diabetic foot ulcerations are secondary to what condition?
    a. hyperglycemia
    b. peripheral neuropathy
    c. peripheral vascular disease
    d. all of the above

11. Which of the following is NOT part of the three "poly's" of hyperglycemia?
    a. polydipsia
    b. polycythemia
    c. polyuria
    d. polyphagia

12. Which of the following does NOT differentiate diabetic ketoacidosis from hyperosmolar nonketonic syndrome?
    a. hyperglycemia
    b. acidosis
    c. ketones
    d. time of onset

13. Which of the following is NOT common for diabetic ketoacidosis?
    a. neurological deficits
    b. nausea and vomiting
    c. abdominal cramps
    d. thirst and dehydration

14. Alcoholic ketoacidosis differs from diabetic ketoacidosis through which of the following?
    a. acidosis
    b. ketones
    c. hyperglycemia
    d. dehydration

15. What is the single largest source of infection that leads to DKA?
    a. upper respiratory infection
    b. pneumonia
    c. urinary tract infection
    d. infected foot ulceration

Short Answer

Write a brief answer to each of the following questions.

16. What are the three characteristics that differentiate the 20-plus varieties of insulin on the market?

    _____

    _____

17. Describe insulin resistance.

    _____

    _____

18. Explain diabetic ketoacidosis.

    _____

    _____

19. Explain hyperosmolar nonketonic syndrome.

    _____

    _____

20. Differentiate DKA from HONKS.

    _____

    _____

Fill in the Blank

Complete each sentence by adding the appropriate word in the provided blanks.

21. A Paramedic's check is called a _____ blood glucose test as opposed to a fasting glucose test.

22. Obesity-induced diabetes is called _____.

23. The device used to measure blood sugar is called a _____.

24. The symptoms of hypoglycemia, the result of epinephrine secretion, are called _____ symptoms.

25. If venous access cannot be obtained in a patient with hypoglycemia, then intramuscular _____ should be used.

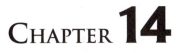

CHAPTER **14**

DISORDERS OF HOMEOSTASIS

Case Study
Chief Concern

"Unit 43, respond to 3 Mountain View for 53-year-old male with severe nausea, vomiting, diarrhea, and confusion. Time out 02:45 hours." Sitting up in the front seat of the ambulance, Joshua nudges Aiden, "Wake up. We got a run."

Rubbing his eyes, Aiden looks at the dispatch information on the computer screen while tapping the call accepted button. "Hmm, nausea and confusion. Well, that narrows it down," he laughs. In evaluating the run history for the location, he recognizes the patient. It's Jim. Jim has chronic obstructive pulmonary disease and is constantly in and out of the hospital, intubated, ventilated, weaned, and sent home on steroids and oxygen. Yet he continues to smoke. However, the complaints of nausea and confusion make Aiden wonder if maybe it isn't Jim, but rather someone visiting Jim, since they are not part of his usual complaints. Then again, maybe Jim has a surprise in store for them.

Critical Thinking Questions

1. What are some of the electrolyte problems associated with nausea, vomiting, and diarrhea?

_____

_____

2. What complications can these electrolyte disturbances produce?

_____

_____

History

Jim has COPD and is on chronic steroids. Unfortunately, since his disease cost him his job at the county jail, he can't afford his COBRA payments and he has not reached Medicaid eligibility yet. Unable to afford all his medications, he has elected to stop taking his steroids. His logic is that since he will stop smoking he will not need the steroids.

Recently he has been put on rifampin as a result of an exposure to tuberculosis at the jail. Although the risk of his contracting tuberculosis was small, the jail staff told him he needed to take the rifampin "prophylactically." He blames his bout of nausea, vomiting, and abdominal pain on the rifampin.

Critical Thinking Questions

1. What are the important elements of the history that a Paramedic should obtain?

_____

_____

2. What is the symptom pattern associated with acute adrenocortical insufficiency?

_____

_____

Examination

Joshua looks at Aiden, who looks at Jim and then back to Joshua. One look confirms that they both concur. Jim is sick. Laid out on the couch, he is pale, diaphoretic, and hot to the touch. His lips are cyanotic and he is confused.

Helping Jim to his feet, so he can transfer to the stretcher, Aiden takes the opportunity to get a second set of vital signs, which he will compare to the first set he took when Jim was supine. Just as he suspected, Jim's heart rate jumped 20 beats per minute while his systolic blood pressure dropped 20 points.

Critical Thinking Questions

1. What are the elements of the physical examination of a patient with suspected adrenocortical insufficiency?

_____

_____

2. Why are orthostatic vital signs a critical element in this examination?

_____

_____

Assessment

Standing outside the rear of the ambulance after loading Jim, Aiden turns to Joshua and asks, "I'm thinking adrenal insufficiency, what do you think?" Joshua says, "I agree, I think it might be Addison's disease. Never thought I would actually see a case like this."

Critical Thinking Questions

1. What diagnosis did the Paramedic announce to the patient?

_____

_____

2. What is Addison's disease?

_____

_____

Treatment

While providing supportive care in the form of fluid resuscitation and oxygen therapy, Aiden calls medical control and gives a detailed history. The physician on the other end of the line orders 100 mg of hydrocortisone and continued fluid resuscitation, warning Aiden to not expect too much response from the fluid bolus.

Aiden questions the doctor about why Jim has peaked T waves on the ECG monitor. The doctor replies that over two-thirds of cases of acute adrenal insufficiency patients have concurrent electrolyte disorders.

Critical Thinking Questions

1. What is the standard of care of patients with suspected acute adrenal insufficiency?

_____

_____

2. What electrolyte disturbances should the Paramedic suspect?

_____

_____

Evaluation

Aiden draws a blood sample for glucose analysis as part of his routine and is surprised when the reading comes back 50 mg/dL. Aiden yells to the front of the ambulance, "His glucose is low but I don't get it! He's awake and alert." Joshua yells back, "Hey, you shouldn't be surprised! It's all part of the crisis." Aiden draws up the dextrose 50% and slowly starts to push it in while thinking he should recheck that glucose in another 10 minutes.

Critical Thinking Questions

1. What are some of the predictable complications?

_____

_____

2. What are other potential complications that could result from excessive vomiting and diarrhea?

_____

_____

Disposition

The ambulance arrives at the hospital and the patient is immediately taken into the resuscitation room. "Doc," Aiden says, "when you get a minute, could you go over this adrenal stuff again? He was really complex and I just want to understand it."

Critical Thinking Questions

1. What is the most appropriate transport decision that will get the patient to definitive care?

_____

_____

2. What key points about the patient's condition should be discussed with the emergency department staff?

_____

_____

Practice Questions
Multiple Choice

Select the best answer for each of the following questions.

1. Which of the following hormones is NOT secreted by the pituitary gland?
   a. antidiuretic hormone
   b. thyroid stimulating hormone
   c. gonad stimulating hormone
   d. adrenocorticotropic hormone

2. The blood sugar may NOT be elevated in which of the following endocrine disorders?
   a. diabetes insipidus
   b. Cushing's syndrome
   c. diabetes mellitus
   d. hyperthyroidism

3. What causes Graves' disease?
   a. radiation
   b. infection
   c. trauma
   d. autoimmune disease

4. Which of the following endocrine disorders is NOT immediately life-threatening?
   a. thyroid storm
   b. myxedema
   c. Graves' disease
   d. Cushing's syndrome

5. Which of the following is NOT a sign or symptom of myxedema?
   a. altered mental status
   b. hypothermia
   c. hyperglycemia
   d. bradycardia

6. Which of the following signs and symptoms is caused by hyperthyroidism?
   a. palpitations
   b. hypothermia
   c. hypertension
   d. exophthalmos

7. Aldosterone affects _____ retention.
   a. sodium
   b. potassium
   c. calcium
   d. magnesium

8. Which endocrine disorder can cause hypernatremia?
   a. diabetes insipidus
   b. Cushing's syndrome
   c. diabetes mellitus
   d. hyperthyroidism

9. Which medical condition can lead to profound and acute dehydration?
   a. diabetes insipidus
   b. Cushing's syndrome
   c. diabetes mellitus
   d. hyperthyroidism

10. What condition can be caused by excessive diarrhea?
    a. hyponatremia
    b. hypokalemia
    c. hypernatremia
    d. hyperkalemia

11. Which of the following ECG changes is NOT seen with hyperkalemia?
    a. shortened QT interval
    b. prolonged PR Interval
    c. U waves
    d. peaked T waves

12. Chronic alcoholics are prone to which condition?
    a. hyponatremia
    b. hypokalemia
    c. hypocalcemia
    d. hypomagnesemia

13. What can cause carpal spasms?
    a. hyponatremia
    b. hypokalemia
    c. hypocalcemia
    d. hypomagnesemia

14. Buffalo hump and moon faces are seen with which condition?
    a. diabetes insipidus
    b. Cushing's syndrome
    c. diabetes mellitus
    d. hyperthyroidism

15. Which condition can be caused by sudden cessation of steroids?
    a. Cushing's syndrome
    b. Addison's disease
    c. thyroid storm
    d. Graves' disease

Short Answer

Write a brief answer to each of the following questions.

16. Differentiate diabetes insipidus from diabetes mellitus.

    _____

    _____

17. What is the mechanism that causes cerebral edema, coma, seizures, and death in the patient with hyponatremia?

    _____

    _____

18. What is the symptom pattern for hyperkalemia?

    _____

    _____

19. What electrolyte disorder can hyperventilation cause and what is the symptom pattern?

    _____

    _____

20. Which endocrine disorder can be mistaken for a psychiatric disorder?

    _____

    _____

Fill in the Blank

Complete each sentence by adding the appropriate word in the provided blanks.

21. Deficiencies in antidiuretic hormone lead to _____ _____.

22. Goiters associated with symptoms of increased thyroid hormones are called _____ goiters.

23. Bilateral protrusion of the eyes, with retraction of the eyelids, is called _____.

24. Facial twitching elicited when tapping on the face in front of the ear is called _____ sign.

25. Torsades de pointes is seen with _____.

CHAPTER 15

ADDICTION DISORDER—ALCOHOLISM

Case Study

Chief Concern

As the snow gently falls outside, the radio crackles, "Ambulance 24, respond to corner of Broadway and Second Street in front of City Mission. Man down, reported seizing. Patient is a known inebriate. Police are en route to assist." As the ambulance lights start to flash, one Paramedic says to the other, "We know that address. Bet that it's Henry again."

Critical Thinking Questions

1. What are some of the possible causes of the patient's convulsions?

   _____

   _____

2. How can intoxication be related to the seizure activity?

   _____

   _____

History

The patient, who did turn out to be Henry, appears to be post-ictal. While one Paramedic starts the physical examination, the other Paramedic starts to question bystanders. One of the bystanders, the day manager for the City Mission, is very familiar with Henry. Despite the fact that he did not witness the seizure, he has some information he wants to share with the Paramedics. It seems that at the end of the month Henry ran out of money from his disability check. Without cash, Henry announced that it was the perfect time to "dry out."

Critical Thinking Questions

1. What are the important elements of the history that a Paramedic should obtain?

   _____

   _____

2. What is the symptom pattern associated with an epileptic seizure?

   _____

   _____

Examination

Henry is slowly recovering, as evidenced by his "colorful" language. "You had another seizure," the Paramedic tells him. "Just lie there for a minute while I check you over." Turning to his partner, he asks if she can check the pulse oximeters for a reading and obtain a quick blood sugar.

Critical Thinking Questions

1. What are the elements of the physical examination of a patient with suspected seizure disorder?

   _____

   _____

2. Why is a rapid trauma exam a critical element in this examination?

   _____

   _____

Assessment

The Paramedics consider how Henry's history of trying to "dry out" is suggestive of an alcohol withdrawal-induced seizure. However, other causes, such as traumatic brain injury and toxicology, cannot be eliminated based on the limited information available.

For Henry's sake, the Paramedics decide to "hope for the best, and treat for the worst" on the assumption that this is a breakthrough seizure and the patient needs supportive care.

Critical Thinking Questions

1. What is the significance of the alcohol withdrawal?

   _____

   _____

2. What diagnosis did the Paramedic announce to the patient?

   _____

   _____

Treatment

The Paramedics know obtaining venous access is critical. Henry might have another seizure, or worse, and need immediate sedation. The Paramedics also prepare to obtain a 12-lead ECG on Henry. "In his agitated and hyperstimulated state, he could be pushing his heart too hard," one Paramedic explains.

Critical Thinking Questions

1. What is the standard of care of patients with suspected seizure disorder?

   _____

   _____

2. Are there any special considerations that the Paramedic should take?

   _____

   _____

Evaluation

Henry starts to "weird out" in the back of the ambulance, talking about spiders crawling on his skin. He picks at his skin, leaving angry red welts. Henry asks the crew to turn off the lights and siren because they are hurting his eyes. One Paramedic politely advises Henry that the lights are not on, but Henry continues to insist that he is seeing flashing lights. Henry is becoming increasingly agitated, alarming the Paramedics. Although the Paramedics suspected Henry might be developing Wernicke–Korsakoff syndrome, since he is often forgetful, they know that these symptoms are from the alcohol withdrawal.

After contacting medical control, the Paramedics agree to administer diazepam and to keep haloperidol ready if Henry's agitation escalates.

Critical Thinking Questions

1. What are some of the predictable complications of alcohol withdrawal?

_____

_____

2. What are some of the predictable complications associated with the treatments for alcohol withdrawal?

_____

_____

Disposition

The diazepam does the trick. Henry is visibly calmer and has stopped picking at his skin. Within moments, the ambulance arrives at the hospital and Henry is brought to triage. At first the triage nurse thinks Henry is being admitted for "detox" (detoxicification) and calls for a wheelchair. The Paramedics explain that the call came for a man seizing and that it may be prudent to put him on a stretcher for observation.

Critical Thinking Questions

1. What is the most appropriate transport decision that will get the patient to definitive care?

_____

_____

2. What are some of the transportation considerations?

_____

_____

Practice Questions
Multiple Choice

Select the best answer for each of the following questions.

1. Which of the following causes of delirium is NOT potentially reversible in the field?
   a. alcohol withdrawal
   b. hypoglycemia
   c. hypoxia
   d. heavy metal poisoning

2. Which of the following is NOT part of alcoholism?
   a. distortions of reasoning
   b. inability to control consumption
   c. adverse personal, social, professional, and/or financial consequences
   d. unwillingness to seek medical care

3. Ethyl alcohol binds to the _____ receptor in the _____.
   a. serotonin, mesolimbic system
   b. dopamine, brainstem
   c. NMDA, cerebral cortex
   d. GABA, central nervous system

4. Which of the following medications can give a disulfiram-like reaction (i.e., cramps, nausea, and vomiting)?
   a. metronidazole (Flagyl®) to treat trichomonas infections
   b. chlorpropamide (Diabinese®), an oral hypoglycemic agent
   c. cefotaxime (Claforan®), a cephalosporin antibiotic
   d. all of the above

5. Acute pancreatitis, secondary to alcoholism, can lead to which condition?
   a. pancreatic cancer
   b. cholecystitis
   c. hyperlipidemia
   d. diabetes

6. All of the following factors, when combined, cause hyperbilirubinemia, EXCEPT _____.
   a. obstructed common bile duct
   b. diminished Kupffer cells
   c. decreased albumin production
   d. reduced bilirubin production

7. What causes esophageal varices?
   a. primary hypertension
   b. impaired coagulopathy
   c. caput medusa
   d. portal hypertension

8. Which classic cerebral syndrome attributed to alcoholism is permanent?
   a. Wernicke's syndrome
   b. Cushing's syndrome
   c. Alzheimer's dementia
   d. Korsakoff psychosis

9. What causes death from hyperammonemia?
   a. lethal dysrhythmia
   b. increased acid load and acidosis
   c. acute renal failure and hyperkalemia
   d. cerebral edema

10. Which of the following alcohols is ethanol or drinking alcohol?
    a. methyl alcohol
    b. ethylene glycol
    c. isopropyl alcohol
    d. ethyl alcohol

11. Which of the following alcohols is most likely to produce blindness?
    a. ethyl alcohol
    b. ethylene glycol
    c. isopropyl alcohol
    d. methyl alcohol

12. Which of the following alcohols could kill a child in an amount as small as 2 tablespoons?
    a. methyl alcohol
    b. ethyl glycol
    c. isopropyl alcohol
    d. ethylene glycol

13. What is the drug of choice to treat alcohol withdrawal?
    a. haloperidol
    b. versed
    c. thiamine
    d. diazepam

14. What is a complication of the administration of sodium bicarbonate to an ethylene glycol poisoning?
    a. hyperkalemia
    b. metabolic acidosis
    c. kidney failure
    d. hypocalcemia

15. What type of alcohol is "rubbing alcohol"?
    a. methyl alcohol
    b. ethylene glycol
    c. isopropyl alcohol
    d. ethyl alcohol

Short Answer

Write a brief answer to each of the following questions.

16. What is the name of the transient delirium seen in alcoholic patients?

    _____

    _____

17. Hematemesis is most closely related to what alcoholism-related abnormality?

    _____

    _____

18. What impact does alcohol have on pregnancy?

    _____

    _____

19. What class of drugs is used to treat alcohol withdrawal?

    _____

    _____

20. The C in the CAGE Alcohol Assessment Tool stands for which question?

    _____

    _____

Fill in the Blank

Complete each sentence by adding the appropriate word in the provided blanks.

21. The other name for alcohol withdrawal is _____ _____.

22. Alcohol is most like the drugs in the _____ classification.

23. The _____ _____ in the brain controls emotions and inhibitions.

24. The medical term for breast enlargement in males secondary to alcoholism is _____.

25. The tremors in the hands, due to hepatic encephalopathy, are called _____ or liver flap.

Chapter 16

TOXICOLOGICAL EMERGENCIES

Case Study
Chief Concern

The call comes in as an "unknown, man down." Dispatch relays that cops on the scene confirm that the man is alive, awake, and agitated. The location is in the downtown area referred to as "the point," which is known to have its share of "druggies, whores, and homeless people." Police advise EMS that the scene is safe and they are to proceed in.

Pulling up to a scene reminiscent of a Christmas tree, because of all the flashing colored lights, Juan and Emmanuel step out of the rig and walk over to a man who is face down, in handcuffs, with a knee in his back. He is yelling something about the devil trying to kill him.

Critical Thinking Questions

1. What are some of the possible causes of delirium?

   _____

   _____

2. Which cause of delirium should be considered last?

   _____

   _____

History

"Let's roll him over," Juan suggests to the officers, "so we can get a look at him." "D'Virgilio!" exclaims Manny (short for Emmanuel). The man, a known psychiatric patient, has a history of bipolar illness. He is on imipramine (Tofranil) and gets medication every morning at a clinic on Green Street. A known pill hoarder, D'Virgilio pretends to swallow the medicine and then regurgitates it later to sell for drugs. D'Virgilio, a street person who is known to have gotten into cocaine, is a notorious heavy drinker.

"Hey V, what's going on tonight?" Juan asks. While Juan is trying to make heads or tails out of D'Virgilio's ramblings, the police are emptying his pockets. Sure enough, several "unidentified pills" are in his pocket in a little plastic baggie. The sergeant on-scene wants to call for the drug identification officer, but Manny says, "I recognize these. This is Tofranil. You can tell by the orange and yellow capsule and the number 40 on it. These are 100 mg capsules."

"Then what is this?" the police sergeant asks as he dangles a rock of crack cocaine in another little baggie. Manny realizes D'Virgilio is suffering from a mixed overdose.

Critical Thinking Questions

1. What are the important elements of the history that a Paramedic should obtain?

   _____

   _____

2. What is the symptom pattern associated with delirium?

   _____

   _____

Examination

After completing the primary assessment—checking the patient out for hypoxia, hypoglycemia, and hypotension—Manny stops to consider "V's" plight. The patient's mental status seems to wax and wane from agitated to somnolent. His pupils are as big as saucers. He is tachycardiac and his blood pressure is elevated. However, Manny's main concern is that he is "dry as a bone and hot as a pistol."

Critical Thinking Questions

1. What are the elements of the physical examination of a patient with suspected overdose?

   _____

   _____

2. Why is blood glucose a critical element in this examination?

   _____

   _____

Assessment

"Let's get him out of here," Manny beseeches the assembled police officers. "He's burning up and I don't know why." Many hands help to lift the patient onto the gurney. His hands are cuffed to each side of the stretcher as the stretcher is lifted into the ambulance. Looking at the officer sitting next to him, Manny asks, "Could you please hold this up?" while he hands him a bag of saline.

Critical Thinking Questions

1. What diagnosis did the Paramedic announce to the patient?

   _____

   _____

2. What are the three causes of delirium that should be evaluated and treated first?

   _____

   _____

Treatment

Fortunately, the agitation from both anticholinergics and sympathomimetics can be treated with benzodiazepines. While placing him on the ECG to monitor for dysrhythmia, Manny considers using ice packs for the extreme hyperthermia. Although the hyperthermia is of concern, he knows that the underlying problem is hypoxia. A combination of acidosis from his agitation and hyperthermia will lead to a rightward shift in the oxyhemoglobin curve.

Critical Thinking Questions

1. What is the standard of care of patients with suspected overdose?

_____

_____

2. What basic care should be provided first?

_____

_____

Evaluation

"Hey!" yells the cop over the screaming siren, "that don't look right." Manny looks over at the monitor. There is a wide complex tachycardia that resembles torsades de pointes. After checking and confirming the patient's carotid pulse, he reaches into the drug bag and pulls out a prefilled ampoule of sodium bicarbonate. "Elixir of the gods," Manny says as he pushes in the bolus while watching the monitor to see if the QRS starts to narrow.

Critical Thinking Questions

1. What are some of the predictable complications associated with a suspected anticholinergic overdose?

_____

_____

2. What are some of the predictable complications associated with a suspected sympathomimetic overdose?

_____

_____

Disposition

Looking out the window, Manny sighs in relief as they pull into the ambulance bay. "This patient is getting a bit hairy for me," Manny announces as Juan pulls out the stretcher. With the cop following, the patient and the crew enter into the emergency department. It appears chaotic, but they know it is a controlled chaos in which someone will get to them shortly.

Critical Thinking Questions

1. What is the most appropriate transport decision that will get the patient to definitive care?

_____

_____

2. Given the choice of hospitals, which one would be preferred?

_____

_____

Practice Questions
Multiple Choice

Select the best answer for each of the following questions.

1. In which route does a poison have the most delayed effect?
   a. inhaled
   b. injected
   c. transdermal
   d. ingested

2. Which toxidrome is associated with vomiting and diarrhea?
   a. sympathomimetics
   b. anticholinergics
   c. cholinergics
   d. opiates

3. Which toxidrome is associated with pinpoint pupils and respiratory depression?
   a. sympathomimetics
   b. anticholinergics
   c. cholinergics
   d. opiates

4. Which toxidromes share a symptom pattern of hyperthermia, tachycardia, and dilated pupils?
   a. sympathomimetics and anticholinergics
   b. anticholinergics and cholinergics
   c. cholinergics and opiates
   d. opiates and sympathomimetics

5. Which toxidromes share a symptom of constricted pupils (miosis)?
   a. sympathomimetics and anticholinergics
   b. anticholinergics and cholinergics
   c. cholinergics and opiates
   d. opiates and sympathomimetics

6. Which toxidromes share a symptom of agitation?
   a. sympathomimetics and anticholinergics
   b. anticholinergics and cholinergics
   c. cholinergics and opiates
   d. opiates and sympathomimetics

7. Which toxidrome is associated with an immediately decreased level of consciousness?
   a. sympathomimetics
   b. anticholinergics
   c. cholinergics
   d. opiates

8. What symptom differentiates the sympathomimetic and anticholinergic toxidromes?
   a. agitation
   b. diaphoresis
   c. tachycardia
   d. hypertension

9. Which of the following substances does NOT induce an anticholinergic toxidrome?
   a. cocaine
   b. tricyclic antidepressants
   c. antihistamines
   d. atropine

10. Which of the following substances does NOT induce an opiate toxidrome?
    a. cocaine
    b. oxycodone
    c. hydrocodone
    d. codeine

11. Which substance that can induce an opiate toxidrome may not induce pinpoint pupils (miosis)?
    a. heroin
    b. morphine
    c. codeine
    d. oxycodone

12. Which toxidromes share a symptom of respiratory depression?
    a. sympathomimetics and anticholinergics
    b. opiates and sedative–hypnotics
    c. cholinergics and opiates
    d. sedative–hypnotics and sympathomimetics

13. Which of the following alcohols is NOT considered a "toxic" alcohol?
    a. methanol
    b. ethanol
    c. isopropyl
    d. ethylene glycol

14. What is the most common material for internal decontamination?
    a. syrup of ipecac
    b. activated charcoal
    c. water
    d. sorbital

15. What is the drug of choice in the treatment of sympathomimetic poisoning?
    a. atropine
    b. metapropol
    c. 2-PAM
    d. diazepam

Short Answer

Write a brief answer to each of the following questions.

16. Define toxicology.

_____

_____

17. Define a toxidrome.

_____

_____

18. Which poisoning produces a flu-like symptom pattern?

_____

_____

19. What is the telephone number for poison control?

_____

_____

20. Describe how hyperbaric oxygen (HBO) helps with carbon monoxide poisoning.

_____

_____

Fill in the Blank

Complete each sentence by adding the appropriate word in the provided blanks.

21. The _____ pesticides can produce an anticholinergic toxidrome.

22. Cocaine can act like lidocaine, lengthening the QT interval. If ventricular tachycardia occurs, the Paramedic should consider the use of _____ _____.

23. A fine muscle twitching due to stimulation of nicotinic receptors is called _____.

24. _____ prevents organophosphates from permanently binding to acetylcholinase.

25. The two main classes of sedative–hypnotics are _____ and _____.

CHAPTER 17

PSYCHIATRIC DISORDERS

Case Study

Chief Concern

As part of their clinical rotations, the Paramedic students are assigned to ride along with the mobile crisis team. Along with a psychiatric nurse specialist and a clinical social worker, the student responds to any psychiatric or behavioral emergency in the community.

The first call is for a mother who called the police about her daughter. They tell her that there is nothing that they can do other than call the mobile crisis team. She agrees.

Apparently her daughter, after an arrest for shoplifting, has gone into a "tailspin," according to her mother. Now her daughter refuses to go to school and sometimes even refuses to get out of bed.

Critical Thinking Questions

1. What are some of the possible causes of the woman's apparent abnormal behavior?

_____

_____

2. What are some medical causes of abnormal behavior?

_____

_____

History

The mother is concerned about her daughter. She relates how her daughter, Julianna, seems cold and distant, even though they had always enjoyed a close mother–daughter relationship. She tells the team that Julianna does not seem to take pleasure from being with either her friends or her family and that several family members, including her grandmother, have expressed concern about this apparent change.

The mother goes on to relate how Julianna would "hole up" in her rooms for days. The mother often found her in bed in the middle of the day, yet she would hear her up on the computer at all hours of the night. Recently she told her mother that she was too sick to go to school, claiming "the flu," but she did not have a fever or other signs or symptoms.

As the nurse approaches the patient, the Paramedic notes that her answers are short and monosyllabic and that she answers even open-ended questions with either short answers or nonsensical answers.

Critical Thinking Questions

1. What are the important elements of the history that a Paramedic should obtain?

_____

_____

2. What is the symptom pattern for acute psychotic reaction?

_____

_____

Examination

While the social worker continues to obtain more information about Julianna's school attendance, social interactions with friends, sports, and hobbies, the nurse and the Paramedic student exam the patient.

The shades in Julianna's bedroom are drawn and the lights are low, creating a depressing atmosphere. When asked if they can talk to her, she giggles inappropriately but then seems to stare off into space. Her one episode of giggling is the only evidence of emotion that the two witness.

Julianna appears to be her stated age of 16 but is remarkably thin. Her clothes literally hang off her frame. Her primary assessment is unremarkable and a quick head-to-toe examination does not reveal any findings, such as slash marks to the wrist or evidence of injection.

Critical Thinking Questions

1. What are the elements of the physical examination of a patient with suspected acute psychotic reaction?

_____

_____

2. Why are pulse oximeter and blood glucose critical elements in this examination?

_____

_____

Assessment

Based on Julianna's appearance, her affect, and her behavior, the team feels that Julianna should be medically evaluated at the emergency department, perhaps followed up by a visit from mental health services. Although the mother agrees, Julianna is not as agreeable.

The presence of a police officer, as well as the encouraging words of the nurse, convince Julianna to go peacefully to the hospital. Only at that point does Julianna confide in the nurse that her "friend" said it was OK to go with the ambulance. Julianna is alone in the room at the time, and is having a muted but earnest conversation with herself.

Critical Thinking Questions

1. What is the significance of the hallucinations?

_____

_____

2. What safety concerns, if any, should the Paramedic have?

_____

_____

Treatment

While en route to the hospital, efforts are made to keep external stimulus to a minimum, so as not to agitate Julianna. The psychiatric nurse specialist develops a one-on-one relationship with Julianna and asks that all other members of the team communicate their requests through her.

Her first order of business is to determine if Julianna's auditory hallucinations are command hallucinations. If they are, the nurse wants to know if Julianna is going to hurt herself or others. She waits patiently, and from a safe distance, for the answers to her questions, which she asks persistently but politely.

Critical Thinking Questions

1. What is the standard of care of patients with suspected acute psychotic disorder?

_____

_____

2. What other safety concerns should the Paramedic have for the patient?

_____

_____

Evaluation

While en route, Julianna starts to become more visibly agitated. The nurse asks her what the voices are telling her. Julianna replies that the voices are telling her that the Paramedic student, a male, is in league with the Devil and that it is her duty to kill him.

While startled at the revelation, the Paramedic student remains calm. The nurse matter of factly asks Julianna if she would like to be restrained so that she can resist the temptations of the voices, to which Julianna responds "Yes." She relates that she doesn't want to hurt anybody and that she is a good person, but the voices are making her do bad things. Julianna is strapped to the gurney and restrained with soft restraints.

Critical Thinking Questions

1. What are some of the predictable complications associated with auditory hallucinations?

_____

_____

2. What is medical restraint?

_____

_____

Disposition

After arriving at the hospital, the mother—who had followed the ambulance with the social worker in the crisis team's van—immediately heads to the back of the ambulance. Dismayed by the sight of her daughter in restraints, the social worker pulls her aside and explains how the protective medical restraints are in her daughter's best interest since she is experiencing an acute psychotic reaction.

Critical Thinking Questions

1. What is the most appropriate transport decision that will get the patient to definitive care?

_____

_____

2. What are the advantages of transporting a patient with suspected acute psychotic disorder to these hospitals, even if that means bypassing other hospitals in the process?

_____

_____

Practice Questions

Multiple Choice

Select the best answer for each of the following questions.

1. What are perceptions that are not based in reality called?
   a. hallucinations
   b. delusions
   c. dementia
   d. delirium

2. What is another name for meaningless phrases?
   a. stilted speech
   b. alogia
   c. avolition
   d. verbigeration

3. What is extremely formal conversation called?
   a. stilted speech
   b. alogia
   c. avolition
   d. verbigeration

4. Negative symptoms of schizophrenia, summed up in the three A's, does NOT include which of the following?
   a. alogia
   b. affective flattening
   c. avolition
   d. absent speech

5. Delusions and hallucinations are rare in _____ schizophrenia.
   a. hebephrenic
   b. catatonic
   c. paranoid
   d. simple

6. _____ schizophrenia often occurs during adolescence.
   a. Hebephrenic
   b. Catatonic
   c. Paranoid
   d. Simple

7. _____ schizophrenia starts subtly and leads to an inability to perform activities of daily living.
   a. Hebephrenic
   b. Catatonic
   c. Paranoid
   d. Simple

8. Delusions and hallucinations are common in _____ schizophrenia.
   a. hebephrenic
   b. catatonic
   c. paranoid
   d. simple

9. Waxy flexibility and mutism are classic signs of _____ schizophrenia.
   a. hebephrenic
   b. catatonic
   c. paranoid
   d. simple

10. Excessive hand washing is an example of what condition?
    a. social phobia
    b. panic attack
    c. post-traumatic stress disorder
    d. obsessive–compulsive disorder

11. Overwhelming anxiety about contact with EMS would be an example of what condition?
    a. social phobia
    b. panic attack
    c. post-traumatic stress disorder
    d. obsessive–compulsive disorder

12. What is the use of rhyming words called?
    a. cognitive slippage
    b. echolalia
    c. clang association
    d. perseveration

13. What is an incoherent string of words called?
    a. thought blocking
    b. flight of ideas
    c. word salad
    d. cognitive slippage

14. Command hallucinations are a form of what condition?
    a. paranoid persecution
    b. visual hallucination
    c. cognitive dissonance
    d. auditory hallucination

15. Which of the following is NOT a first rank symptom?
    a. auditory hallucinations
    b. paranoid persecution
    c. thought blocking
    d. broadcasting

Short Answer

Write a brief answer to each of the following questions.

16. Compare and differentiate the psychogenic and somatogenic theories of mental illness.

   _____

   _____

17. Describe post-traumatic stress disorder.

   _____

   _____

18. List the potentially reversible causes of delirium.

_____

_____

19. Differentiate delirium from dementia.

_____

_____

20. Describe a simple Romberg's test.

_____

_____

Fill in the Blank

Complete each sentence by adding the appropriate word in the provided blanks.

21. _____ _____ is an example of a genetic-based mental illness.

22. Externalizing internal psychiatric pain, in the form of medical complaints, is called _____.

23. Another name for manic–depressive illness is _____ disease.

24. A _____ _____ is a sudden overwhelming fear.

25. Intermittent, spasmodic muscular contractions are called _____ _____ _____.

CHAPTER 18

BEHAVIORAL DISORDERS

Case Study

Chief Concern

"University Ambulance Five, respond to the Yellowstone building, Rocky Mountain quad, room 212 for a female, despondent, threatening suicide." The lights come on in the dayroom as the bell starts ringing, waking the crew from their slumber.

The crew knows that, since it is the end of the semester, suicide rates skyrocket as students prepare to go home for the holidays, especially among those who have to explain to Mom and Dad why they weren't invited back to the university for the spring semester.

Critical Thinking Questions

1. What are some of the possible causes of this behavior?

_____

_____

2. What safety measures should the Paramedics consider on approaching the emotionally disturbed patient?

_____

_____

History

The crew arrives to find university police, led by Officer Dale, standing outside the door to the dorm room. Officer Dale, who is cross-trained as a Paramedic, is well-known to the crew as a compassionate caregiver. The patient has apparently barricaded herself in the room and refuses to come out. Officer Dale tries to convince her to take down the barricade while he obtains a medical history.

The patient, Gillian, has had a bad semester between a breakup with her high school sweetheart and a grade point average that didn't add up to make a whole number. Her voice sounds as if she's been drinking.

She keeps saying that she just wants to be left alone. However, Officer Dale explains that she is among friends that want to help. When there is no response from the other side of the door, the university police elect to breach the door.

Critical Thinking Questions

1. What are the important elements of the history that a Paramedic should obtain?

_____

_____

2. What factors could exacerbate the situation, making it more dangerous?

_____

_____

Examination

As they burst into the room, Officer Dale is startled at what he sees. The room is a mess. Gillian had wedged the dresser up against the door and overturned the bed, which allowed her to hide behind it. Unable to see what, if anything, she has in her hands, he carefully proceeds into the room.

Gillian's eyes have streams of mascara running from them from tears, but she is awake. Her pupils are as big as saucers. Her pale skin glistens with sweat and she just plain looks "wild." He cannot see any blood or source for bleeding. By the way she screams at the crew, Dale estimates that her airway must be patent and, from the volume of the screams, she is moving good air. She gets to her feet, suggesting to Officer Dale that her blood pressure must be reasonable.

Out in the hall, another officer is in communication with university health services. They indicate Gillian sought medical attention for an unplanned pregnancy, she is not a diabetic, and otherwise she is a picture of health for a young woman of her age.

Critical Thinking Questions

1. What are the elements of the physical examination of a patient with a suspected behavioral emergency?

_____

_____

2. Why is a rapid trauma assessment a critical element in this examination?

_____

_____

Assessment

"Get out of here! Leave me alone! I just want to die!" Gillian yells. Officer Dale motions for the crew to stand outside the hall as he tries to reason with Gillian. "Keep back," Gillian cries. Officer Dale respects her wishes, stating, "OK, I will stand here if you promise me you don't have a weapon." In this way, the dialogue begins. As the minutes start to add up, Officer Dale notices that Gillian is becoming less agitated. Is she calming down, he wonders, or is this the effect of some drugs she has taken?

Realizing the end game is to get Gillian to cooperate and accept treatment, Officer Dale finally gives Gillian her options. She can walk out of the room on her own or she can be carried out. He explains that they have already talked to a physician and she has ordered a medical restraint, if necessary.

Critical Thinking Questions

1. What is the significance of the patient's statements?

_____

_____

2. What are the elements of a suicide threat?

_____

_____

Treatment

While listening to Officer Dale, the crew assembles in the hallway and devises a plan. Each member is given an assignment, a soft restraint, and instructions to enter the room on Officer Dale's signal. He decides to make one more plea for cooperation. If that fails, Dale will pick up his radio to call "Code 5," which will signal the crew to enter the room, surround the patient, and begin the restraint.

Critical Thinking Questions

1. What is the standard of care of patients with a behavioral emergency?

_____

_____

2. What are some of the patient-specific concerns and considerations that the Paramedic should consider when applying this plan of care that is intended to treat a broad patient population presenting with a behavioral emergency?

_____

_____

Evaluation

Although Gillian is remarkably agile, the crew manages to get her onto the stretcher. One crew member tries to get a "submission hold," but the crew's leader instructs him to stay with the plan: to place her on the stretcher face-up, with her major muscle groups weakened by strategic placement of restraints in opposing directions and a spit mask applied.

Once Gillian grasps the situation, she becomes remarkably calm. Although some see this as good, Officer Dale wants a complete examination, including ECG monitor, pulse oximeter, blood glucose, and even end-tidal CO_2, to ensure she is being compliant and not exhausted. Officer Dale is familiar with excited delirium and has heard of other cases of in-custody deaths.

Critical Thinking Questions

1. What is the standard of care of patients for the medical restraint of an emotionally disturbed person?

_____

_____

2. What are some of the patient-specific concerns and considerations that the Paramedic should consider when applying this plan of care to the emotionally disturbed person?

_____

_____

Disposition

En route to the hospital, Officer Dale recontacts the physician contacted earlier to give her an update. After consultation, they agree sedation is not needed. Gillian stops showing any aggressive behavior. For a moment, Officer Dale's heart goes out to the young woman whose first steps into the "adult world" seemed to be a series of missteps.

Critical Thinking Questions

1. What is the most appropriate transport decision that will get the patient to definitive care?

_____

_____

2. If in an either/or situation (i.e., medical facility or psychiatric hospital), to which hospital should the patient be transported?

_____

_____

Practice Questions
Multiple Choice

Select the best answer for each of the following questions.

1. What is the first of the four S's of medical restraint?
   a. support
   b. structure
   c. symptom management
   d. safety

2. Which of the following is NOT considered a medical therapeutic device?
   a. straight jacket
   b. safety belts
   c. cervical immobilization collar
   d. stretcher strap

3. Which of the following is NOT an antipsychotic?
   a. haloperidol
   b. droperidol
   c. diazepam
   d. Haldol®

4. What is involuntary rotational movement of the eyes called?
   a. acute dystonic reaction
   b. oculogyric crisis
   c. nystagmus
   d. trismus

5. Involuntary spasmodic contractions of the neck (wry neck) is an example of what situation?
   a. acute dystonic reaction
   b. oculogyric crisis
   c. nystagmus
   d. trismus

6. What is clenched teeth, secondary to administration of neuroleptic medications, called?
   a. acute dystonic reaction
   b. oculogyric crisis
   c. nystagmus
   d. trismus

7. Extrapyramidal symptoms are treated in the field with which medication?
   a. cogentin
   b. benadryl
   c. valium
   d. ativan

8. Which medication used in a behavioral emergency has been associated with a prolonged QT interval?
   a. diazepam
   b. ativan
   c. droperidol
   d. haloperidol

9. Aggression has been most closely connected to which situation?
   a. increased serotonin levels
   b. increased dopamine levels
   c. decreased norepinephrine levels
   d. decreased serotonin levels

10. Which of the following medical conditions can cause aggressive behavior?
   a. stroke
   b. hypoglycemia
   c. hypoxia
   d. all of the above

11. What is the best indicator of a person who will have a successful suicide?
    a. sex
    b. age
    c. previous attempts
    d. unpredictability

12. What is the focus of the patient interview?
    a. gain the patient's cooperation
    b. talk the patient out of suicide
    c. reinforce the patient is safe
    d. inform the patient of the need for physical restraint

13. Which of the following is NOT considered counterproductive in the patient interview?
    a. improper show of force
    b. reinforcing the patient is safe
    c. use of confrontation
    d. patronizing the patient

14. Which of the following is an acceptable restraint device for Paramedics to use?
    a. leather restraints
    b. tasers
    c. handcuffs
    d. batons

15. Improper medical restraint can lead to _____.
    a. positional asphyxia
    b. strangulation
    c. aspiration of vomitus
    d. all of the above

Short Answer

Write a brief answer to each of the following questions.

16. What is a functional definition of abnormal behavior?

    _____

    _____

17. Define a behavioral emergency.

    _____

    _____

18. Define a medical restraint.

    _____

    _____

19. What are the three levels of medical restraint?

    _____

    _____

20. When is physical restraint acceptable?

    _____

    _____

Fill in the Blank

Complete each sentence by adding the appropriate word in the provided blanks.

21. An in-custody death of a restrained patient with a behavioral emergency is called _____ _____.

22. The interpersonal space between people is described by the theory of _____.

23. Using clarifying questions, paraphrasing, and summarizing is an example of _____ _____.

24. Any device intended for medical purposes that limits the patient's movements is considered a _____ _____.

25. Placing the patient in the prone position, with arms and legs tied together, is called _____-_____.

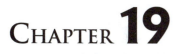

CHAPTER 19

DISORDERS: ABDOMINAL HEMORRHAGE

Case Study

Chief Concern

A 9-1-1 call comes in from a grandmother whose 1-year old granddaughter has abdominal pain and blood in the stool. While en route to the call, the Paramedics—using the intercom system in the Paramedic pumper—discuss the possible reasons why a 1-year-old would have blood in her stool.

Arriving on-scene, the Paramedics are met by the grandmother, who is standing on the porch and waving them on into the house. As they make their way up the steps, the grandmother anxiously explains that her granddaughter is in a great deal of pain and she couldn't stand to wait for her daughter to get home from work, so she called 9-1-1. The Paramedics reassure her that she did the right thing and they are there to help.

Critical Thinking Questions

1. What are some of the possible causes of gastrointestinal bleeding?

_____

_____

2. Why should the Paramedic be concerned about blood in the stool of a 1-year-old infant?

_____

_____

History

While looking at the infant, who appears to be writhing in the crib, the grandmother explains that her granddaughter appears to have intermittent abdominal pain that she describes as "colic." The pain seems to come in waves every 10 or 20 minutes, after which the baby seems fine.

She is trying to soothe the baby, who refuses the bottle she had prepared. "Oh, and she vomited," the grandmother adds.

Critical Thinking Questions

1. What are the important elements of the history that a Paramedic should obtain?

_____

_____

2. Does the patient's vomiting have any relationship to the gastrointestinal bleeding?

_____

_____

Examination

The infant is crying and active in the crib. The primary assessment is unremarkable; however, the infant's tense belly and abdominal pain on palpation let the Paramedic know she needs immediate medical attention. "Could you please tell me how many diapers she has gone through in the past 24 hours?" one Paramedic asks. The grandmother produces a diaper containing what looks like red currant jelly.

Critical Thinking Questions

1. What are the elements of the physical examination of a patient with suspected acute GI bleed?

_____

_____

2. Why would a diaper count be important?

_____

_____

Assessment

The two Paramedics confer as the infant is placed in a car seat for the trip to the hospital. "It could be a volvulus," suggests one Paramedic. The other replies, "Nope, I bet it's an intussusception. Regardless, this kid's got a hot belly and we need to get to the hospital. And don't forget the diaper with the poo."

Critical Thinking Questions

1. What diagnosis did the Paramedic announce to the patient's grandmother?

_____

_____

2. How does the Paramedic explain an intussusception or volvulus to the grandmother in lay terms?

_____

_____

Treatment

With the infant secured to the car seat, the car seat secured to the stretcher, and the stretcher locked in place, the Paramedics place the pulse oximeter probe on the infant's big toe. This provides both the infant's heart rate and oxygen saturation. One Paramedic places an oxygen mask on the infant's chest to provide blow-by oxygen, while the other lays out his intravenous equipment and looks for venous access on the chubby baby.

Critical Thinking Questions

1. What is the standard of care of patients with suspected gastrointestinal bleeding?

_____

_____

2. What issues are different when caring for a child with suspected gastrointestinal bleeding versus an adult?

_____

_____

Evaluation

Between two bouts of abdominal pain, each lasting two minutes and coming 10 minutes apart, the infant looks angelic, smiles, and babbles as infants do. The grandmother, seat belt in place, sits on the bench seat and tries to distract her granddaughter from all the activity that is going on around her.

Critical Thinking Questions

1. What are some of the predictable complications associated with acute GI bleed?

2. What should the Paramedic do if these complications arise?

Disposition

Arriving at the emergency department entrance, the mother greets her infant daughter. As they move down the hallway, the Paramedics try to explain that the baby seems alright but that, as a precaution, they thought it best to have the baby examined in the emergency department. The mother agrees.

Critical Thinking Questions

1. What is the most appropriate transport decision that will get the patient to definitive care?

2. Why would surgery be necessary?

Practice Questions
Multiple Choice

Select the best answer for each of the following questions.

1. Which of the following is NOT part of Mackler's triad, differentiating Boerhaave syndrome from a Mallory–Weiss tear?
   a. acid reflux
   b. vomiting
   c. lower chest pain
   d. subcutaneous emphysema

2. A college student has been binge drinking. Intoxicated, the patient has been violently vomiting and now is vomiting bright red blood. What is the likely cause of the bloody vomiting?
   a. Boerhaave syndrome
   b. gastroesophageal reflux disease
   c. esophagitis
   d. Mallory–Weiss tear

3. Which of the following will NOT cause chest pain?
   a. hiatus hernia
   b. gastroesophageal reflux disease
   c. hepatorenal syndrome
   d. Boerhaave syndrome

4. Which of the following is NOT associated with violent vomiting following intoxication?
   a. gastroesophageal reflux disease
   b. hiatus hernia
   c. Mallory–Weiss tear
   d. esophageal varices

5. Which of the following is NOT associated with vomiting blood?
   a. Boerhaave syndrome
   b. hiatus hernia
   c. Mallory–Weiss tear
   d. esophageal varices

6. Which of the following may actually be an inferior wall myocardial infarction in evolution?
   a. gastroesophageal reflux disease
   b. hiatus hernia
   c. Mallory–Weiss tear
   d. esophageal varices

7. The patient should not self-medicate, with antacids, which of the following?
   a. gastroesophageal reflux disease
   b. hiatus hernia
   c. Mallory–Weiss tear
   d. esophagitis

8. Which of the following is due to an infection in the lower GI tract?
   a. angiodysplasia
   b. Crohn's disease
   c. ulcerative colitis
   d. dysentery

9. Which of the following is inclusive of the others?
   a. Crohn's disease
   b. regional enteritis
   c. ulcerative colitis
   d. inflammatory bowel disease

10. Which of the following is NOT considered an autoimmune disorder?
    a. irritable bowel syndrome
    b. Crohn's disease
    c. ulcerative colitis
    d. regional enteritis

11. Which condition is associated with cancer?
    a. polyps
    b. volvulus
    c. diverticulosis
    d. Meckel's diverticulum

12. Bright red blood per rectum (BRBPR) is associated with which condition?
    a. volvulus
    b. diverticulosis
    c. hemorrhoids
    d. Meckel's diverticulum

13. Which condition would create melena?
    a. Mallory–Weiss tear
    b. Crohn's disease
    c. irritable bowel syndrome
    d. hemorrhoids

14. Which of the following medications is NOT associated with black stools?
    a. Pepto–Bismol®
    b. TUMS®
    c. iron supplements
    d. aspirin

15. Which of the following would NOT be a sign of developing peritonitis?
    a. nausea and vomiting
    b. fever and chills
    c. crampy abdominal pain
    d. bright red blood per rectum

Short Answer

Write a brief answer to each of the following questions.

16. Describe hepatorenal syndrome.

    _____

    _____

17. What other conditions are confused with irritable bowel syndrome?

    _____

    _____

18. Differentiate volvulus from intussusception.

    _____

    _____

19. Describe orthostatic vital signs.

    _____

    _____

20. Describe the optimal position for an abdominal examination.

    _____

    _____

Fill in the Blank

Complete each sentence by adding the appropriate word in the provided blanks.

21. The _____ of _____ divides upper and lower abdominal bleeding.

22. Subcutaneous emphysema secondary to Boerhaave syndrome is called _____ _____.

23. _____ _____ is due to cirrhosis of the liver.

24. _____ is the common thread among most causes of lower GI bleeding.

25. Black tarry stools are called _____.

CHAPTER 20

DISORDER: ABDOMINAL PAIN

Case Study

Chief Concern

"Please send help," pleads the voice on the other end of the telephone. The dispatcher replies, "Help is on the way. Again, you are 19 years old and you have right lower abdominal pain that came on all of a sudden, correct?" As the dispatcher queries the patient, she types the information into the alert screen. The closest ambulance, in this case A–4–8, will get the alert via their mobile on-board data terminal. All of the pertinent information, including address, shortest route to the scene, and call history for that location, will be displayed.

Critical Thinking Questions

1. What are some of the possible causes of right lower quadrant abdominal pain?

   _____

   _____

2. Which of these causes of right lower quadrant abdominal pain are specific to women?

   _____

   _____

History

The ambulance is on-scene in less than five minutes. Dick, the chief Paramedic, and his partner, Renee, walk up the stairs of the second floor walkup. Renee announces their arrival, to which she hears a faint voice yelling, "In here."

"Hello," Renee says as she enters the bathroom. The patient, a young woman, is lying on the bathroom floor in the fetal position. The sink and toilet are clean. "What's going on today?" Renee asks. Following the mnemonic OPQRST, Renee asks the patient questions, carefully noting her answers. All the while, she compares her knowledge of abdominal illness to the patient's symptoms.

The patient states the pain came on very sudden, "like a lightning bolt hit me," and is intense, 10 on 10 pain. The pain does not radiate anywhere. She is nauseous but hasn't vomited. She is due for her period, which should have come two weeks ago. Although she is sexually active, she and her boyfriend use condoms "like religion" she tells Renee.

Critical Thinking Questions

1. What are the important elements of the history that a Paramedic should obtain?

   _____

   _____

2. What history beyond the standard OPQRST AS/PN should the Paramedic obtain?

   _____

   _____

Examination

After assuring the patient's modesty, Renee starts the physical examination, beginning with inspection and leaving palpation for last. The patient has lower right abdominal pain. She does not have referred pain when the left lower quadrant is palpated. She does not have rebound tenderness nor does she appear to have a fever. The examination is periodically interrupted as the patient sits up as if to vomit. However, she only grabs her abdomen and quickly lies down without vomiting.

Critical Thinking Questions

1. What are the elements of the physical examination of a patient with acute abdominal pain?

_____

_____

2. Why are orthostatic vital signs a critical element in the patient's examination?

_____

_____

Assessment

The patient stops Renee and asks what's wrong. Renee patiently explains that there are several possible explanations but for now they are going to focus on treating the abdominal pain.

Critical Thinking Questions

1. What is the significance of the abdominal pain?

_____

_____

2. What diagnosis did the Paramedic give to the patient?

_____

_____

Treatment

The patient's pain seems to worsen when she attempts to vomit, so Renee elects to treat the patient's nausea as the first order of business. To improve the speed of delivery, Renee starts a peripheral intravenous access and delivers the antiemetic as a bolus.

Renee places the patient on high-flow, high-concentration oxygen; places two large bore intravenous access lines in each antecubital space; and places her on the cardiac monitor and pulse oximeter. She also performs a noninvasive blood pressure monitoring.

Critical Thinking Questions

1. What is the standard of care for treating patients with acute abdominal pain?

_____

_____

2. What is the concern in this case?

_____

_____

Evaluation

As the patient is being moved into the ambulance, her monitor shows a drop in blood pressure and rise in heart rate. Checking the patient, Renee and Dick find her pulse is consistent with the monitor and she is less responsive than before.

"Time to turn up the juice," exclaims Dick. "Let's get moving!" Renee, climbing into the back of the ambulance, puts on the headphones while she opens up the hanging saline bags. "Medical center, this is A–4–8, how do you copy?" Soon a voice comes on over the headphones. Using the voice-activated microphone, Renee gives report while she is reassessing the patient.

Critical Thinking Questions

1. What are some of the predictable complications associated with acute abdominal emergencies?

_____

_____

2. What are some of the predictable complications associated with the treatments for abdominal emergencies?

_____

_____

Disposition

The patient is rapidly transported to the emergency department. The receiving doctor concurs with the Paramedics' thoughts that she may have an ectopic pregnancy but agrees that, regardless of the cause of her condition, the Paramedics did well to treat her for hypoperfusion.

Critical Thinking Questions

1. What is the most appropriate transport decision that will get the patient to definitive care?

_____

_____

2. What key information should the Paramedic pass along to the emergency department and why?

_____

_____

Practice Questions
Multiple Choice

Select the best answer for each of the following questions.

1. Which of the following is NOT found in the "true abdomen"?
   a. pancreas
   b. uterus
   c. urinary bladder
   d. intestines

2. Which of the following is in both the abdominal cavity and the retroperitoneal cavity?
   a. pancreas
   b. aorta
   c. rectum
   d. liver

3. Which of the following is NOT in the retroperitoneal cavity?
   a. kidneys
   b. aorta
   c. pancreas
   d. liver

4. Which of the following is NOT protected by the thoracic cage?
   a. pancreas
   b. liver
   c. spleen
   d. kidneys

5. Which of the following does NOT cause peritonitis?
   a. ruptured appendix
   b. perforated ulcer
   c. ruptured spleen
   d. perforated intestine

6. What is another name for gallstones?
   a. uroliths
   b. lilyliths
   c. choleliths
   d. bilyliths

7. What is the most common cause of hepatomegaly?
   a. backward heart failure
   b. hepatitis
   c. liver cancer
   d. cirrhosis

8. Which of the following does NOT cause upper quadrant abdominal pain?
   a. appendicitis
   b. gastroenteritis
   c. hepatitis
   d. pancreatitis

9. Which of the following does NOT cause pancreatitis?
   a. gallstones
   b. alcohol abuse
   c. appendicitis
   d. cancer

10. What is the most common cause of peptic ulcer disease?
    a. Helicobacter pylori
    b. nonsteroidal anti-inflammatory drugs
    c. stress
    d. Zollinger–Ellison syndrome

11. Which abdominal disorder is primarily a pediatric disease?
    a. volvulus
    b. Crohn's disease
    c. hernia
    d. intussusception

12. Which bowel obstruction is most common in children?
    a. Ogilvie syndrome
    b. Hirschsprung's disease
    c. Crohn's disease
    d. volvulus

13. What test is used to check for cholecystitis, pressure on the right upper quadrant during inhalation producing pain during exhalation?
    a. obturator sign
    b. Rovsing's sign
    c. Murphy's sign
    d. dancer's sign

14. Periumbilical pain is a form of referred pain seen in which condition?
    a. liver abscess
    b. cholecystitis
    c. splenic rupture
    d. appendicitis

15. What is the most common cause of left lower quadrant abdominal pain in the elderly?
    a. paralytic ileus
    b. appendicitis
    c. volvulus
    d. diverticulitis

Short Answer

Write a brief answer to each of the following questions.

16. In broad terms, what are the three etiologies of paralytic ileus?

    _____

    _____

17. Describe the test for the obturator sign.

    _____

    _____

18. What are some causes of an acute abdomen (i.e., hot belly)?

    _____

    _____

19. Describe the etiology of visceral abdominal pain.

    _____

    _____

20. What are the effects of a large bowel obstruction?

    _____

    _____

Fill in the Blank

Complete each sentence by adding the appropriate word in the provided blanks.

21. Gallbladder pain is called _____ _____.

22. Yellowing of the skin and yellowing of the whites of the eyes is called _____.

23. The location of the appendix, called _____ _____, is found two-thirds of the distance on an imaginary line drawn from the umbilicus to the anterior superior iliac crest.

24. Pain in the right lower quadrant when the left lower quadrant is palpated is called _____ _____.

25. _____ occurs when the bowel twists on itself.

CHAPTER 21

LOSS OF RENAL FUNCTION

Case Study

Chief Concern

The Paramedic unit is called to Mrs. Washington's residence. Mrs. Washington complains of feeling weak and dizzy. The crew recognizes the address. Abdullah remarks, "This is not the usual time for Mrs. Washington's dialysis. She should have been in dialysis this morning."

Critical Thinking Questions

1. What are some of the possible causes of weakness and dizziness in the dialysis patient?

   _____

   _____

2. How is the time of the call related to the weakness and dizziness?

   _____

   _____

History

Mrs. Washington is a heavy-set African American woman with a history of diabetes and hypertension. These two factors led to her kidney failure and eventual dependence on dialysis. However, she never lets her dialysis get in the way of her family responsibilities. To her, family comes first and she tends to her grandchildren at every opportunity, even to the neglect of her dialysis. However, didn't happen this time, as she went to dialysis as scheduled and came home on time.

Mrs. Washington complains of headache and a little nausea and thinks she might be coming down with the flu. However, when her vision starts to blur she knows that something is wrong.

Critical Thinking Questions

1. What are the important elements of the history that a Paramedic should obtain?

   _____

   _____

2. What is the symptom pattern for disequilibrium syndrome?

   _____

   _____

Examination

Abdullah quickly performs a Cincinnati Stroke Scale following the primary assessment. The CSS is negative, reducing the likelihood of stroke, but her vital signs and mental status are suggestive of increased intracranial pressure. Abdullah also notes a peculiar tremor in Mrs. Washington's hands when she performs the pronator test.

Critical Thinking Questions

1. What are the elements of the physical examination of a patient with suspected disequilibrium syndrome?

_____

_____

2. Why is a Cincinnati Stroke Scale a critical element in this examination?

_____

_____

Assessment

Abdullah decides to quickly transport Mrs. Washington, as he is concerned about the possibility of increased intracranial pressure. While he suspects disequilibrium syndrome, he doesn't want to take any chances.

Critical Thinking Questions

1. Why does Abdullah suspect disequilibrium syndrome?

_____

_____

2. What would be some signs of increased intracranial pressure?

_____

_____

Treatment

Once on-board, Abdullah continues the routine advanced life support treatments including oxygen as needed, venous access, and ECG monitoring. With an eye toward signs of increasing intracranial pressure, Abdullah looks for Cushing's triad. All reports (i.e., pulse oximeter, noninvasive blood pressure, ECG, etc.) indicate Mrs. Washington is stable.

Abdullah then tries to obtain venous access. He considers accessing her shunt but reconsiders, remembering that shunt access is only allowed in "life-or-death" situations. However, Mrs. Washington's venous "options" are extremely limited.

Critical Thinking Questions

1. What is the standard of care of patients with suspected increased intracranial pressure?

_____

_____

2. Are there any concerns about fluid resuscitation?

_____

_____

Evaluation

As Abdullah unsuccessfully attempts venous access, he realizes this must be considered a life-threatening emergency. He elects to gain venous access using the AV graft. He has already assessed the AV graft, feeling a thrill and auscultating a healthy bruit. After gaining access, he administers the diazepam which immediately resolves the crisis. However, he knows that this is the lull before the storm.

Critical Thinking Questions

1. What is the process used for obtaining venous access via an AV graft?

_____

_____

2. What are some of the predictable complications associated with fluid resuscitation?

_____

_____

Disposition

At the emergency department, Abdullah turns Mrs. Washington over to the emergency nurses. After a short conversation with the emergency department attending, they agree that the situation warrants emergency access of the AV fistula.

Critical Thinking Questions

1. What is the most appropriate transport decision that will get the patient to definitive care?

_____

_____

2. What are the advantages of transporting a patient with suspected uremia to a hospital with a dialysis center, even if that means bypassing other hospitals in the process?

_____

_____

Practice Questions
Multiple Choice

Select the best answer for each of the following questions.

1. Which of the following medications has NOT been implicated as a cause of hematuria?
   a. furosemide
   b. Plavix®
   c. rifampin
   d. penicillin

2. What is the most common kidney stone?
   a. caffeine stone
   b. purine stone
   c. xanthine stone
   d. calcium stone

3. What are the largest kidney stones, the ones unable to pass through the ureter, called?
   a. caffeine stone
   b. purine stone
   c. xanthine stone
   d. calcium stone

4. Which stones appear more commonly with patients who have chronic diarrhea?
   a. caffeine stone
   b. purine stone
   c. xanthine stone
   d. calcium stone

5. Which stones are the result of a genetic inborn error of metabolism?
   a. caffeine stone
   b. purine stone
   c. cystine stone
   d. calcium stone

6. Which of the following is NOT part of the triad of symptoms for kidney stones?
   a. urinary urgency
   b. hematuria
   c. suprapubic pain
   d. dysuria

7. What is an ascending urinary tract infection called?
   a. pyonephrosis
   b. cystitis
   c. pyelonephritis
   d. bacteriuria

8. The patient with which of the following conditions will not see gross blood in the urine?
   a. bladder cancer
   b. urinary tract infection
   c. kidney stone
   d. cystitis

9. Which of the following is NOT a primary cause of end-stage renal disease?
   a. diabetes
   b. hypertension
   c. polycystic kidney disease
   d. kidney stones

10. Which of the following is NOT part of the symptom pattern associated with dialysis disequilibrium syndrome?
    a. hypertension
    b. confusion
    c. headache
    d. blurred vision

11. What is the sound of turbulent blood flow in an AV graft called?
    a. thrill
    b. murmur
    c. gallop
    d. bruit

12. What is the feel of blood running through an AV graft called?
    a. thrill
    b. murmur
    c. gallop
    d. bruit

13. What is the drug of choice to use during a hyperkalemic-induced cardiac arrest?
    a. calcium gluconate
    b. sodium bicarbonate
    c. calcium chloride
    d. sodium chloride

14. T waves on the ECG start to peak at which blood potassium level?
    a. 3.5 mEq/L
    b. 4.5 mEq/L
    c. 5.5 mEg/L
    d. 6.5 mEq/L

15. What is the connection of an artery to a vein, for dialysis, called?
    a. end-to-end anastomosis
    b. AV fistula
    c. AV graft
    d. Udall procedure

Short Answer

Write a brief answer to each of the following questions.

16. What are the two mechanisms that account for kidney stone formation?

_____

_____

17. How does hemodialysis work?

_____

_____

18. What is disequilibrium syndrome?

_____

_____

19. Describe the difference between carotenodermia and jaundice.

_____

_____

20. Why do patients with kidney failure look pale?

_____

_____

Fill in the Blank

Complete each sentence by adding the appropriate word in the provided blanks.

21. Blood in the urine that is not visible to the naked eye is called _____ blood.

22. _____ _____ has a similar symptom pattern as a urinary tract infection.

23. Total body edema, secondary to kidney failure, is called _____.

24. The medical term for liver flap, seen with disequilibrium syndrome, is _____.

25. The droplets of urine around the facial hair is called _____ _____.

CHAPTER 22

VASCULAR DISORDERS

Case Study

Chief Concern

Liam and Maud have been assigned to Zone B in the heights. Largely consisting of suburban neighborhoods, Zone B is a favored assignment. After being up all night working on the city fire, Liam and Maud are both looking forward to some "light duty."

The call comes in as a "private" call, meaning that the party calling either called the company directly or his or her doctor's office had called for an ambulance transport. These private calls were rarely an emergency, and if they turned out to be more than they were billed the ambulance had the option to call the city fire department for backup.

The patient, Velma, is an adolescent with unexplained swelling in her right arm. Although Liam and Maud know that this is not an emergency, loss of use of a limb can be devastating for an adolescent. Therefore, they take the call seriously.

Critical Thinking Questions

1. What are some of the possible causes of a swollen, painful deformity?

    _____

    _____

2. How is the patient's age related to these causes?

    _____

    _____

History

Liam and Maud are met at the door by an anxious mother who ushers them into a den that looks more like a clinic than a den. In the middle of the room is a hospital bed, and in that bed is Velma. She broke her leg in a biking accident and is recuperating at home. She has home health aides as well as her mother to care for her. Her broken leg, set in a long cast, is up in the air, suspended in a hammock-like device. Her right arm is extended straight out on a board.

From the doorway Liam and Maud can see the central venous line, a peripheral inserted central catheter (PICC), and a "mini-bag" of antibiotics hanging next to it. Apparently Velma was sent home with intravenous antibiotics for a wound infection with secondary osteomyelitis.

Critical Thinking Questions

1. What are the important elements of the history that a Paramedic should obtain?

    _____

    _____

2. What additional history would be helpful?

    _____

    _____

Examination

While Liam obtains the history from the mother—which is typed out and has extensive notes about Velma's history—Maud starts the physical examination. She obtains a set of vital signs on the unaffected side, including a temperature, and then proceeds to her focused examination of the right arm.

Velma has significant swelling to the right arm, proximal to the PICC line and extending into the axilla. Although she has a positive radial pulse, the red streaks from the insertion site into the axilla concern Maud. Although Velma does not complain of joint pain, Maud elects not to test that theory.

Critical Thinking Questions

1. What are the elements of the physical examination of a patient with suspected deep vein thrombus?

_____

_____

2. Why was the patient's temperature important?

_____

_____

Assessment

Maud runs the "5 P's" in her head. The presence of a pulse and absence of pain makes her think that this is not an acute arterial occlusion. Based on the history and physical findings, she suspects either a venous occlusion or perhaps a deep vein thrombus (DVT).

Critical Thinking Questions

1. What potential diagnoses are considered in Velma's case?

_____

_____

2. What diagnosis seems most likely based on the patient's presentation?

_____

_____

Treatment

After placing the limb in a position of comfort, the Paramedics transfer Velma to the stretcher for the trip to the hospital. She is offered pain medication, for either her leg or her arm, which she accepts.

Liam wisely chooses to start venous access on the unaffected limb rather than risk using the PICC line and disrupting a clot or fibrin plug. Velma's PICC line was put in because the antibiotics she was being given were particularly caustic to veins, not because she lacked veins. Therefore, Liam is able to easily gain venous access. The morphine makes Velma visibly more comfortable and makes Liam feel better about the bumpy roads in the city.

Critical Thinking Questions

1. What is the standard of care of patients with suspected acute venous occlusion or deep vein thrombus?

_____

_____

2. What is a PICC line?

_____

_____

Evaluation

Sitting back to complete his paperwork on the tablet computer, Liam is taken by surprise when the monitor alarms go off. The monitor shows that Velma's heart rate has skyrocketed and her oxygen saturation is plummeting.

Velma looks visibly anxious and complains of shortness of breath. Her oxygen saturation remains low despite the administration of high-flow, high-concentration oxygen.

Liam auscultates her lung sounds and finds them to be clear. That leads him to think she must have thrown a pulmonary embolism. "Maud, let's light it up!" he calls to the forward cab as he reaches for the microphone to contact medical control for instructions.

Critical Thinking Questions

1. What are some of the predictable complications associated with acute venous occlusion or deep vein thrombus?

   _____

   _____

2. What are some signs of a pulmonary embolism?

   _____

   _____

Disposition

So much for a slow day in Zone B, Maud sighs as she reaches down to flip the switches that activate the warning lights. Although it may have been possible to meet up with the city fire department Paramedics, she decides to proceed directly to the hospital, reasoning that it is closer.

Critical Thinking Questions

1. What is the most appropriate transport decision that will get the patient to definitive care?

   _____

   _____

2. What happens if the Paramedic suspects that the patient will need surgical intervention?

   _____

   _____

Practice Questions

Multiple Choice

Select the best answer for each of the following questions.

1. Which cause of nontraumatic extremity pain is NOT vascular in origin?
   a. venous occlusion
   b. rhabdomyolysis
   c. arterial occlusion
   d. gangrene

2. Which of the following is NOT one of the five "P's" of acute arterial occlusion?
   a. pain
   b. pallor
   c. pulselessness
   d. pitting edema

3. Which acute arterial occlusion is NOT the result of processes remote from the extremity?
   a. plaque rupture
   b. atrial fibrillation
   c. aortic aneurysm
   d. aortic embolism

4. The signs and symptoms of acute arterial occlusion are most similar to which other condition?
   a. crush injury
   b. compartment syndrome
   c. stroke
   d. peripheral edema

5. Which group is NOT prone to plaque-induced rupture?
   a. smokers
   b. obese people
   c. runners
   d. hypertensive people

6. The Paramedic must suspect _____ for a nontraumatic fracture in middle-aged females.
   a. osteoporosis
   b. kidney failure
   c. cancer
   d. brittle bone disease

7. What differentiates necrotizing fasciitis from cellulitis?
   a. severe pain
   b. erythema
   c. lymphangitis
   d. edema

8. Which of the following is NOT a cause of chronic extremity pain?
   a. arterial occlusion
   b. arthritis
   c. fibromyalgia
   d. tendonitis

9. Which of the following is NOT a form of arthritis?
   a. osteoarthritis
   b. rheumatoid arthritis
   c. gout
   d. bursitis

10. Which musculoskeletal disorder tends to affect the elderly more frequently than other groups?
    a. osteoarthritis
    b. rheumatoid arthritis
    c. gout
    d. bursitis

11. What condition is suggested by fever and chills?
    a. cellulitis
    b. rheumatoid arthritis
    c. tendonitis
    d. bursitis

12. What is the most frequent cause of acute arterial occlusion in the upper extremity?
    a. atrial fibrillation
    b. pathological fractures
    c. central venous lines
    d. disability

13. If a patient suffers joint dislocation from minor trauma, what condition should the Paramedic suspect?
    a. osteoarthritis
    b. rheumatoid arthritis
    c. gout
    d. bursitis

14. Which of the following is NOT typically caused by repetitive motion?
    a. tenosynovitis
    b. arthritis
    c. bursitis
    d. tendonitis

15. Which musculoskeletal disorder is associated with headaches?
    a. fibromyalgia
    b. rheumatoid arthritis
    c. bursitis
    d. gout

Short Answer

Write a brief answer to each of the following questions.

16. Differentiate acute distal arterial occlusion from venous occlusion.

    _____

    _____

17. Describe the nontraumatic causes and pathophysiology of rhabdomyolysis.

    _____

    _____

18. What is arthritis?

    _____

    _____

19. What venereal disease is associated with a musculoskeletal disease?

    _____

    _____

20. What is fibromyalgia?

    _____

    _____

Fill in the Blank

Complete each sentence by adding the appropriate word in the provided blanks.

21. A nontraumatic fracture affecting adolescents is called a _____ _____ _____ _____.

22. Streaking up a leg, secondary to cellulitis, is called _____.

23. A cutaneous abscess under a nail bed is called a _____.

24. The five "P's" of acute arterial occlusion are pain, paresthesia, paralysis, pallor, and _____.

25. Inflammation of the bursa sac, with accumulation of fluid, is called _____.

CHAPTER 23

BLEEDING DISORDERS

Case Study

Chief Concern

200 Rosewood Manor, a rest home with a skilled nursing unit, calls requesting a transport for an 87-year-old male patient with a history of dementia. The only information that the caller provides is that the doctor ordered the patient to be taken to the hospital and she thinks it is for a bloody nose.

"I hate those third-party callers," says Andrea. "You never know what you're getting." With those words, she turns on the lights and siren and works her way into traffic.

Critical Thinking Questions

1. What are some of the possible causes of nosebleeds?

   _____

   _____

2. What potentially life-threatening conditions could cause a nosebleed?

   _____

   _____

History

Andrea introduces herself to the nurse on duty, who is dutifully copying the nursing transfer forms, including a MOLST form. As she does so, she explains to Andrea that Jake is a recent transfer from the hospital to Rosewood Manor. He has an impressive history including multiple admissions for alcohol rehabilitation and a recent admission for esophageal varices.

Jake's nosebleed came on suddenly and spontaneously, without any trauma. He was simply lying in bed. She notes that the nursing aid reported bleeding from his gums when he performed routine oral hygiene this morning.

Critical Thinking Questions

1. What are the important elements of the history that a Paramedic should obtain?

   _____

   _____

2. What specific medication history should the Paramedic obtain?

   _____

   _____

Examination

Although Andrea remembers that the nurse reported Jake was demented, she did not report that Jake was also obtunded. Although he is maintaining his airway independently, everything else is in decline. His respirations are markedly shallow, pulse oximeter SpO$_2$ 85%, pulse bradycardiac at the carotid, the radial pulse is absent, and the blood pressure, as her partner puts it, is "in the toilet."

Andrea works to start resuscitation, keeping in mind the instructions on the MOLST form (e.g., oxygen but no ventilation). Moving him over to the stretcher, she notes that he has very large and diffuse bruises. The nurse explains that elderly patients bruise very easily. Although Andrea understands this, these bruises are in areas that are not typically used for lifting and other tasks.

Jake also has an indwelling catheter, "in him since he left the hospital," the nurse explains. "We have been meaning to change it but we are short-handed and nobody had time." Andrea notes blood on his nightgown and lifts up his gown to discover blood at the meatus of his penis, proximal to his indwelling catheter.

She also notes, as she makes a mental survey of him from head to toe, that his toes are gangrenous. The nurse explains that was due to Jake's diabetes and that they were scheduled to be amputated later in the week.

Critical Thinking Questions

1. What are the elements of the physical examination of a patient with suspected bleeding disorder?

   _____

   _____

2. Why is a neurological assessment a critical element in this examination?

   _____

   _____

Assessment

Andrea suspects that Jake is in end-stage sepsis and that he also has disseminated intravascular coagulation. Somewhat frustrated, as the MOLST form severely limits her options for treatment and resuscitation, Andrea elects to transport Jake immediately and perform the limited supportive care she can while on the way to the hospital.

Critical Thinking Questions

1. What is the significance of the widespread bruising?

   _____

   _____

2. If disseminated intravascular coagulation, secondary to sepsis, is suspected, what other workups are needed?

   _____

   _____

Treatment

Frustrated that she cannot help Jake with his breathing, Andrea maintains the high-flow, high-concentration oxygen. However, it isn't appreciably changing the SpO$_2$. Concentrating on obtaining venous access, the MOLST form says she can give fluids but cannot give medications. Therefore, she hopes that a fluid bolus might boost his blood pressure.

Critical Thinking Questions

1. What is the standard of care of patients with suspected DIC secondary to sepsis?

   _____

   _____

2. Assuming the MOLST form did not prohibit administration of any medications, what medication would be given to support the blood pressure?

   _____

   _____

Evaluation

Jake is quickly deteriorating. His blood pressure is extremely low and his heart rate is even lower. Andrea notes that there is blood coming from around the venous site and she knows that is not a good sign. If he is bleeding on the outside, she reasons as she blots the blood with a bandage, he is most certainly bleeding on the inside as well.

Critical Thinking Questions

1. What are some of the predictable complications associated with DIC?

_____

_____

2. Beyond vasopressor support, what else can a Paramedic due to help the patient with end-stage sepsis?

_____

_____

Disposition

As the ambulance pulls into Rosewood Manor, Andrea sees Jake take his last breath. Looking at the monitor, he still shows an agonal rhythm but she understands that he probably bled to death internally.

Electing to advise the emergency department first, she grabs the nursing notes and the MOLST form and proceeds into the ambulance while her partner waits outside with Jake.

Critical Thinking Questions

1. What is the most appropriate transport decision that will get the patient to definitive care?

_____

_____

2. What special hospital services may the patient need beyond intensive care?

_____

_____

Practice Questions

Multiple Choice

Select the best answer for each of the following questions.

1. Which of the following is NOT part of primary hemostasis?
   a. von Willebrand factor
   b. coagulation cascade
   c. fibrinogen
   d. platelets

2. Which clotting disorder is the most common?
   a. von Willebrand disease
   b. hemophilia A
   c. hemophilia B
   d. sickle cell disease

3. Which clotting disorder is a problem with factor IX?
   a. von Willebrand disease
   b. hemophilia A
   c. hemophilia B
   d. sickle cell disease

4. Hemarthrosis is rare in which population of patients?
   a. von Willebrand disease
   b. hemophilia A
   c. hemophilia B
   d. sickle cell disease

5. Which of the following is an autoimmune condition?
   a. idiopathic thrombocytopenic purpura
   b. heparin–induced thrombocytopenia
   c. hemolytic anemia
   d. disseminated intravascular coagulation

6. What is widespread arterial and venous thrombosis due to sepsis called?
   a. purpura fatalis
   b. idiopathic thrombocytopenic purpura
   c. purpura fulminans
   d. thrombocytopenia

7. Disseminated intravascular coagulation is seen with which condition?
   a. systemic inflammatory response syndrome (SIRS)
   b. idiopathic thrombocytopenic purpura (TIP)
   c. venous thrombus embolism (VTE)
   d. von Willebrand disease (vWF)

8. Which population is NOT affected by sickle cell disease?
   a. Africans
   b. Indians
   c. Mediterranean
   d. Inuits

9. Who is sickle cell disease inherited from?
   a. mother
   b. father
   c. either
   d. both

10. Which condition occurs due to a blood transfusion?
    a. immune-mediated hemolytic anemia
    b. alloimmune hemolytic anemia
    c. thrombotic thrombocytopenic purpura
    d. autoimmune hemolytic anemia

11. Which condition affects the mother during pregnancy?
    a. immune-mediated hemolytic anemia
    b. alloimmune hemolytic anemia
    c. thrombotic thrombocytopenic purpura
    d. hemolytic, elevated liver enzymes and low platelets

12. Which disorder has been associated with smoking?
    a. hemolytic anemia
    b. thrombotic thrombocytopenic purpura
    c. methemoglobinemia
    d. polycythemia

13. Epistaxis (nosebleed) is seen most commonly in which condition?
    a. von Willebrand disease
    b. hemophilia A
    c. hemophilia B
    d. sickle cell disease

14. Abdominal pain is seen most commonly in which condition?
    a. von Willebrand disease
    b. hemophilia A
    c. hemophilia B
    d. sickle cell disease

15. Hemarthrosis (blood in the joints) is seen most commonly in which condition?
    a. von Willebrand disease
    b. hemophilia A
    c. hemophilia B
    d. sickle cell disease

Short Answer

Write a brief answer to each of the following questions.

16. What is disseminated intravascular coagulation?

    _____

    _____

17. Describe how polycythemia can lead to heart failure.

    _____

    _____

18. Describe the pathophysiology of autoimmune hemolytic anemia.

    _____

    _____

19. Name the three nutrients necessary for red blood cell production.

    _____

    _____

20. What is von Willebrand disease?

    _____

    _____

Fill in the Blank

Complete each sentence by adding the appropriate word in the provided blanks.

21. _____ is a term used to describe any bleeding disorder due to problems with the coagulation cascade.

22. _____ is the term used to describe decreased hemoglobin.

23. Erythroblastosis fetalis, a life-threatening neonatal condition caused by the mixing of fetal blood with maternal blood, is a form of _____ _____ _____.

24. A blood syndrome from undercooked meats, called hamburger syndrome, that affects kidneys is called _____ _____ _____.

25. _____ is the cause of the most common infection-related hemolytic anemia in the world.

CHAPTER 24

BACK PAIN

Case Study

Chief Concern

"Rescue One to Communications, we are on-scene." Communications acknowledges the arrival of Rescue One. The call is for a 50-year-old female with severe lower back pain and weakness in her legs. Responding to the call, the two Paramedics discuss some atraumatic reasons why a fiftysomething-year-old female would have lower back pain and weakness in the legs.

Critical Thinking Questions

1. What are some of the possible musculoskeletal causes of back pain?

_____

_____

2. What are some nontraumatic, nonmusculoskeletal causes of back pain?

_____

_____

History

The crew members, Mark and Matt, arrive to find the patient lying on the living room floor. "Good morning," Mark proclaims as he gets down to one knee. "What have we here?" The patient, Pat, explains that she has had increasingly severe back pain for the last two weeks and this morning she had trouble with her legs. Sensing this was more than a backache, she called 9-1-1.

While Matt obtains vital signs, Mark continues with the questioning. Pat is adamant that the pain is not due to trauma; she has not fallen, been in a car crash, or endured anything similar. That disclosure leads Mark down another set of questions.

Critical Thinking Questions

1. What are the important elements of the history that a Paramedic should obtain?

_____

_____

2. What are the important elements of the patient's past medical history?

_____

_____

Examination

Matt obtains a full set of vitals and starts a physical examination, starting anteriorly then proceeding to the patient's posterior side, as the patient is log-rolled onto a backboard. The anterior abdomen is soft and nontender, with no evidence of a pulsating mass at the midline. Log-rolling the patient, Matt cannot elicit any tenderness at the costovertebral angle with a kidney tap.

Pat's vital signs are slightly elevated but within the normal range for an adult. A brief focused physical examination shows that Pat does not have any localized spinal tenderness, but has a lot of muscle spasm around the spinal column in the lower lumbar area. Any leg movement seems to increase the pain, and the sensation and strength in her legs seem to be decreased.

Critical Thinking Questions

1. What are the elements of the physical examination of a patient with back pain?

_____

_____

2. Why is a peripheral neurological examination a critical element in this examination?

_____

_____

Assessment

Mentally reviewing the symptom complex, Mark remembers that Pat does not have abdominal pain. However, Pat does have difficulty in urinating. The physical examination also reveals that Pat does not have very much motor strength or sensation in either of her lower legs.

Mark and Matt confer and agree that they can probably exclude a ruptured aortic aneurysm as there is no abdominal pain, tenderness, masses, or circulation issue in the lower extremities. Furthermore, Pat does not have any fever or weight loss, which makes cancer or an infection less likely. Pat's history and physical condition is consistent with acute cord compression. In addition, the muscle weakness and decreased sensation point toward an acute cord compression.

Critical Thinking Questions

1. What is the significance of the leg weakness?

_____

_____

2. What diagnosis did the Paramedic announce to the patient?

_____

_____

Treatment

Pat is moved to the ambulance on a backboard but complains bitterly of the pain the backboard is causing her. After consultation with medical control, Matt and Mark remove Pat from the backboard for the trip into the hospital, although they elect to keep her supine. The medical director also authorizes analgesia as needed for Pat's back pain in order to make the trip to the hospital tolerable.

Critical Thinking Questions

1. What is the standard of care of patients with suspected acute cord compression?

_____

_____

2. What analgesia might be used in this case?

_____

_____

Evaluation

Pat remains relatively stable throughout the transport. Mark elects to re-dose Pat before unloading her at the hospital because of her stable vital signs. His therapeutic goal is have Pat's pain a 0 on the 0–10 scale.

Critical Thinking Questions

1. What are some of the predictable complications associated with acute cord compression?

   _____

   _____

2. How would an aortic aneurysm present?

   _____

   _____

Disposition

At the hospital, report is given to the attending physician. The physician confirms the history and physical examination findings, orders a stat MRI, and calls the neurosurgeon on call. The MRI shows an acute cord compression from a central disk herniation between the L4 and L5 vertebrae.

Pat expresses her thanks to Matt and Mark for treating her so well and making her comfortable.

Critical Thinking Questions

1. What is the most appropriate transport decision that will get the patient to definitive care?

   _____

   _____

2. What special hospital services might be needed?

   _____

   _____

Practice Questions
Multiple Choice

Select the best answer for each of the following questions.

1. Which of the following is NOT associated with aging?
   a. spinal stenosis
   b. diskitis
   c. osteoporosis
   d. all of the above

2. Which of the following is an atypical, atraumatic, nonmusculoskeletal cause of back pain?
   a. constipation
   b. kidney stones
   c. pyelonephritis
   d. abdominal aortic aneurysm

3. Which of the following atraumatic, nonmusculoskeletal causes of back pain is more common in women?
   a. constipation
   b. kidney stones
   c. pyelonephritis
   d. abdominal aortic aneurysm

4. Which of the following organs is NOT found in the retroperitoneal space?
   a. kidneys
   b. spleen
   c. aorta
   d. ovaries

5. What differentiates traumatic back pain from atraumatic back pain?
   a. location of the pain
   b. specific event leading to pain
   c. numbness in the extremities
   d. severity of the pain

6. Which of the following is NOT suggestive of an aortic aneurysm?
   a. syncope
   b. headache
   c. lightheadedness
   d. orthostatic hypotension

7. What differentiates atraumatic, musculoskeletal back pain from renal calculi?
   a. location of the pain
   b. specific event leading to pain
   c. migration of the pain
   d. severity of the pain

8. Numbness in the perineum is from compression of _____ to _____ nerves.
   a. T12 to L1
   b. L3 to L4
   c. L6 to L7
   d. S4 to S5

9. Which of the following causes of atraumatic, musculoskeletal back pain is associated with night sweats?
   a. tuberculosis
   b. pyelonephritis
   c. osteoporosis
   d. diskitis

10. Which of the following signs is NOT associated with aortic aneurysm rupture?
    a. bilateral leg weakness
    b. cold legs
    c. saddle anesthesia
    d. pain on urination

11. Which of the following is NOT a nonspecific sign of an infection in the spine?
    a. urinary incontinence
    b. night sweats
    c. fever
    d. unintended weight loss

12. Which of the following is NOT one of the listed signs and symptoms of a surgical emergency for nontraumatic back pain?
    a. night sweats
    b. abdominal pain
    c. syncope
    d. incontinence

13. Which condition is rarely produced by a herniated disk?
    a. shooting pains down a leg
    b. unilateral numbness
    c. pins and needles in a foot
    d. bilateral weakness

14. What is spinal cord compression in the lumbar spine called?
    a. lumbaritis
    b. acute diskitis
    c. spinal stenosis
    d. cauda equina syndrome

15. It is important to obtain _____ for a patient with nontraumatic back pain.
    a. analgesia history
    b. surgical history
    c. last stool
    d. all of the above

Short Answer

Write a brief answer to each of the following questions.

16. Describe the pathophysiology of diskitis.

    _____

    _____

17. Describe saddle anesthesia.

    _____

    _____

18. What is stool incontinence?

    _____

    _____

19. Why is back pain with associated abdominal pain a "red flag"?

    _____

    _____

20. Describe the physical examination of the patient with atraumatic, musculoskeletal back pain.

    _____

    _____

Fill in the Blank

Complete each sentence by adding the appropriate word in the provided blanks.

21. Back pain from _____ is usually due to urinary tract infection.

22. A narrowing of the spinal canal is called _____ _____.

23. Loss of sensation in the perineum is called _____ _____.

24. _____ tend to cause constipation, a source of back pain, leading to more back pain.

25. An infection of the disk between the spinal vertebrae is called _____.

CHAPTER 25

DISORDERS OF CENTRAL CIRCULATION

Case Study
Chief Concern

"This headache is killing me!" exclaims Joe, a large framed, heavy set, elderly, African American male in obvious distress, who is cradling his head in his hands. When Joe looks up at Sara, the Paramedic in charge, she can see a tear running down his cheek and thinks to herself, "I'll bet that this bear of a man never cried a day in his life. He must be in real pain."

Critical Thinking Questions

1. What are some of the primary causes of Joe's headache?

_____

_____

2. What are some of the secondary causes of a headache?

_____

_____

History

Although Joe's headache is a bad headache, the worst in his life, it did not come on suddenly. The headache has been progressively worsening this morning. Tylenol® isn't even coming close to helping. Several times he has felt nauseous but he didn't vomit. He also tells Sara that he is having some trouble seeing but he cannot find his glasses. Joe denies passing out and, although he is in too much pain to work, he doesn't feel weak. (Joe relates that he worked every day of his life.)

"I am late to work now," Joe states, "but I can't work with my head like this. I can't concentrate." Joe drives busses for the city and county transit authority and prides himself on his nearly flawless attendance.

Joe relates a history of hypertension and diabetes. Both conditions are controlled by medication that he admits he "sometimes forgets" to take. He was a smoker for 30 plus years, two packs a day, until the authority banned smoking on busses.

Critical Thinking Questions

1. What are the important elements of the history that a Paramedic should obtain?

_____

_____

2. What are some of the important elements of the past medical history that a Paramedic should obtain?

_____

_____

Examination

While Sara continues to obtain a medical history, her EMT partner obtains a set of vital signs. In mid-sentence, she feels a tap on her elbow. Looking down, she sees her partner's notepad with the numbers 220/120 written down. Looking at her partner, he nods. She asks him to take a blood pressure in the other arm, and then looks back at Joe. "Joe," she says, "let's get you to the hospital."

Critical Thinking Questions

1. What are the elements of the physical examination of a patient with suspected hypertensive emergency?

_____

_____

2. Why is a cardiovascular examination, including a12-lead ECG, a critical element in this examination?

_____

_____

Assessment

"What's going on? I can't go to the hospital. I've got to go to work. Isn't there something you can give me so I don't have to go to the hospital?" Joe asks. "Joe," Sara patiently explains, "your blood pressure is high, dangerously high. I don't know why it's so high, but there are some potentially life-threatening reasons why someone's blood pressure is so high. If you don't get it fixed you could have a stroke or a heart attack!"

Critical Thinking Questions

1. What diagnosis did the Paramedic announce to the patient?

_____

_____

2. Why would the patient not be aware of the seriousness of the illness?

_____

_____

Treatment

While on the way to the hospital, Sara turns down the interior lights, and turns off the ambulance siren and lights, all in an effort to keep Joe calm. She considers sedation but dismisses the idea. She obtains venous access, just in case, and then calls medical command at the resource hospital. After consulting with an ED attending physician, they decide to continue to monitor Joe and withhold any pharmacological treatment for the present.

Critical Thinking Questions

1. What is the standard of care of patients with suspected hypertensive crisis?

_____

_____

2. Why are nitrates preferred in the prehospital treatment of suspected hypertensive crisis?

_____

_____

Evaluation

In mid-sentence, Joe starts slurring his words. "What did you say, Joe?" Sara asks, hoping to get Joe to repeat what he had just said. Joe must know something is wrong, because he refuses to talk. "Look, Joe, you've got to talk to me!" Sara protests. Joe looks at her and smiles a crooked smile.

Critical Thinking Questions

1. What are some of the predictable complications associated with acute hypertensive crisis?

   _____

   _____

2. What are some of the predictable complications associated with the treatments for acute hypertensive crisis?

   _____

   _____

Disposition

Joe is transferred immediately to the stroke unit within the emergency department for immediate evaluation upon his arrival. His neurological status continues to deteriorate. His words are slurred, his answers nonsensical, and his facial droop is obvious even when he isn't smiling. And he isn't smiling much now.

Sara finishes her report to the nurse at the bedside and turns to say goodbye to Joe. He reaches out and grabs her arm, smiles his crooked smile, and mouths the words "Thank you."

Critical Thinking Questions

1. What is the most appropriate transport decision that will get the patient to definitive care?

   _____

   _____

2. What specialty hospitals have these capabilities?

   _____

   _____

Practice Questions
Multiple Choice

Select the best answer for each of the following questions.

1. Stage I hypertension is defined as a diastolic blood pressure greater than _____ mmHg.
   a. 70
   b. 80
   c. 90
   d. 100

2. Stage II hypertension is defined as a diastolic blood pressure greater than _____ mmHg.
   a. 70
   b. 80
   c. 90
   d. 100

3. An "acceptable" blood pressure is defined as a diastolic blood pressure less than _____ mmHg
   a. 70
   b. 80
   c. 90
   d. 100

4. Signs and/or symptoms of end-organ damage is seen with which situation?
   a. hypertensive emergency
   b. acute hypertensive episode
   c. hypertensive urgency
   d. Stage II hypertension

5. Which of the following is the least common manifestation of an acute hypertensive emergency?
   a. acute pulmonary edema
   b. non-STEMI
   c. acute renal failure
   d. aortic aneurysm

6. Which of the following is the most difficult end-organ dysfunction to detect in the field?
   a. hypertensive encephalopathy
   b. renal failure
   c. heart failure
   d. myocardial infarction

7. Peripheral vascular insufficiency, secondary to hypertension, can result in what condition?
   a. extremity pain
   b. peripheral nerve damage
   c. erectile dysfunction
   d. all of the above

8. Rarely, acute systemic hypertension can lead to what condition?
   a. ventricular rupture
   b. heart failure
   c. aortic aneurysm
   d. ventricular hypertrophy

9. Hypertension-induced seizures can occur during which stage of pregnancy?
   a. second term
   b. third term
   c. up to two weeks postpartum
   d. all of the above

10. In the prehospital setting, what is the most common treatment for hypertensive emergencies?
    a. nitrates
    b. beta blockers
    c. diuretics
    d. transport

11. What is the drug of choice for eclampsia-induced hypertension?
    a. beta blockers
    b. diuretics
    c. magnesium
    d. beta blockers

12. Hypertension is NOT implicated in which of the following conditions of pregnancy?
    a. pregnancy-induced hypertension
    b. pre-eclampsia
    c. eclampsia
    d. hyperemesis gravidarum

13. Patients with chronic hypertension are at risk for what condition?
    a. stroke
    b. renal failure
    c. heart attack
    d. all of the above

14. What percentage of Paramedics think that health education is part of their job?
    a. 10%
    b. 25%
    c. 50%
    d. 80%

15. Shear forces in the bloodstream, caused by hypertension, cause aortic aneurysms because the aorta is _____.
    a. dilated
    b. thinner
    c. irregular
    d. all of the above

Short Answer

Write a brief answer to each of the following questions.

16. What are the effects of chronic hypertension on the brain?

    _____

    _____

17. What are the effects of chronic hypertension on the heart?

    _____

    _____

18. What are the effects of chronic hypertension on the kidneys?

    _____

    _____

19. What are the essential historical elements that a Paramedic should gather for a patient manifesting with neurological symptoms?

    _____

    _____

20. What are the essential historical elements that a Paramedic should gather for a patient manifesting with cardiac symptoms?

    _____

    _____

Fill in the Blank

Complete each sentence by adding the appropriate word in the provided blanks.

21. Altered mental status, seizures, and visual disturbances are signs of _____ _____.

22. The gray zone between hypertension and hypertensive emergency is called _____ _____.

23. Generalized itching is a sign of _____.

24. Seizures induced by hypertension in a pregnant patient are due to _____.

25. Renal hypotension, secondary to systemic hypertension, activates the _____ –_____ –_____ _____.

CHAPTER 26

DISORDERS OF THE HEAD, EYES, EARS, NOSE, AND THROAT

Case Study
Chief Concern

The portable chirps "Medic zone one, respond to a man with blurred vision, 21 Havana Avenue, time out 0930." Stuffing their mouths with the last of a half-eaten breakfast, the Paramedics get up from their booth and run toward the door. "Keep it warm until we get back, Shirley," they call. "Sure, sure, I will keep it warm." Shirley replies as she scrapes the dish into the garbage.

Alamar considers possible causes for the man's blurry vision. "Something in his eyes. That's pretty broad. And that is a residential neighborhood, so I am thinking this isn't industrial." Mayra responds, "Yeah, but what could it be then?"

Critical Thinking Questions

1. What are some potential causes of eye injury?

_____

_____

2. What are some "secondary" or indirect causes of blurred or lost vision?

_____

_____

History

When the Paramedics arrive, Amanda greets them and explains what happened. Her husband, Mark, was nearly done with the prep work for his new deck. He was proud of his newest "work." However, when he put down a bag of cement he was going to use for the footing, the bag exploded, sending a plume of cement dust into the air. Amanda found Mark on his knees covered in cement dust and screaming in pain as he rubbed his eyes furiously. Amanda had advised, "Stop rubbing your eyes, here's a hose, get some water into them."

Critical Thinking Questions

1. What are the properties of cement dust?

_____

_____

Case Studies & Practice Questions   **143**

© 2011 Cengage Learning. All Rights Reserved. May not be scanned, copied or duplicated, or posted to a publicly accessible website, in whole or in part.

2. Was Amanda's advice correct?

_____

_____

Examination

"Nice work, Mark, the irrigation is incredibly important. How does your eye feel?" Alamar asks while donning protective gloves. "Let's take a look at your eyes." The sclera is reddened and inflamed but the iris is already opaque. "Can you see how many fingers I have up, Mark?" Alamar asks.

Critical Thinking Questions

1. What are the elements of the physical examination of a patient with an ocular burn?

_____

_____

2. What are the elements of the eye exam?

_____

_____

Assessment

"Am I going to go blind?" Mark asks.

Mayra replies, "It's too early to tell, but you are doing the right thing by irrigating your eyes."

"That was Amanda's idea," Mark comments. "Thank you, baby!"

Critical Thinking Questions

1. What diagnosis does the Paramedic tell the patient?

_____

_____

2. What is the prognosis for a burn to the eye?

_____

_____

Treatment

"Mark," Alamar explains, "I am going to roll your eyelids up, then down, both top and bottom, and put this Morgan lens® in."

"What's a Morgan lens®?" Mark asks

"It's like a contact lens with an IV attached to it. It doesn't actually touch your eye—that would hurt. Instead, it will float above the eye on a cushion of water."

Critical Thinking Questions

1. What is the standard of care for patients with ocular burns?

_____

_____

2. What device might be helpful with irrigation?

_____

_____

Evaluation

Mark's eyes stop burning on the way into the hospital. "Do I still need this?" Mark asks, pointing to the irrigation setup.

"Yes," Mayra replies, "at least until the doctor looks at your eyes."

Critical Thinking Questions

1. Is the irrigation still needed?

_____

_____

2. When should the irrigation stop?

_____

_____

Disposition

"Well, we're here," Mayra states. "Mark, I want you to lean your head back and just relax." With Amanda walking next to the stretcher, holding Mark's hand, he sits back onto the stretcher.

Stopping the stretcher, Mayra steps to the side and explains the case to the triage nurse. "To the ENT room, stat." the triage nurse directs the patient care associates, "and keep the irrigation going with lactated Ringer's."

Critical Thinking Questions

1. What is the most appropriate transport decision that will get the patient to definitive care?

_____

_____

2. What specialty hospital may be preferred?

_____

_____

Practice Questions
Multiple Choice

Select the best answer for each of the following questions.

1. Which of the following is NOT a primary headache?
    a. hypoglycemia
    b. cluster
    c. tension
    d. migraine

2. Which of the following is NOT a physiologic cause of dizziness?
    a. dehydration
    b. infection
    c. vertigo
    d. amusement park ride

3. Which cranial nerve is responsible for providing the brain with information needed for balance?
    a. III
    b. V
    c. VIII
    d. X

4. Peripheral vertigo is a problem of which area of the body?
   a. inner ear
   b. vestibular system
   c. cranial nerves
   d. cerebellum

5. Central vertigo, versus peripheral vertigo, is usually _____.
   a. gradual
   b. moderate to intense
   c. associated with hearing loss
   d. associated with nausea

6. Which of the following is NOT a cause of peripheral vertigo?
   a. benign paroxysmal positional vertigo
   b. stroke
   c. Ménière disease
   d. labyrinthitis

7. The patient complains of lightheadedness and dizziness. Which of the following causes of lightheadedness and dizziness is NOT a precursor to a more severe medical condition?
   a. labyrinthitis
   b. carotid artery stenosis
   c. concussion
   d. dysrhythmia

8. Unilateral blurred vision and tearing of the eye should suggest what condition to the Paramedic?
   a. corneal abrasion
   b. acute angle glaucoma
   c. retinal detachment
   d. stroke

9. Which symptoms accompany ocular migraines?
   a. blurred vision
   b. nausea
   c. headache
   d. all of the above

10. Which of the following is NOT a common cause of epistaxis?
    a. hypertension
    b. nose-picking
    c. infection
    d. dried nasal passages

11. Patients who want to keep their heads in slight flexion with little movement may have what condition?
    a. peritonsillar abscess
    b. retropharyngeal abscess
    c. epiglottis
    d. Ludwig's angina

12. What condition refers to swelling and infection of the floor of the mouth?
    a. peritonsillar abscess
    b. retropharyngeal abscess
    c. epiglottis
    d. Ludwig's angina

13. A deviated uvula may be a sign of which condition?
    a. peritonsillar abscess
    b. retropharyngeal abscess
    c. epiglottis
    d. Ludwig's angina

14. The classic triad of drooling, dysphagia, and distress (respiratory) are signs of which condition?
    a. peritonsillar abscess
    b. retropharyngeal abscess
    c. epiglottis
    d. Ludwig's angina

15. What instrument is used to examine the eye?
    a. otoscope
    b. ophthalmoscope
    c. obamoscope
    d. oculoscope

Short Answer

Write a brief answer to each of the following questions.

16. Explain the origins of dizziness.

    _____

    _____

17. What is the difference between peripheral vertigo and central vertigo?

    _____

    _____

18. What is disequilibrium?

    _____

    _____

19. What is acute angle–closure glaucoma?

    _____

    _____

20. What is more dangerous to the eye, an alkali burn or an acid burn?

    _____

    _____

Fill in the Blank

Complete each sentence by adding the appropriate word in the provided blanks.

21. Ringing in the ears is called _____.

22. A feeling of "spinning around" is called _____.

23. A feeling of being "off-balance" is called _____.

24. Pink eye is also called _____.

25. The medical term for nosebleed is _____.

CHAPTER 27

INFECTIOUS DISEASES: FEVER

Case Study
Chief Concern

The call comes in for a man spitting up blood. He calls the private ambulance and insists that they not use the lights or siren. Arriving in the gated community of Oakwood Estates, as instructed, the crew shuts down the lights and siren. Arriving at the home, Andre can't help but notice the place looks like a mansion. Donning his HEPA mask, Andre's muffled voice is barely audible, "What do you think?" Jay, his partner, turns to him and shrugs his shoulders. "Policy says if they cough, we mask."

Critical Thinking Questions

1. What are some of the possible pulmonary causes of hemoptysis?

   _____

   _____

2. What are some of the extrapulmonary causes of hemoptysis?

   _____

   _____

History

Mr. Wentworth is a foreign service agent who has worked for the past 30 years in "the bush" in South Africa fighting the triple threat of malaria, AIDS, and tuberculosis. He was sent home after a diagnosis of prostate cancer. His treatment consists of radiation and chemotherapy. He has experienced some night sweats and weight loss, but he attributes them both to his cancer as well as his chemo.

What alarms Mr. Wentworth is the hemoptysis. "I've never spit up blood before. That's not natural," he says. "I would have taken myself to the hospital but, to be honest, I feel too weak to drive." Further questioning reveals that he also has a low grade fever and some "rigors." Again, he assumes these are part of the side effects of the chemotherapy.

Critical Thinking Questions

1. What are the important elements of the history that a Paramedic should obtain?

   _____

   _____

2. Why should the patient's overseas travel be explored in more depth?

   _____

   _____

Examination

Mr. Wentworth looks feeble and frail, not like the picture of the robust man standing with Nelson Mandela that is on the fireplace mantle. His breathing is labored and he appears exhausted. Auscultation of his breath sounds reveals diffuse loud rales (crackles) in the upper lobes. He is also warm to the touch.

While examining his chest, Andre notices the raised purple lesions on his neck along the carotid groove as well as some supraclavicular ones. These lesions are red, almost cyanotic, rubbery, and cold to the touch. Mr. Wentworth also complains of a sharp chest pain located in the right upper chest that worsens with a deep breath.

Critical Thinking Questions

1. What are the elements of the physical examination of a patient with suspected tuberculosis?

2. Why is a 12-lead ECG a critical element in this examination?

Assessment

Despite the fact that Mr. Wentworth got the Bacillus Calmette—Guerin (BCG) 30 years ago, it would appear he has contracted tuberculosis. Andre thinks his tuberculosis is advanced as evidenced by the lymphadenopathy.

"Mr. Wentworth," asks Andre, "which hospital would you like to go to?" Mr. Wentworth replies, "Any hospital, St. Mary's, the Medical Center, Community, your choice, but please don't use that bloody siren in the neighborhood, kids are trying to sleep."

Critical Thinking Questions

1. What diagnosis did the Paramedic announce to the patient?

2. What other medical conditions could cause the symptom complex?

Treatment

Jay puts Mr. Wentworth in oxygen and Andre places him on the ECG monitor for the trip. After establishing venous access, Andre elects to try a gentle trial of saline solution. Mr. Wentworth is both tachycardiac and a little hypotensive.

Critical Thinking Questions

1. What is the first priority of care for the Paramedic treating the patient with suspected tuberculosis?

2. What is the next priority of care for the Paramedic treating the patient with suspected tuberculosis?

Evaluation

Mr. Wentworth becomes increasingly less responsive. Andre elects to use medication-facilitated intubation to help assist ventilation for the obviously exhausted Mr. Wentworth. After successfully intubating Mr. Wentworth, Jay starts a dopamine drip to help support his pressure on the way to the hospital.

Critical Thinking Questions

1. What are some of the predictable complications associated with suspected tuberculosis?

_____

_____

2. What advanced complications can be expected for the patient with tuberculosis?

_____

_____

Disposition

Pulling into the Medical Center driveway, Andre whispers into Mr. Wentworth's ear, "We are at the Medical Center. I am going to give you some more medicine to help you relax. Let us do all the work."

As the stretcher is unloaded, several old men in suits and topcoats walk over. "Is this Mr. Wentworth?" they ask.

"Yes," replies Andre. One of the men comes over, puts his hand on Mr. Wentworth's hand, and says, "We are all here for you."

Critical Thinking Questions

1. What is the most appropriate transport decision that will get the patient to definitive care?

_____

_____

2. What specialty hospital might be preferred in this case?

_____

_____

Practice Questions

Multiple Choice

Select the best answer for each of the following questions.

1. What is the least common cause of infection in the elderly?
   a. meningitis
   b. pneumonia
   c. bedsores
   d. urinary tract infections

2. Which of the following is a helminth?
   a. tapeworm
   b. flea
   c. tick
   d. lice

3. Which of the following is a single-cell lifeform?
   a. protozoa
   b. bacteria
   c. fungus
   d. helminth

4. Which lifeform is a true parasite?
   a. bacterium
   b. protozoa
   c. virus
   d. fungus

5. Which of the following would NOT be considered a "zoonotic" carrier?
   a. cattle
   b. dogs
   c. people
   d. birds

6. Infectivity is a function of all of the following EXCEPT _____.
   a. mode of transfer
   b. dose
   c. virulence
   d. host resistance

7. Which of the following is NOT part of the innate immune system?
   a. cytokines
   b. histamine
   c. antibodies
   d. leukotrienes

8. Which of the following is NOT a leukocyte?
   a. mast cells
   b. lymphocytes
   c. basophils
   d. neutrophils

9. Antibodies in mother's milk are a form of which type of immunity?
   a. acquired passive immunity
   b. acquired active immunity
   c. naturally acquired immunity
   d. artificially acquired immunity

10. Vaccines are a form of which type of immunity?
    a. acquired passive immunity
    b. acquired active immunity
    c. naturally acquired immunity
    d. artificially acquired immunity

11. Which of the following is an endotoxin?
    a. cytotoxin
    b. enterotoxin
    c. neurotoxin
    d. none of the above

12. During which time period is a disease most communicable?
    a. incubation/prodromal phase
    b. prodromal/infectious phase
    c. infectious /recovery phase
    d. incubation/recovery phase

13. Which of the following is NOT considered a constitutional sign of an infection?
    a. sore throat
    b. fever
    c. muscle aches
    d. malaise

14. Which diseases can cause hemoptysis?
    a. tuberculosis
    b. Yersinia pestis
    c. cancer
    d. all of the above

15. What is the most common pediatric respiratory disease?
    a. laryngotracheobronchitis
    b. epiglottis
    c. pertussis
    d. tuberculosis

Short Answer

Write a brief answer to each of the following questions.

16. What is a carrier?

_____

_____

17. What is turbidity in urine?

_____

_____

18. Define virulence.

_____

_____

19. What are the four stages of infection?

_____

_____

20. What is a residual? What is a sequela?

_____

_____

Fill in the Blank

Complete each sentence by adding the appropriate word in the provided blanks.

21. Prevention of an infection, by the presence of another microbe, is called _____ _____.

22. A disease capable of being transmitted to others is considered _____.

23. Contaminated surfaces containing pathogens are called _____.

24. A virus that is weakened, and incapable of pathogenecity, is _____.

25. The peak of infection is called its _____.

CHAPTER 28

INFECTIOUS DISEASES: RASH

Case Study

Chief Concern

"How long has Viktoria had the rash?" Willow asks. Willow is a brand new Paramedic who is on her first run, accompanied by Erik, her field training officer. Before they arrive on-scene, Erik drills Willow on the possible causes of a rash for a 10-year-old girl.

Critical Thinking Questions

1. What are some of the possible infectious causes of pediatric rashes?

   _____

   _____

2. What infectious disease(s) would be a problem for the Paramedic if she were pregnant?

   _____

   _____

History

Viktoria is the 10-year-old daughter of a foreign officer from Nigeria. She is in the United States visiting her father before returning to Africa. Her father feels it is important to expose her to the world outside of the village in which she was brought up and home-schooled. He had the privilege of visiting New York City and the United Nations when his dad was a representative.

Viktoria's rash appeared quite suddenly and without any of the typical prodrome of muscle aches, anorexia, or headache. She had a low-grade fever that did not alarm her father. What did alert her father to the problem was her reluctance to go to his office. In fact, she didn't even want to eat, which he felt was curious because she had a ravenous appetite for Western food.

Critical Thinking Questions

1. What are the important elements of the history that a Paramedic should obtain?

   _____

   _____

2. What specific questions beyond the standard SAMPLE history should the Paramedic ask?

   _____

   _____

Examination

Viktoria has a rash that covers her body, but the greatest numbers of vesicles are on her face and arms. Willow notes that the rash seems to spare her hands and there are scant vesicles on her trunk and legs. The rash must be itchy, as Viktoria has clearly dug her fingernails into her skin to relieve the itch.

Viktoria denies any of the classic meningeal signs such as nuchal rigidity, photophobia, or headache. Other than a fever, Viktoria seems fine.

Critical Thinking Questions

1. What are the elements of the physical examination of a patient with suspected infection?

_____

_____

2. What would a limited number of vesicles around a wrist, for example, suggest?

_____

_____

Assessment

"What is going on with little Viktoria?" her father asks in an English accent. "Does she need to go to the hospital?" Although Willow knows that Viktoria is infected, she isn't sure if transporting her to the emergency department—and potentially exposing other, more vulnerable patients to the infection—is wise. Willow decides to speak to Erik, who applauds her thinking and suggests she contact medical control.

Critical Thinking Questions

1. What diagnosis did the Paramedic announce to the patient's father?

_____

_____

2. Is the location of the rash important to the diagnosis?

_____

_____

Treatment

While Willow is trying to raise the attending physician Erik provides oxygen. When he suggests intravenous access, both the father and child resist, stating they would like the doctor's opinion first. Erik agrees and awaits word from Willow.

Critical Thinking Questions

1. What is the standard of care of patients with a suspected communicable disease?

_____

_____

2. What are some of the patient-specific concerns and considerations that the Paramedic should consider when applying this plan of care that is intended to treat a broad patient population presenting with communicable disease?

_____

_____

Evaluation

During the assessment, Viktoria remains essentially stable. Other than the persistent itching, she seems like a happy kid. A careful immunization history reveals that, although Viktoria has received the required MMR, DtP, Hep A and B, and polio vaccinations, the chickenpox vaccination was not needed and therefore she did not receive it prior to traveling to the United States.

Critical Thinking Questions

1. What are some of the predictable complications associated with a suspected communicable disease?

_____

_____

2. What symptom pattern would alert the Paramedic to this complication?

_____

_____

Disposition

After ascertaining that Viktoria is essentially a healthy kid with a rash, medical control suggests that her father take her to a pediatric clinic at the hospital and to apply some calamine lotion to relieve the itch in the interim.

Willow and Erik are happy to provide Viktoria a "ride" to the hospital in the ambulance, which seems to brighten up the 10-year-old's day!

Critical Thinking Questions

1. What is the most appropriate transport decision that will get the patient to definitive care?

_____

_____

2. What are some of the transportation considerations?

_____

_____

Practice Questions
Multiple Choice

Select the best answer for each of the following questions.

1. Which of the following diseases is transmitted by the fecal–oral route?
   a. chickenpox
   b. measles
   c. polio
   d. tuberculosis

2. Which of the following diseases is not bloodborne?
   a. syphilis
   b. gonorrhea
   c. human immunodeficiency virus
   d. hepatitis B

3. Which of the following diseases has NOT been linked to congenital birth defects?
   a. chickenpox
   b. German measles
   c. measles
   d. mumps

4. Which of the following is NOT one of the "three C's" of measles?
   a. catarrhal signs
   b. conjunctivitis
   c. cough
   d. coryza

5. Which childhood infection does NOT have catarrhal symptoms?
   a. chickenpox
   b. roseola
   c. measles
   d. mumps

6. Which childhood disease typically affects children between 6 months and 2 to 3 years, versus 2 to 12 years?
   a. roseola
   b. measles
   c. mumps
   d. rubella

7. Which sexually transmitted disease causes chancres?
   a. syphilis
   b. gonorrhea
   c. chlamydia
   d. human immunodeficiency virus

8. A person may submit a writ of *habeas corpus* to prevent this form of rapid containment.
   a. isolation
   b. quarantine
   c. movement restrictions
   d. protect in place

9. Which sign is most specific for meningitis?
   a. headache
   b. fever
   c. nuchal rigidity
   d. photophobia

10. Which of the following childhood vaccinations is NOT universally required?
    a. measles, mumps, and rubella
    b. diphtheria, tetanus, and pertussis
    c. polio
    d. human papilloma virus

11. What rash proceeds in a cephalocaudal fashion?
    a. measles
    b. mumps
    c. smallpox
    d. chickenpox

12. What is the most dangerous (i.e., lethal) form of meningitis?
    a. pneumococcal
    b. meningococcal
    c. haemophilius
    d. neisseria

13. Which of the following diseases will cause a nonblanching rash?
    a. measles
    b. meningitis
    c. mumps
    d. smallpox

14. Which infection will cause trismus and risus sardonicus?
    a. measles
    b. meningitis
    c. tetanus
    d. pertussis

15. To which disease is tuberculosis a secondary disease?
    a. smallpox
    b. AIDS
    c. meningitis
    d. pertussis

Short Answer

Write a brief answer to each of the following questions.

16. What is a cluster?

_____

_____

17. What is social distancing?

_____

_____

18. What is ring vaccination?

_____

_____

19. What is targeted vaccination?

_____

_____

20. What is mass vaccination?

_____

_____

Fill in the Blank

Complete each sentence by adding the appropriate word in the provided blanks.

21. _____ _____ _____ was formerly known as venereal disease.

22. _____ is an itching sensation.

23. Finding out which individual infected another is called _____ _____.

24. Most rashes can be described as _____.

25. The most common sexually transmitted infection is _____.

CHAPTER 29

DISORDERS OF THE IMMUNE SYSTEM

Case Study

Chief Concern

The crew is called to transport a 20-year-old co-ed from the university health center to the medical center for evaluation of nontraumatic joint pain in both hands. Jessica and Randy, from the campus ambulance, are alerted by the tones and head to the station to pick up the ambulance. While en route to the health center, they discuss nontraumatic joint pain.

Critical Thinking Question

1. What are some of the possible causes of nontraumatic joint pain?

   _____

   _____

History

The pair arrive at the health center and are met at the door by the nurse. "Imani has had pain in her fingers for several days. Today she spiked a fever and decided to come to the university health center. The nurse practitioner gave her a complete physical and cannot find a source for the infection. Imani does not have any cold symptoms, no cough, and her lungs are clear. She denies any symptoms of a urinary tract infection, and our urine analysis of her clean-catch urine sample supports her claims. Imani denies any trauma to her hands and we were very careful to get any history of trauma. The nurse practitioner is stumped and with our limited diagnostic capabilities she wants Imani transported to the medical center for further diagnostic workup. Here are all of her papers," the nurse states.

Critical Thinking Questions

1. What are the important elements of the history that a Paramedic should obtain?

   _____

   _____

2. Why should the Paramedic take a careful medication history?

   _____

   _____

Examination

Randy and Jessica introduce themselves to Imani and start a preliminary examination. Imani appears to have swelling of the proximal interphalangeal joint (PIP) and metacarpophalangeal joints (MIP) in both hands. The joints appear as swollen and tender. However, that is the extent of the signs of inflammation. More proximal joints appear to be untouched.

Jessica remarks about the unusual facial rash. Although it is not unusual for a young college co-ed to have "skin problems," owed to all the stress, change of diet, and so forth, this breakout appears to be a rash that extends over the bridge of the nose to both cheeks.

Critical Thinking Questions

1. What are the elements of the physical examination of a patient with suspected autoimmune disorder?

_____

_____

2. What signs would suggest systemic lupus erythematosus?

_____

_____

Assessment

Imani relates to Jessica that she has just started the fever but has had the joint pain for almost a week. When Jessica inquires about the rash on her face, she summarily dismisses it as her skin "breaking out." Jessica listens intently as Imani is placed on the stretcher and prepared for transport.

Critical Thinking Questions

1. What diagnosis would be probable in this case?

_____

_____

2. What diagnosis did the Paramedic announce to the patient?

_____

_____

Treatment

Jessica speaks with the nurse practitioner before leaving and asks what should be done to help Imani. The nurse practitioner suggests that all that is needed is obtaining venous access and monitoring her. Jessica asks if 125 mg of methylprednisolone will help. Although the nurse practitioner agrees that it might be helpful, she suggests that Jessica withhold the steroid until after they have a complete workup and can rule out infectious etiology for the fever.

Critical Thinking Questions

1. What is the standard of care of patients with suspected autoimmune disorders?

_____

_____

2. Why would the Paramedic withhold the steroid?

_____

_____

Evaluation

Before leaving the university health clinic, Imani asks if she can take her ibuprofen, which has apparently given her some relief from the discomfort. Jessica asks Imani if she can wait until she talks to the physician on-line. After conferring with medical authority at the medical center, she permits Imani to take 400 mg of ibuprofen.

Critical Thinking Questions

1. What are some predictable complications of systemic lupus erythematosus (SLE)?

_____

_____

2. What is the cause of death for patients with SLE?

_____

_____

Disposition

The rheumatology resident meets Imani and the crew at the door. Apparently the nurse practitioner called ahead to the triage nurse and explained the situation. After conferring with the emergency department attending, the rheumatology resident is called to the emergency department to "workup" the patient.

"Hi, my name is Baasim," Dr Premjii says. "What seems to be the problem today, Imani?"

Critical Thinking Questions

1. What is the most appropriate transport decision that will get the patient to definitive care?

_____

_____

2. What important assessment information should the Paramedic relay to the emergency department staff?

_____

_____

Practice Questions
Multiple Choice

Select the best answer for each of the following questions.

1. Which of the following is NOT considered a passive barrier to infection?
    a. skin
    b. mucous membranes
    c. stomach acid
    d. antibodies

2. Which of the following antigens stimulate an antibody response?
    a. dust and pollen
    b. bacteria and virus
    c. antibiotics and medications
    d. all of the above

3. Which of the following is the primary surveillance cell?
    a. lymphocytes
    b. T cells
    c. B cells
    d. cytokines

4. Which of the following plays a primary and initial role in immune response?
   a. cytokines
   b. leukotrienes
   c. heparin
   d. histamine

5. What is the effect of these "immune chemicals"?
   a. increased nasal secretions (rhinorrhea)
   b. increased bronchial secretions (bronchorrhea)
   c. increased stomach acid
   d. all of the above

6. Which of the following is a symptom of an allergic reaction?
   a. coughing
   b. vomiting
   c. diarrhea
   d. all of the above

7. Which of the following is a sign of a localized reaction?
   a. erythema
   b. urticaria
   c. pruritus
   d. all of the above

8. Which of the following is an autoimmune disease?
   a. systemic lupus erythematosus
   b. rheumatoid arthritis
   c. ankylosing spondylitis
   d. all of the above

9. Which of the following produces a characteristic "butterfly mask" rash on the face?
   a. systemic lupus erythematosus
   b. rheumatoid arthritis
   c. ankylosing spondylitis
   d. fibromyalgia

10. Which of the following autoimmune diseases does not primarily affect the joints?
    a. systemic lupus erythematosus
    b. rheumatoid arthritis
    c. ankylosing spondylitis
    d. fibromyalgia

11. Which of the following is NOT an "artificial" immunodeficiency?
    a. acquired immunodeficiency disease
    b. leukemia
    c. immunomodulating drugs
    d. chemotherapy

12. Swelling of the tongue is an example of what condition?
    a. erythema
    b. urticaria
    c. pruritus
    d. angioedema

13. Which of the following is a sign of potential airway compromise?
    a. stridor
    b. wheezes
    c. tonsillar swelling
    d. all of the above

14. Systemic lupus erythematosus is common among which group?
    a. women from age 15 to 40
    b. women from age 40 to 65
    c. men from age 15 to 40
    d. men from age 40 to 65

15. Which of the following is a symptom of complications related to immunosuppression?
    a. fever and chills
    b. rash
    c. cough
    d. all of the above

Short Answer

Write a brief answer to each of the following questions.

16. What do mast cells secrete?

_____

_____

17. What are the signs and symptoms of mast cell stimulation?

_____

_____

18. What are the two most common autoimmune diseases?

_____

_____

19. How does the human immunodeficiency virus cause AIDS?

_____

_____

20. What is acute transplant rejection?

_____

_____

Fill in the Blank

Complete each sentence by adding the appropriate word in the provided blanks.

21. Particles that stimulate an immune response are called _____.

22. The medical term for hives is _____.

23. A patient with a low neutrophil count is said to be _____.

24. Swelling of the lips, tongue, and upper airway is called _____.

25. Patients who develop antibodies to their own body's cells is an _____ response.

CHAPTER 30

ANAPHYLAXIS

Case Study

Chief Concern

The call comes in for a man with difficulty breathing. Medcom (medical communications) gives scant information other than a 40-year-old male with trouble breathing is semiconscious. The address is also unfamiliar to the responders. Most of the Paramedics know the "regulars," those patients with chronic obstructive pulmonary disease who often "crash" and need EMS.

The radio then crackles out the message "Patient's wife thinks it's a medication reaction." The Paramedic on the crew, Dale, starts to ponder the factors and possibilities: difficulty breathing, 40-year-old man, semiconscious, medication reaction.

Critical Thinking Questions

1. What are some of the possible causes of anaphylaxis caused by injection?

   _____

   _____

2. What are some of the possible causes of anaphylaxis caused by ingestion?

   _____

   _____

History

Mrs. Reed meets the crew as they pull into the driveway. Waving frantically, she yells, "Hurry up, hurry up! I think he stopped breathing!" Entering the residence, the crew is immediately taken aback by the rather large man with a rather large tongue protruding from his mouth.

The crew immediately tries ventilating the patient with a bag–mask assembly while Dale asks the wife a quick series of questions. "When did this happen? Was he stung? What did he eat last? Did it occur suddenly or over a period of time?" He stops the questions long enough to take a breath, giving the wife a chance to answer.

Critical Thinking Questions

1. What are the important elements of the history that a Paramedic should obtain?

   _____

   _____

2. What important additional information should a Paramedic try to obtain?

   _____

   _____

Examination

Dale takes a quick moment to inspect the patient's oropharynx. His swollen tongue, coupled with tonsillar edema, appear to almost occlude the airway. The stridor is audible without any stethoscope, and Dale is surprised to hear faint but clear lung sounds.

Opening the patient's shirt completely, Dale inspects for urticaria. There is none! The entire team can tell Dale is puzzled. The expression on his face says it all. The EMT on the team also reports that the patient's vital signs are a little elevated but acceptable.

Critical Thinking Questions

1. What is the first priority in the physical examination of a patient with suspected anaphylaxis?

_____

_____

2. What is the next priority in the physical examination of the patient with suspected anaphylaxis?

_____

_____

Assessment

"What's happening to my husband?" Mrs. Reed pleads. Dale calmly explains that her husband is having trouble breathing because his airway is closing and that the team is doing everything it can to re-establish his airway.

Critical Thinking Questions

1. What is the significance of stridor?

_____

_____

2. What diagnosis did the Paramedic announce to the patient?

_____

_____

Treatment

Dale knows that this is a complex patient that will need a coordinated team effort to treat. Turning to the EMT on the team, he instructs her to get the EpiPen and to administer 0.3 mg epinephrine intramuscularly. Next, he addresses the advance EMT and asks him to attempt venous access. If venous access is not available—and Dale suspects that it might not be—then the intraosseous kit should be prepared.

Dale turns his attention to the patient's airway. The EMT is able to ventilate the patient using the bag–mask assembly but is not able to introduce an oropharyngeal airway.

Critical Thinking Questions

1. What is the first priority in the care of the patient with suspected anaphylaxis?

_____

_____

2. What is the next priority in the care of the patient with suspected anaphylaxis?

_____

_____

Evaluation

Fortunately, Dale is able to intubate the patient, even though the endotracheal tube is much smaller than he expected for such a large man. Just as Dale starts to relax, the EMT advises him that the patient's blood pressure is dropping.

Dale thinks this might be the result of the accumulation of carbon dioxide that leads to an increased acid load and subsequent vasodilation. However, he cannot wait for the ventilation to reverse the respiratory acidosis because the patient's blood pressure has dropped so low that the patient is losing consciousness. He elects to insert intraosseous access and to administer epinephrine via an infusion.

Critical Thinking Questions

1. What are some of the predictable complications associated with anaphylaxis?

   _____

   _____

2. What are some of the predictable complications associated with the treatments for anaphylaxis?

   _____

   _____

Disposition

Between the ventilation and the epinephrine infusion, the patient starts to become more responsive. The team collectively sighs in relief and starts to load the patient for the trip to the hospital.

Dale realizes this is one of the more complex cases he has had lately, and is quite happy the team pulled together to make it work. The wife is obviously pleased. Dale decided to alert the medical director and ask him to speak to the team.

Critical Thinking Questions

1. What is the most appropriate transport decision that will get the patient to definitive care?

   _____

   _____

2. What important patient information should be shared with the emergency department staff?

   _____

   _____

Practice Questions
Multiple Choice

Select the best answer for each of the following questions.

1. Which immunoglobulin is responsible for the allergic reaction?
   a. IgA
   b. IgD
   c. IgE
   d. IgM

2. Which of the following conditions can cause wheezing similar to the wheezing in anaphylaxis?
   a. asthma
   b. aspiration
   c. airway obstruction
   d. all of the above

3. Which chemical is similar to histamine?
   a. bradykinin
   b. leukotriene
   c. angiotensin
   d. urticarine

4. If the patient is on beta blockers, the Paramedic should consider using _____ first line.
   a. glucagon
   b. intravenous epinephrine
   c. diphenhydramine
   d. albuterol

5. Which medication is a corticosteroid?
   a. albuterol
   b. methylprednisolone
   c. diphenhydramine
   d. epinephrine

6. Which medication has been implicated in anaphylaxis?
   a. penicillin
   b. aspirin
   c. cephalosporins
   d. all of the above

7. What is the first sign of bronchoconstriction?
   a. increased respiratory rate
   b. bilateral wheezing
   c. diminished breath sounds at bases
   d. visible retractions

8. Which of the following will NOT swell in angioedema?
   a. face
   b. lips
   c. hands
   d. tongue

9. What is the red flag indicating severe anaphylaxis?
   a. tachycardia
   b. tachypnea
   c. hypotension
   d. angioedema

10. What is the side effect of diphenhydramine?
    a. sedation
    b. tachycardia
    c. hypotension
    d. tachypnea

11. What is the dose of epinephrine for moderate reactions?
    a. 0.3 to 0.5 mg IM
    b. 0.3 to 0.5 mg IV
    c. 0.3 to 0.5 mg SQ
    d. 0.3 to 0.5 mg bolus

12. Which medication cannot be given via small volume nebulizer?
    a. epinephrine
    b. albuterol
    c. diphenhydramine
    d. methylprednisolone

13. What is the most immediate life threat in anaphylaxis?
    a. airway constriction
    b. bronchoconstriction
    c. vasodilation
    d. diaphoresis

14. Histamine is released from which of the following?
    a. mast cells
    b. IgE
    c. immunoglobulins
    d. antigens

15. Which medication classification is known for causing an atypical allergic reaction?
    a. ACE inhibitors
    b. beta blockers
    c. calcium channel blockers
    d. diuretics

Short Answer

Write a brief answer to each of the following questions.

16. Compare the pharmacological properties of subcutaneous epinephrine to intramuscular epinephrine.

_____

_____

17. Why should the Paramedic be cautious when administering epinephrine to the elderly?

_____

_____

18. What are the signs of poor perfusion that would lead a Paramedic to think that severe anaphylaxis may occur?

_____

_____

19. What other conditions are included in the differential for anaphylaxis?

_____

_____

20. What is the drug of choice for anaphylaxis?

_____

_____

Fill in the Blank

Complete each sentence by adding the appropriate word in the provided blanks.

21. A red raised rash is called _____.

22. An allergic-like reaction is called a(n) _____ reaction.

23. The medical term for itching is _____.

24. Reddened skin is called _____.

25. The substance that causes an immune reaction is called an _____.

CHAPTER 31

BARIATRIC MEDICINE

Case Study

Chief Concern

"Can you help us over here?" the waitress asks. Hanna and her partner, Alfonso (everyone calls him Al), have stopped at the Western diner for a quick bite to eat. They hear a commotion in the back of the restaurant but cannot see what happened. Apparently a rather large man (Hanna estimates he must weigh 500 pounds) fell out of his chair. He is again upright, thanks to the help of several patrons, but is having obvious trouble breathing.

Critical Thinking Questions

1. What are some of the possible medical conditions that would cause a fall?

   _____

   _____

2. How is trouble breathing related to the patient's obesity?

   _____

   _____

History

Witnesses report that the patient was eating with his wife, Consuela, when he appeared to "just fall asleep before he fell." As Al starts an assessment on Rafael (everyone calls him Rafa), Hanna starts to ask his wife questions. "Tell me again what happened, Consuela."

Consuela reports that Rafa has bouts of daytime sleepiness. This is the first time they have been out of the house in quite some time because of it. She also reports that, despite the use of CPAP at home, Rafa is still experiencing restless nights and sleep apnea. She denies seeing any seizure activity following the fall, nor does Rafa have any complaints. He states he simply fell out of his chair, breaking the arm of the chair in the process.

His past medical history includes type 2 diabetes and hypertension. Both conditions are well controlled with medications including insulin and a beta blocker.

Critical Thinking Questions

1. What past pulmonary history should the Paramedic obtain?

   _____

   _____

2. What past cardiac history should the Paramedic obtain?

   _____

   _____

Examination

Rafa is a large man who, by his own admission, weighs 525 pounds. He is awake and alert at the moment and maintains an adequate airway independently.

His body habitus makes it hard for Al to do a complete assessment. Unable to visualize jugular venous distention, Al proceeds to the chest wall where he is met by distant heart sounds and faint rales (crackles) at the bases. Rafa's abdomen is protuberant and nontender to palpation. His legs are wrapped in soaked dressings that suggest Rafa has weeping pedal edema. In addition, the smell is suggestive of MRSA.

Critical Thinking Questions

1. What confounds the physical examination of the obese patient with suspected respiratory failure?

   _____

   _____

2. What confounds the physical examination of the obese patient with suspected heart failure?

   _____

   _____

Assessment

Though Rafa is hyperdynamic (i.e., elevated heart rate and blood pressure), Hanna feels it is important for Rafa to be seen in the emergency department.

Rafa asks, "Why do I have to go? I feel fine. Just a little short of breath." As he pants, Hanna can see his pulse rate climb and his oxygen saturation fall.

"Well," starts Hanna, "for one thing, you passed out and that's not natural."

"But, I just fell asleep," protests Rafa.

Critical Thinking Questions

1. What is the significance of the falling oxygen saturation?

   _____

   _____

2. What is the significance of the syncope in the obese patient?

   _____

   _____

Treatment

With Consuela's help, Hanna convinces Rafa to go get checked out to be sure he didn't hurt himself in the fall. Al has already called ahead to have the bariatric ambulance, and additional help, brought to the scene.

Rafa is greatly relieved when he finds out that they can take him out the emergency exit and not through the main dining room. In preparation for the transfer, Hanna places Rafa on CPAP with high-flow, high-concentration oxygen.

However, Hanna is concerned about this transfer. She doesn't trust the pulse oximeter because the readings are fluctuating wildly and Al isn't able to get a satisfactory ECG tracing. She feels a little blind.

Critical Thinking Questions

1. What are some of the patient-specific cardiac concerns and considerations that the Paramedic should consider when applying a plan of care to a morbidly obese patient?

   _____

   _____

2. What are some of the patient-specific respiratory concerns and considerations that the Paramedic should consider when applying a plan of care to a morbidly obese patient?

_____

_____

Evaluation

As Hanna suspects, Rafa's condition deteriorates by the time he gets in the back of the ambulance. His respiratory rate has climbed and his level of consciousness has fallen. "POPE," says Hanna.

"What?" asks Al.

"Post-obstructive pulmonary edema," explains Hanna. "Let's get the suction, oxygen, airways, and venous access for drugs." Hanna elects to perform a conscious intubation using the ultra–short-acting medication etimodate. Standing behind Rafa, who is in the semi-Fowler's position, she introduces the Robert–Shaw blade. Visualizing the glottic opening, she captures the floppy epiglottis. With Al's use of the BURP technique during external laryngeal manipulation, she intubates Rafa.

Almost immediately, a wall of pink frothy sputum comes rushing up the tube. "Suction!" she calls. After clearing the endotracheal tube, she gets an end-tidal capnography reading. "65," Hanna reports. "Al, he's retaining. Let's increase the rate but not the volume on the transport ventilator to try to blow off some of that carbon dioxide."

Critical Thinking Questions

1. What are some of the predictable complications associated with having a bariatric patient lie flat?

_____

_____

2. What are some treatments that could help prevent post-obstructive pulmonary edema?

_____

_____

Disposition

Rafa is transported aboard the bariatric ambulance to Shady Oaks Hospital. Shady Oaks is known for its bariatric care and prides itself on being a bariatric surgery center.

Critical Thinking Questions

1. What are the advantages of transporting a bariatric patient to these hospitals, even if that means bypassing other hospitals in the process?

_____

_____

2. What patient information should be shared with the emergency department staff while en route?

_____

_____

Practice Questions
Multiple Choice

Select the best answer for each of the following questions.

1. What is the most reliable weight calculation, medically speaking?
   a. Broselow tape
   b. body mass index
   c. Met Life tables
   d. bathroom scale

2. Obesity starts at a BMI greater than what value?
   a. 28
   b. 32
   c. 35
   d. 40

3. Morbid obesity starts at a BMI greater than what value?
   a. 28
   b. 32
   c. 35
   d. 40

4. Approximately _____ of patients with type 2 diabetes are obese.
   a. one-third
   b. one-half
   c. two-thirds
   d. all

5. The patient with shortness of breath while lying flat is said to have which condition?
   a. paroxysmal nocturnal dyspnea
   b. orthopnea
   c. exertional dyspnea
   d. dependent dyspnea

6. The shortness of breath experienced by an obese patient can be attributed to which condition?
   a. backward heart failure
   b. cor pulmonale
   c. restrictive lung defect
   d. all of the above

7. Which of the following is NOT considered a cardinal sign of heart failure?
   a. jugular venous distention
   b. angina
   c. ventricular gallop
   d. dependent peripheral edema

8. Which heart sound is heard in heart failure?
   a. ventricular gallop
   b. murmur of aortic stenosis
   c. pericardial friction rub
   d. murmur of mitral regurgitation

9. Obese patients are at risk for liver failure because of what condition?
   a. hepatitis
   b. steatohepatitis
   c. lipid-induced hepatic failure
   d. hepatomegaly

10. Restrictive lung disease, secondary to obesity, leads to which condition?
    a. hypercarbia
    b. carbon dioxide narcosis
    c. sleep apnea
    d. all of the above

11. A large abdomen, or panniculus, can cause a loss of up to _____ of functional residual lung capacity.
    a. one-third
    b. one-half
    c. two-thirds
    d. complete

12. What is the preferred blade to use when intubating the obese patient?
    a. Miller
    b. Macintosh
    c. Robert–Shaw
    d. Wis-Hipple

13. Which of the following is NOT a "hook and toss" method of moving a patient?
    a. stand and pivot
    b. cradle lift
    c. draw sheet pull
    d. shoulder lift

14. What is the best way to prevent post-obstructive pulmonary edema?
    a. positive pressure ventilation
    b. high-flow, high-concentration oxygen
    c. continuous positive airway pressure
    d. intubation with positive end-expiratory pressure

15. The obese patient will have a decreased clearance of _____ medications.
    a. acidotic
    b. hydrophobic
    c. lipophilic
    d. polarized

Short Answer

Write a brief answer to each of the following questions.

16. What is the BMI?

_____

_____

17. What is cardiac remodeling?

_____

_____

18. Explain physiologic polycythemia in obesity.

_____

_____

19. What is a useful definition of obesity?

_____

_____

20. What is a "lift team?"

_____

_____

Fill in the Blank

Complete each sentence by adding the appropriate word in the provided blanks.

21. Inhibition of glucose utilization is called _____ _____.

22. Carbon dioxide narcosis, secondary to obesity, is called _____ _____.

23. A physique that suggests certain medical conditions is called a _____ _____.

24. The large abdominal mass is called a _____.

25. Sudden backward heart failure as a result of lying flat is called _____-_____ _____ _____.

CHAPTER **32**

DISORDERS OF UNEXPLAINED WEIGHT LOSS

Case Study

Chief Concern

"That's odd," Aiden comments as he walks from the dispatcher's office with the trip ticket. "The caller said that the patient is bleeding from every orifice and doesn't want lights or siren in the neighborhood."

The call is for a 48-year-old female requesting transportation to St. Vincent's hospital. However, the patient wants to go to the hospice unit, not the emergency department. The patient is reportedly too weak to walk and the family has no other means to get her to the hospital.

Critical Thinking Questions

1. What are some of the possible causes of the patient's bleeding?

   _____

   _____

2. Why did the patient request "no lights or siren?"

   _____

   _____

History

Mrs. Jancin has been diagnosed with breast cancer. She had been in remission for about five years; however, the cancer recently reappeared. She underwent a bilateral mastectomy with lymph node stripping plus chemotherapy and radiation. However, the cancer has advanced into her liver, lungs, and bones. She is T1, N4, and M1 in the TNM cancer staging system.

Mrs. Jancin has stopped eating, stating that she simply is not hungry anymore. After eating as little as a cracker, she says she's full. As a result, she has lost a dramatic amount of weight.

Critical Thinking Questions

1. What are the important elements of the history that a Paramedic should obtain?

   _____

   _____

2. Why isn't Mrs. Jancin eating?

   _____

   _____

Examination

Aiden is awestruck by Mrs. Jancin's gaunt appearance. Her skin is hanging off her bones and covered in large purple splotches. Her eyes are half-opened as she surveys those that enter the room. Unable to even lift a hand, she utters a feeble hello.

Aiden recalls that his mother has breast cancer, but it has been in remission after successful rounds of chemotherapy and radiation. His heart jumps to his throat when he realizes that his mother could have been like this.

Going to Mrs. Jancin's side, Aiden introduces himself as he holds her arm. It is so pale and tiny that just the act of putting on the pediatric blood pressure cuff has caused a skin tear. Although Aiden is visibly shaken, Mrs. Jancin reassures him that that happens all the time and it isn't his fault.

Mrs. Jancin is literally weeping blood. Her bedclothes and bedding are stained with blood. She has lost all of her strength, and is unable to stand, even with assistance.

Critical Thinking Questions

1. What are the elements of the physical examination of a patient with suspected paraneoplastic syndrome?

2. Why is a blood glucose level a critical element in this examination?

Assessment

Mrs. Jancin's nurse confirms the dramatic weight loss, some 75 pounds, plus the anorexia. An examination of Mrs. Jancin's abdomen reveals a swollen belly owed to the ascites secondary to her liver failure.

Mrs. Jancin weakly points to the headboard. Above her head is a "do not attempt resuscitation" order neatly pinned to the wall. Looking at Mrs. Jancin, Aiden responds, "I understand. Are you in any pain?"

Critical Thinking Questions

1. What is the Paramedic's primary concern for the terminally ill patient?

2. What are some of the Paramedic's concerns about analgesia?

Treatment

Aiden offers Mrs. Jancin oxygen, which she promptly dismisses. "How can I talk to you with that mask on, dear boy?" Mrs. Jancin asks. She likewise refuses an ECG monitor or an IV. She does consent to the pulse oximeter, which reads 95%. Aiden is sure all three of the red blood cells she has left are well-oxygenated, but he also knows that neither intravenous solutions nor supplemental oxygen will make a difference.

Critical Thinking Questions

1. What is the standard of care of patients with suspected paraneoplastic syndrome?

2. What is the nature of the special Paramedic–patient relationship for the patient with paraneoplastic syndrome?

Evaluation

Mrs. Jancin complains of feeling a little nauseous on the ride into the hospital. Aiden is at a crossroads. He has an anti-emetic to offer, but Mrs. Jancin's muscle wasting is so severe that she doesn't have an acceptable injection site. In addition, Mrs. Jancin is adamant about not wanting an IV. Therefore, Aiden contacts his medical director on the cell phone. The doctor explains that ondansetron can be given intranasally and with about the same effects as intravenous administration. Aiden is relieved that he can still care for Mrs. Jancin.

Critical Thinking Questions

1. What is the most predictable complication associated with paraneoplastic syndromes?

_____

_____

2. What would be the preferred treatment for this complication?

_____

_____

Disposition

Bypassing the emergency department, the ambulance pulls into the building across the street which is specifically dedicated to breast cancer and designed to look homey. It contains none of the usual entrapments of a hospital. In fact, the waiting area to the hospice unit looks more like a living room than a waiting room.

A hospice nurse meets Mrs. Jancin at the door and immediately takes her hand. "Thank you," she says to Aiden.

"But I didn't do anything." Aiden remarks.

"Dear," Mrs. Jancin says, "I will not forget your kindness."

Critical Thinking Questions

1. What is the most appropriate transport decision that will get the patient to definitive care?

_____

_____

2. What is the difference between hospice care and hospital care?

_____

_____

Practice Questions
Multiple Choice

Select the best answer for each of the following questions.

1. Which one of the following diseases is NOT typically associated with extreme weight loss?
   a. cancer
   b. tuberculosis
   c. acquired immunodeficiency disease
   d. myocardial infarction

2. Pott's disease is tuberculosis of what body area?
   a. kidneys
   b. lungs
   c. spine
   d. adrenal glands

3. Night sweats are seen in AIDS and some other disorders. Which of the following is NOT known for night sweats?
   a. cancer
   b. tuberculosis
   c. hypoglycemia
   d. myocardial infarction

4. What is the most common area affected by cancer in women?
   a. breast
   b. lung
   c. colorectal
   d. ovarian

5. Which type of cancer is the most common cause of mortality in women?
   a. breast
   b. lung
   c. colorectal
   d. ovarian

6. What is the most common area affected by cancer in men?
   a. prostate
   b. lung
   c. colorectal
   d. bladder

7. Which type of cancer is the most common cause of mortality in men?
   a. prostate
   b. lung
   c. colorectal
   d. bladder

8. A T2N1M0 staged cancer would be _____.
   a. localized without metastasis or lymph node involvement
   b. localized with axillary (sentinel) node involvement but without metastasis
   c. disseminated cancer with extensive lymph node and metastasis.
   d. disseminated cancer with one lymph node involvement and extensive metastasis

9. Which of the following is NOT a form of complementary medicine?
   a. megavitamins
   b. massage
   c. hypnosis
   d. acupuncture

10. What is another name for sleep hyperhidrosis?
    a. paroxysmal nocturnal dyspnea
    b. night terrors
    c. sleep apnea
    d. night sweats

11. The patient with exclusive dependence on opiates for pain relief would be on the _____ tier pain plan.
    a. first
    b. second
    c. third
    d. fourth

12. Which of the following is NOT part of the triad of symptoms associated with terminal cancer?
    a. anorexia
    b. unexplained weight loss
    c. malaise
    d. night sweats

13. Use of chemotherapy and aromatherapy is an example of what type of medicine?
    a. complementary medicine
    b. integrative medicine
    c. alternative medicine
    d. traditional medicine

14. What is the most common childhood cancer?
    a. bladder
    b. lymphoma
    c. leukemia
    d. melanoma

15. Which cancer has been positively linked to genetics?
    a. breast
    b. prostate
    c. lung
    d. colorectal

Short Answer

Write a brief answer to each of the following questions.

16. What is hospice?

_____

_____

17. Compare anorexia with anorexia nervosa.

_____

_____

18. What is cachexia?

_____

_____

19. What are the signs of pancytopenia?

_____

_____

20. How does HIV kill?

_____

_____

Fill in the Blank

Complete each sentence by adding the appropriate word in the provided blanks.

21. The new name for pneumocystis carinii is pneumocystis _____.

22. The specialized branch of pharmacology for cancer treatment is called _____.

23. Using megavitamins for the treatment of cancer is a form of _____ medicine.

24. When cancer goes into a disease-free state it is called _____.

25. Care directed toward relieving pain and suffering, and not curing disease, is called _____ care.

CHAPTER 33

MEDICAL RESUSCITATION

Case Study

Chief Concern

Mr. McIvor collapses at the local off-track betting parlor. When Paramedics arrive, he is barely conscious. Many of the Paramedics know Mr. McIvor, as he is a "frequent flyer," so named for his many hospital visits.

Mr. McIvor's past problems include intoxication, seizures, hypoglycemia, and shortness of breath owing to his COPD. He is a medical student's dream and a Paramedic's nightmare. The Paramedics start by immediately stabilizing his head and neck manually while witnesses are questioned.

Critical Thinking Questions

1. What are some key concerns that a Paramedic should address when confronted with a critically ill patient?

_____

_____

2. What is the "order of resuscitation"?

_____

_____

Disposition

Witnesses describe seizure activity, stating that Mr. McIvor had "fallen out" and fell from his chair to the floor. Faced with a potentially post-ictal patient, the Paramedics elect to maintain the manual cervical spine stabilization while his airway and ventilatory status are assessed. Unlike his seizures in the past, Mr. McIvor did not spontaneously awaken. Concerned, the Paramedics elect to package Mr. McIvor after ensuring the "basics."

Critical Thinking Questions

1. What is the most appropriate transport decision that will get the patient to definitive care?

_____

_____

2. What is the minimum standard of care for an ALS-worthy patient?

_____

_____

Practice Questions

Multiple Choice

Select the best answer for each of the following questions.

1. What is the primary goal of resuscitation?
   a. delivery of oxygen
   b. elimination of carbon dioxide
   c. provision of glucose
   d. support of circulation

2. Which of the following is NOT a stated goal of oxygenation?
   a. maximum oxygen saturation
   b. decreased acidosis
   c. increased partial oxygen pressure
   d. nitrogen washout

3. Carbon dioxide retention leads to which situation?
   a. increased acidosis
   b. decreased oxygenation
   c. oxyhemoglobin shift
   d. all of the above

4. Which of the following is NOT one of the top three priorities for resuscitation?
   a. hypoxia
   b. infection
   c. hypoglycemia
   d. hypotension

5. Snoring can be a sign of which condition?
   a. partially obstructed airway
   b. unconsciousness
   c. foreign matter aspiration
   d. all of the above

6. Hypoxia may be evidenced by which symptom?
   a. cyanosis
   b. pallor
   c. mottled skin
   d. snoring respirations

7. Which of the following provides ventilation?
   a. nonrebreather oxygen mask
   b. bag–mask assembly
   c. endotracheal intubation
   d. supraglottic airway

8. Which device does NOT "stent" the lower airway open?
   a. CPAP
   b. nonrebreather oxygen mask
   c. bag–mask assembly
   d. oxygen-powered, flow-restricted ventilation device

9. Which device "drives" the most oxygen into the plasma (i.e., partial oxygen pressure is increased)?
   a. CPAP
   b. nonrebreather oxygen mask
   c. bag–mask assembly
   d. oxygen-powered, flow-restricted ventilation device

10. A patient with which condition should be intubated?
    a. facial trauma
    b. medical cardiac arrest
    c. hypoglycemic diabetes
    d. opiate overdose

11. What is a sign of inadequate perfusion?
    a. ashen skin
    b. pallor
    c. mottling
    d. all of the above

12. What is one of the first signs of decompensation in a young patient?
    a. widening pulse pressure
    b. tachycardia
    c. tachypnea
    d. lowered mean arterial pressure

13. Primary cardiogenic shock is best treated with which process?
    a. large fluid infusion
    b. dopamine drip
    c. dobutamine drip
    d. epinephrine infusion

14. What is the optimal care for a patient with a STEMI?
    a. balloon pump
    b. angioplasty
    c. fibrinolytics
    d. vasopressor infusion

15. What is the therapeutic goal for fluid resuscitation in hypovolemia?
    a. systolic blood pressure of 90 to 100 mmHg
    b. 2 liters of saline infused
    c. increased systolic pressure by 20 mmHg
    d. saline infusion for adequate urine output

Short Answer

Write a brief answer to each of the following questions.

16. What are the substrates that the brain needs to survive?

    _____

    _____

17. What are the four main components for adequate delivery of oxygen?

    _____

    _____

18. What is the look test, sick vs. not sick test, and doorway diagnosis?

    _____

    _____

19. What risk is attendant with multiple intubation attempts?

_____

_____

20. What are the three components to be considered during resuscitation of hypoperfusion?

_____

_____

Fill in the Blank

Complete each sentence by adding the appropriate word in the provided blanks.

21. Increased carbon dioxide leads to _____ which impairs epinephrine effectiveness.

22. The _____ _____ mechanically augments the heart.

23. The Paramedic can actually worsen bleeding with _____.

24. A standardized treatment algorithm with an end goal is called early _____-_____ _____.

25. _____ increases the partial pressure of oxygen in the blood.

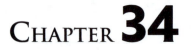

CHAPTER **34**

GYNECOLOGICAL DISORDERS

Case Study

Chief Concern

"I think I'm losing the baby!" Xian-Lun cries. The call comes to dispatch as a 9-1-1 hang up. When the dispatcher calls back, all he can make out is a woman sobbing, so he sends the police. Officers on-scene report that the scene is safe and that the woman is alone.

Critical Thinking Questions

1. What are some of the possible causes of vaginal bleeding in women of child-bearing age?

   _____

   _____

2. What is the implication of the comment, "I think I'm losing the baby!"?

   _____

   _____

History

Arriving on-scene, the Paramedics are led into a back bedroom of an apartment. The many boxes—some opened and some still sealed—suggest that the woman has just moved into the apartment.

Xian-Lun is obviously pregnant, nearing the third trimester. She states this is her first pregnancy and the bleeding started last night, becoming heavier this morning.

She relates that she called 9-1-1 but changed her mind. She had some bleeding earlier in the pregnancy. In addition, she doesn't have any health insurance. She has been getting advice from her maternal grandmother who lives in another city now. She has not seen a doctor for prenatal care, preferring to follow her grandmother's advice.

Critical Thinking Questions

1. What are the important elements of the history that a Paramedic should obtain?

   _____

   _____

2. What additional history should the Paramedic obtain?

   _____

   _____

Examination

Xian-Lun consents to an abdominal examination after the Paramedic explains that it will not be necessary to "expose" her in front of the police officers. Her abdomen shows obvious signs of pregnancy and the baby has not dropped yet. Inspection does not reveal any masses, abnormal distention, or ecchymosis.

Xian-Lun has a sanitary napkin in place and admits to changing the pad at least every hour for the last four hours. The Paramedic gives Xian-Lun time and privacy to change the pad in the bathroom before the trip to the hospital, after confirming that she is not passing clots.

As she stands, the Paramedics elect to obtain a set of orthostatic vital signs. However, she complains of feeling light-headed and is immediately placed on the stretcher.

Critical Thinking Questions

1. What are the elements of the physical examination of a patient with vaginal bleeding?

2. What is a "pad count"?

Assessment

Xian-Lun is told to seek medical attention for her pregnancy. At first she resists, preferring instead to contact her maternal grandmother. However, she is ultimately convinced by the Paramedics to go to the hospital to "at least be checked out." The Paramedics reinforce that the emergency department will see her regardless of her ability to pay. Trusting the Paramedics, to whom she has developed a rapport, she agrees.

Critical Thinking Questions

1. What is the significance of the vaginal bleeding?

2. What is the risk with vaginal bleeding during pregnancy?

Treatment

The Paramedics package Xian-Lun for transportation to the hospital. Obtaining venous access is easier than they anticipated, and she agrees to wear an oxygen mask. The Paramedics place an abdominal pad under her buttocks to absorb any excess blood that might spill from the sanitary napkin.

Critical Thinking Questions

1. What is the standard of care of patients with vaginal bleeding?

2. When is fluid resuscitation necessary?

Evaluation

While en route to the hospital, Xian-Lun starts to complain of lower abdominal cramps that are labor-like. When questioning Xian-Lun about the onset of these cramps, she admits that her boyfriend is unhappy with the pregnancy. She tells the Paramedics that the real reason she hung up is that she was afraid he would be angry if the "authorities" came to the apartment.

Following her lead, the Paramedics ask if he struck her in the abdomen. With her head lowered, in a barely audible voice, she admits, "Yes."

Critical Thinking Questions

1. What are the implications of domestic violence in this case?

_____

_____

2. What responsibilities does a Paramedic have to report domestic violence?

_____

_____

Disposition

Xian-Lun is transported to the "birthing center" at the hospital where she is immediately rushed to ultrasound by the nurses. The Paramedics pass off the report to the nurses, taking one of them aside and explaining that domestic violence may be at the core of this case.

Critical Thinking Questions

1. What is the most appropriate transport decision that will get the patient to definitive care?

_____

_____

2. What should the Paramedic report to the emergency department staff?

_____

_____

Practice Questions
Multiple Choice

Select the best answer for each of the following questions.

1. What is the cause of the most immediately life-threatening abdominal pain in women of child-bearing age?
   a. ovarian cysts
   b. ovarian torsion
   c. ectopic pregnancy
   d. pelvic inflammatory disease

2. Which condition is related to sexually transmitted infections?
   a. ovarian cysts
   b. ovarian torsion
   c. ectopic pregnancy
   d. pelvic inflammatory disease

3. Which condition is most likely to occur in older women?
   a. endometriosis
   b. uterine prolapse
   c. pelvic inflammatory disease
   d. vulvovaginitis

4. What is most likely the cause of painless, bright red blood from the vagina in the third trimester?
   a. spontaneous abortion
   b. threatened abortion
   c. placenta previa
   d. placental abruption

5. What is most likely the cause of painful bright red blood from the vagina in the third trimester?
   a. spontaneous abortion
   b. threatened abortion
   c. placenta previa
   d. placental abruption

6. What is most likely the cause of painless bright red blood from the vagina, with tissue?
   a. spontaneous abortion
   b. threatened abortion
   c. placenta previa
   d. placental abruption

7. What is premature separation of the placenta from the uterine wall called?
   a. spontaneous abortion
   b. threatened abortion
   c. placenta previa
   d. placental abruption

8. What is obstruction of the cervical os by the placenta called?
   a. spontaneous abortion
   b. threatened abortion
   c. placenta previa
   d. placental abruption

9. What is another name for painful menses?
   a. dysmenorrhea
   b. menorrhagia
   c. metrorrhagia
   d. metromenorrhagia

10. What is another name for heavy menstrual flow?
    a. dysmenorrhea
    b. menorrhagia
    c. metrorrhagia
    d. metromenorrhagia

11. What is another name for irregular menses?
    a. dysmenorrhea
    b. menorrhagia
    c. metrorrhagia
    d. metromenorrhagia

12. Which of the following is associated with exercise or trauma and causes severe abdominal pain?
    a. ruptured ovarian cysts
    b. ovarian torsion
    c. ectopic pregnancy
    d. pelvic inflammatory disease

13. Which of the following causes a loss of blood to the ovaries and subsequent infarction?
    a. ruptured ovarian cysts
    b. ovarian torsion
    c. ectopic pregnancy
    d. pelvic inflammatory disease

14. Which of the following is NOT dysfunctional uterine bleeding?
    a. dysmenorrhea
    b. menorrhagia
    c. metrorrhagia
    d. metromenorrhagia

15. Which condition can block the urinary meatus, preventing urination?
    a. uterine prolapse
    b. herpes
    c. Bartholin gland abscess
    d. vulvovaginitis

Short Answer

Write a brief answer to each of the following questions.

16. The saying goes, "Any woman of child-bearing age who has lower abdominal pain is pregnant until proven otherwise." To what is this referring?

    _____

    _____

17. How should a Paramedic respond to a "foreign body" lodged in the vagina?

    _____

    _____

18. What is considered severe vaginal bleeding?

    _____

    _____

19. Which conditions can cause vaginal itching and odorous discharge?

    _____

    _____

20. Name the four conditions that can cause vaginal bleeding.

    _____

    _____

Fill in the Blank

Complete each sentence by adding the appropriate word in the provided blanks.

21. An irregular and heavy menses is called _____.

22. A pregnancy outside of the uterus is called a _____ pregnancy.

23. Small amounts of blood, called _____, is common in 25% of pregnancies.

24. The medical term for the vaginal opening is the _____.

25. The lay term for abortion is _____.

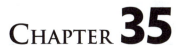

CHAPTER 35

NORMAL PREGNANCY

Case Study
Chief Concern

Karri and Jon are just about to bite into their juicy burgers when the tones go off and the dispatcher announces, "27-year-old female, 6 months pregnant with abdominal pain." They both swallow hard. Pregnancy calls—not childbirth calls, but pregnancy-related calls—make them both crazy. However, they both understand that the physiology of a woman changes dramatically when she is pregnant.

Critical Thinking Questions

1. What are some of the possible causes of the patient's abdominal pain?

   _____

   _____

2. How can the pregnancy and the abdominal pain be related?

   _____

   _____

History

The patient is an obviously pregnant woman who is sitting at the dining room table in obvious discomfort. After the Paramedics introduce themselves, the patient relates her present dilemma. Her pain started shortly after she had eaten at the local burger joint—ironically, the same one Karri and Jon had just visited!

She describes the pain as severe, 8 on a scale of 1 to 10, that comes in waves and worsens with deep inspiration. "Exactly where is the pain?" Karri asks. "Could you point with one finger of one hand to where it hurts the most?"

Both Karri and Jon sigh in relief when she points to the right upper quadrant. "Tell us more," Jon implores. She says this is her second pregnancy. She has one child who is living with his father at this time.

Karri delves further into the patient's past medical history. It turns out the patient has been having trouble with this pregnancy. Early in the pregnancy, she had "high enema."

Puzzled, Karri asks, "Hyperemesis?"

"Yes," the patient confirms. She goes on to say she sometimes gets abdominal pain when she rolls over in bed or even when she is just coughing. She is due June 30th.

Critical Thinking Questions

1. What are the elements of the history of pregnancy?

   _____

   _____

2. What is the probable explanation for the abdominal pain when coughing?

_____

_____

3. Using Naegle's rule, calculate the patient's last menstrual period.

_____

_____

Examination

Jon asks the patient to sit on the stretcher, which is reclined at a 45-degree angle. He knows that if he lays her flat that she will become short of breath. The abdomen appears round and shows no evidence of contusions. Her pain is greatest in the upper right quadrant when he palpates during a deep inspiration. "Murphy's sign," he mumbles to himself.

Using Leopold's maneuvers, he appreciates the lie of the infant. After estimating the position of the spine, he auscultates for heart sounds. Although he is unable to hear the fetal heart tones, which is not an uncommon situation, he does feel fetal movement under the stethoscope head. Next, Jon goes on to to estimate the fundal height.

Critical Thinking Questions

1. What are the elements of the physical examination of a patient with suspected tachydysrhythmia?

_____

_____

2. Why is the fundal height a critical element in this examination?

_____

_____

Assessment

Karri and Jon tell the patient that they cannot tell her the cause of her abdominal pain. However, they feel confident that it is not related to the pregnancy. This is a great relief to the mother.

Critical Thinking Questions

1. What diagnosis did the Paramedic announce to the patient?

_____

_____

2. Are there any non-pregnancy-related causes for the abdominal pain?

_____

_____

Treatment

While en route to the childbirth center, Karri offers the patient high-flow, high-concentration oxygen. At first she declines, but finally accepts after Karri explains that it might help the baby.

Next, Karri obtains venous access, which is rarely a problem in young mothers as they tend to be hypervascular.

Critical Thinking Questions

1. What is the standard of care of patients with potential pregnancy-related abdominal pain?

_____

_____

2. How can the Paramedic ascertain if the fetus is in distress and how can it be treated?

_____

_____

Evaluation

After the patient has been loaded in the ambulance, she tells Karri that she feels lightheaded. Without thinking, Karri lays the patient down. The patient immediately feels more faint. Karri grabs a radial pulse, which is faint, weak, and very rapid. In addition, the patient's skin is cool and clammy.

"Jon!" Karri yells to the driver's compartment, "I think she is going to pass out. I laid her flat and put her feet up and that seemed to make her worse." Jon yells back through the open compartment door, "Did you lay her on her side?"

Critical Thinking Questions

1. What are some of the predictable complications associated with laying a pregnant woman flat?

_____

_____

2. What is the treatment for this condition?

_____

_____

Disposition

After being placed on her side, the patient seems to stabilize as they pull into the hospital. Even though she is pregnant, the triage nurse sends her to the main emergency department instead of the birthing unit. The story that Jon and Karri provide lead her to believe that her abdominal pain is not pregnancy-related.

Critical Thinking Questions

1. What is the most appropriate transport decision that will get the patient to definitive care?

_____

_____

2. Would the destination change if the patient were to become unconscious?

_____

_____

Practice Questions

Multiple Choice

Select the best answer for each of the following questions.

1. What is the second most common cause of acute abdominal pain during pregnancy?
   a. cholecystitis
   b. appendicitis
   c. gastroenteritis
   d. peritonitis

2. Which anti-nausea medication has NOT been cleared for use in nausea and vomiting during pregnancy?
   a. promethazine
   b. chlorpromazine
   c. diphenhydramine
   d. ondansetron

3. What is a woman who is pregnant for the first time called?
   a. nullipara
   b. primigravida
   c. paragravida
   d. primipara

4. What is a woman who is a first-time mother called?
   a. nullipara
   b. primigravida
   c. paragravida
   d. primipara

5. Which of the following is NOT associated with fetal alcohol syndrome?
   a. smooth philtrum
   b. flattened bridge of nose
   c. Down syndrome
   d. epicanthal folds

6. Which of the following could be a teratogen?
   a. cytomegalovirus
   b. toxoplasmosis
   c. alcohol
   d. all of the above

7. Which of the following dangerous-to-pregnancy diseases is carried by cats?
   a. cytomegalovirus
   b. toxoplasmosis
   c. erythroblastosis fetalis
   d. methicillin-resistance Staph aureus

8. In which situation would measuring the fundal height (centimeters above pubis equals weeks) be most accurate?
   a. first trimester
   b. first stage of labor
   c. twins
   d. third trimester

9. If the fundus is at the umbilicus, then the gestation is about _____ weeks.
   a. 12
   b. 20
   c. 30
   d. 40

10. At how many weeks of pregnancy should the Paramedic be able to hear fetal heart sounds and appreciate fetal movement?
    a. 12
    b. 20
    c. 30
    d. 40

11. What is the long axis of the fetus called?
    a. fetal lie
    b. fetal attitude
    c. fetal position
    d. fetal stance

12. What is a pregnancy-induced convulsion called?
    a. pre-eclampsia
    b. pregnancy-induced hypertensive crisis
    c. toxemia of pregnancy
    d. eclampsia

13. What is the drug of choice for pregnancy-induced convulsions?
    a. magnesium sulfate
    b. sodium bicarbonate
    c. calcium chloride
    d. diazepam

14. A woman with a history of previous pregnancy and cesarean section(s) is at risk for which condition?
    a. placenta previa
    b. placenta accreta
    c. uterine rupture
    d. all of the above

15. What is the only sure guarantee of sterilization?
    a. tubal ligation
    b. total hysterectomy
    c. oophorectomy
    d. pelvic inflammatory disease

Short Answer

Write a brief answer to each of the following questions.

16. Explain supine hypotensive syndrome.

   _____

   _____

17. List some extrauterine causes of abdominal pain in a pregnant woman.

   _____

   _____

18. What is round ligament pain?

   _____

   _____

19. Describe the GPA system for notation of obstetrical history.

   _____

   _____

20. Describe the TPAL system for obstetric history.

   _____

   _____

Fill in the Blank

Complete each sentence by adding the appropriate word in the provided blanks.

21. The mother's first appreciation of fetal movement is called the _____.

22. The most common surgical emergency in pregnancy is _____.

23. The use of medications to slow labor is called _____.

24. Extreme morning sickness is called _____ _____.

25. _____ _____ is used to estimate the date of delivery.

CHAPTER 36

COMPLICATIONS OF PREGNANCY

Case Study
Chief Concern

The roads are slick from the first rain in 10 days. Looking down the highway, Leann can see the oil beading up on the road surface, making the highway look as smooth as glass with the sun shining. Her daydreaming is interrupted by the scratchy voice from under the dash.

"Medic 32, police units on the scene of a motor vehicle crash. Interstate 887, mile marker 215, personal injury. One patient, seven months pregnant." Wheeling around, Leann lights up the fly car and murmurs to herself, "Motor vehicle collision and pregnant woman. Not a good combination."

Pulling up to the scene, Leann can see the "Mommy taxi" off the embankment. Worse, no one is out of the car. From her vantage point, she can see the backs of two car seats.

Critical Thinking Questions

1. How might a pregnant woman experience shock trauma differently from others?

_____

_____

2. How would the pregnancy affect the patient's breathing?

_____

_____

History

Mudiwa, the patient, is seated in the car and is complaining of severe abdominal pain. While the rescue squad works at immobilizing her spine and extricating her from the vehicle, Leann asks her questions. She discovers that Mudiwa's pain is not intermittent and does not radiate. In addition, she has four other children, two by cesarean section, and she claims this pain is worse than the labor for any of them. She admits to not wearing a seat belt. The seat belt doesn't fit, she claims, and it is uncomfortable as well. Mudiwa warns one of the rescue squad EMTs who is putting a strap under her legs that she is wet "down there."

Critical Thinking Questions

1. What are the important elements of the history that a Paramedic should obtain?

_____

_____

2. What implication does the pain have along with vaginal discharge in a woman who is 28 weeks' pregnant?

_____

_____

Examination

Once Mudiwa is out of the car and on the backboard, Leann does a quick assessment. Her blood pressure is low and her heart rate is slightly elevated. Leann asks herself if this is the result of the patient's pregnancy or a sign of early shock. She decides to treat it as shock, telling the crew, "Hope for the best, treat for the worst."

Mudiwa's abdomen is board-like, the pain persistent and severe, and Leann can palpate the outline of the fetus. The last, the outline of the fetus, concerns her, as does the copious amount of vaginal bleeding.

Critical Thinking Questions

1. What are the elements of the physical examination of a pregnant patient with trauma?

_____

_____

2. What are the elements of the physical examination of the fetus of a pregnant woman who has experienced trauma?

_____

_____

Assessment

Electing to contact medical control earlier rather than later, Leann receives an order for an inhaled beta/adrenergic agent. Leann advises the physician that the patient's pain is constant and not like the patient's previous labor. The physician understands and advises Leann to prepare four (4) grams of magnesium sulfate in 250 mL of saline for administration over 15 minutes if the patient starts to experience labor. Leann repeats the order, with the understanding that she is to hold the bolus until the patient labors. Leann is worried about the vasodilation that accompanies magnesium sulfate and the effect it might have on a patient with suspected hemorrhagic shock (i.e., hypotension).

Critical Thinking Questions

1. What are the possible obstetric causes of bleeding in a pregnant woman involved in a motor vehicle collision at 28 weeks?

_____

_____

2. What are the possible non-obstetric causes of bleeding in a pregnant woman involved in a motor vehicle collision?

_____

_____

Treatment

After ensuring the provision of high-flow, high-concentration oxygen, Leann has the "tech" aboard obtain venous access while she completes her physical examination. One EMT is manually displacing the gravid uterus to the side while another one is stuffing pillows to try to achieve a 15-degree angle on the backboard.

Critical Thinking Questions

1. What is supine hypotensive syndrome and how is it treated?

_____

_____

2. What is the standard of care for patients with bleeding during pregnancy?

_____

_____

Evaluation

Mudiwa tells Leann that the pain has stopped and she thinks she will be alright. Leann wonders, "Was the earlier pain actually labor?" She asks the EMT for a repeated blood pressure before she starts the magnesium bolus. The EMT announces that Mudiwa's blood pressure is dropping.

Leann turns to Mudiwa to ask if she is alright, but she can't get a response. She quickly reaches for a carotid pulse and finds none. Although the ECG monitor still shows a sinus tachycardia, Leann orders that CPR begin immediately while she reconnects with the physician.

Critical Thinking Questions

1. Why is treating the mother important to fetal survival?

_____

_____

2. What safeguards does the fetus have against trauma?

_____

_____

Disposition

Mudiwa is wheeled into the first trauma bed in the resuscitation room. Physicians, nurses, and respiratory therapists stream into the room, as a result of the hastily called trauma alert, to perform their various tasks. The trauma resident has not arrived and the attending physician decides that he cannot wait. The physician performs an emergency perimortem cesarean section while the neonatal resuscitation team from the neonatal intensive care unit prepares to receive the newborn.

Critical Thinking Questions

1. What is the most appropriate transport decision that will get the patient to definitive care?

_____

_____

2. What special procedures are going to be carried out in the case of a pregnant woman who is in trauma arrest?

_____

_____

Practice Questions
Multiple Choice

Select the best answer for each of the following questions.

1. What is retention of all the products of conception called?
   a. spontaneous abortion
   b. complete abortion
   c. incomplete abortion
   d. missed abortion

2. What is the approximate percentage of pregnancies that end in spontaneous abortion?
   a. 1 in 5 pregnancies
   b. 1 in 50 pregnancies
   c. 1 in 100 pregnancies
   d. 1 in 1,000 pregnancies

3. Which of the following is NOT a risk factor for ectopic pregnancy?
   a. pelvic inflammatory disease
   b. prior ectopic pregnancy
   c. venereal warts
   d. assisted fertility

4. Vaginal bleeding during pregnancy is most common in the _____ trimester.
   a. first
   b. second
   c. third
   d. any

5. Didelphys refers to which condition?
   a. double vagina
   b. double uterus
   c. bicornate uterus
   d. absent uterus

6. Preterm labor and premature rupture of membranes are associated with which condition?
   a. placenta previa
   b. placental abruption
   c. uterine rupture
   d. ectopic pregnancy

7. Which of the following is NOT a risk factor for placenta previa?
   a. alcohol consumption
   b. tobacco smoking
   c. cesarean section
   d. grand multiparity

8. What is premature separation of a normally implanted placenta from the uterine wall called?
   a. placenta previa
   b. placental abruption
   c. uterine rupture
   d. ectopic pregnancy

9. What is the most common presenting symptom of placental abruption?
   a. vaginal bleeding
   b. abdominal pain
   c. fetal bradycardia
   d. premature labor

10. Which of the following is NOT associated with placental abruption?
    a. tobacco smoking
    b. maternal hypertension
    c. cocaine use
    d. trauma

11. What creates the greatest risk for uterine rupture?
    a. alcohol consumption
    b. tobacco smoking
    c. cesarean section
    d. grand multiparity

12. What is the most common cause of trauma in pregnancy?
    a. intimate partner violence
    b. falls
    c. motor vehicle collisions
    d. assault

13. What is the most significant finding in placental abruption following a motor vehicle collision?
    a. vaginal bleeding
    b. abdominal pain
    c. absence of fetal heart sounds
    d. abdominal ecchymosis

14. What is the extreme consequence of pregnancy-induced hypertension?
    a. headaches
    b. visual changes
    c. epigastric pain
    d. convulsions

15. Which of the following is NOT part of the triad of pre-eclampsia?
    a. proteinuria
    b. edema
    c. hypertension
    d. hyperglycemia

Short Answer

Write a brief answer to each of the following questions.

16. What is the adage about women with abdominal pain?

_____

_____

17. What is meant by "hidden bleeding"?

_____

_____

18. What are the risks for women with gestational diabetes?

_____

_____

19. What is the "bloody show"?

_____

_____

20. What are three agents used to slow labor?

_____

_____

Fill in the Blank

Complete each sentence by adding the appropriate word in the provided blanks.

21. A damaged cervix that bleeds during pregnancy is called a(n) _____ cervix.

22. A _____ _____ is a degenerative process within the chorionic villi of the placenta.

23. Visual changes related to pregnancy-induced hypertension are called _____.

24. HELLP, in HELLP syndrome, stands for _____ _____, _____ _____ _____, and _____ _____ _____ syndrome.

25. Suppression of labor is called _____.

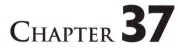
NORMAL CHILDBIRTH

Case Study

Chief Concern

The earthquake only lasted 90 seconds, but it destroyed most of the standing medical facilities. Although government help was on the way, every available home resource was put into use in the interim.

The Paramedics have been assigned to a temporary hospital that used to be a high school gym. To create rooms, the gym is divided into sections by hanging sheets from overhead ropes placed just for that purpose.

It is three in the morning, and Paramedics Romano and Rodriquez are informed, by overhead speaker, of an impending arrival. The patient is a 16-year-old woman in labor. The two Paramedics look at each other and down at the single, prepackaged delivery kit.

Critical Thinking Questions

1. How would a Paramedic assess a pregnant woman to see if she is ready to deliver?

   _____

   _____

2. How would the Paramedic ask about the woman's labor?

   _____

   _____

History

Romano, the more experienced of the two Paramedics, offers to support Rodriquez while she obtains a patient history. The patient, Leila, explains that her contractions are now minutes apart, as she is transferred from the stretcher to the cot by the firefighters.

Leila confirms that she has "broken water," and that this is her first child. Her labor has been less than six hours. Romano whispers into Rodriquez's ear, "We got time."

Critical Thinking Questions

1. What are the important elements of the history that a Paramedic should obtain?

   _____

   _____

2. How would a Paramedic obtain an obstetric history?

   _____

   _____

Examination

Leila asks if she can go to the bathroom. "Why?" asks Rodriquez. "I think I have to move my bowels," replies Leila. Rodriquez shoots Romano a look. "Do you mind if I just check you very quickly?" Sure enough, she can see a tuft of black hair from the baby's head.

"Paramedic Romano, would you mind handing me the birth kit and please close the curtains as you leave to go boil water?" Rodriquez smiles. Romano, red-faced, offers to stay and assist.

Critical Thinking Questions

1. What are the elements of the predelivery physical examination of a pregnant patient?

_____

_____

2. What are the elements of the predelivery physical examination of the fetus?

_____

_____

Assessment

Leila remarks that she really has to go to the bathroom, to which Paramedic Rodriquez replies, "That pressure you feel means you are about to have a baby."

Both Paramedic Romano and Leila are surprised—Paramedic Romano because he has been taught that it may take three hours of pushing to give birth. Leila is experiencing a "precipitous birth," which is altogether unexpected in a 16-year-old patient.

"Leila," Paramedic Rodriquez asks, "which position would you find most comfortable?" Rodriquez describes several positions, including lateral recumbent and squatting.

Critical Thinking Questions

1. What is the significance of the crowning and urge to move the bowels?

_____

_____

2. Why did the Paramedic ask the mother what position she would prefer to be in for the delivery?

_____

_____

Treatment

Paramedic Rodriquez expertly assists with the delivery while Paramedic Romano encourages Leila to pant and blow to control the speed of delivery. Within minutes, the childbirth is complete and Paramedic Rodriquez hands Leila her newborn daughter.

Critical Thinking Questions

1. What equipment will be needed to deliver a baby?

_____

_____

2. Explain the process of assisting with delivery.

_____

_____

Evaluation

Paramedic Romano takes the time to reassure Leila and assist with putting the newborn to her breast while he is determining the APGAR score. Except for the point lost for acrocyanosis, which is expected, the first score is nine. That score is excellent for a newborn born under such trying conditions.

A crowd has assembled outside the curtains and Leila, relieved that everything worked out all right, invites everyone in to see her new daughter, Lilith.

Critical Thinking Questions

1. What are the initial steps in neonatal resuscitation/newborn care?

_____

_____

2. What is the APGAR score?

_____

_____

Disposition

After approximately five minutes, the labor pains start again, but they are much milder. Shortly thereafter, Leila asks for a sanitary napkin, as she feels a trickle of blood. Paramedic Rodriquez explains that she is about to deliver her placenta. The placenta is then closely examined for defects and placed in a rip-proof plastic bag so that the physician can examine it when she arrives.

Critical Thinking Questions

1. What is the last stage of labor?

_____

_____

2. What should the Paramedic observe on the placenta?

_____

_____

Practice Questions
Multiple Choice

Select the best answer for each of the following questions.

1. Which layer of the uterus provides nutrients to the fetus?
   a. perimetrium
   b. epimetrium
   c. osteometrium
   d. endometrium

2. Effacement, thinning of the cervix, occurs in which stage of labor?
   a. first
   b. second
   c. third
   d. fourth

3. What is the first sign of the latent phase of the first stage of labor?
   a. bloody show
   b. ruptured membranes
   c. cervical dilation
   d. delivery of the newborn

4. The delivery of the newborn occurs at the end of which stage of labor?
   a. first
   b. second
   c. third
   d. fourth

5. What is the normal interval of time between the birth of the baby and delivery of the placenta?
   a. 10 minutes
   b. 15 minutes
   c. 20 minutes
   d. 30 minutes

6. In the "cardinal movements of labor," what is the first movement?
   a. engagement
   b. descent
   c. internal rotation
   d. extension

7. What is the greatest concern for premature rupture of membranes?
   a. premature labor
   b. meconium aspiration
   c. infection
   d. premature infant

8. The McRoberts maneuver is used for which situation?
   a. shoulder dystocia
   b. breech delivery
   c. frank delivery
   d. footling presentation

9. The majority of breech deliveries are _____ breeches.
   a. frank
   b. complete
   c. incomplete
   d. footling

10. What is gentle pressure to the occiput to slow flexion called?
    a. Ritgen maneuver
    b. Lovset's maneuver
    c. Mauriceau's maneuver
    d. Apgar maneuver

11. What is the first action taken during a delivery with a prolapsed cord?
    a. cut the cord
    b. pull slack on the cord
    c. slip the cord over the head
    d. deliver through the cord

12. Lovset's maneuver is used for which type of delivery?
    a. frank
    b. complete
    c. incomplete
    d. footling

13. Mauriceau's maneuver helps to ensure what situation?
    a. patent airway
    b. delivery of shoulders
    c. passage of meconium
    d. delivery of hips

14. Most infants lose points on the APGAR for which condition?
    a. acrocyanosis
    b. bradycardia
    c. bradypnea
    d. weak cry

15. To control maternal hemorrhage, what is the first action taken?
    a. fluid bolus
    b. 10 units of oxytocin IM
    c. uterine massage
    d. 10 units of oxytocin IV at 30 mL/hr

Short Answer

Write a brief answer to each of the following questions.

16. What is the first priority during preparations for childbirth?

_____

_____

17. What equipment is needed for delivery?

_____

_____

18. How can a Paramedic prevent a perineal tear?

_____

_____

19. Describe the first actions after the delivery of the newborn.

_____

_____

20. Describe fundal massage.

_____

_____

Fill in the Blank

Complete each sentence by adding the appropriate word in the provided blanks.

21. Excessive amniotic fluid is called _____.

22. Preparatory contractions (i.e., false labor) are called _____-_____ _____.

23. Green-tinged fluid is suggestive of _____ staining.

24. _____ _____ is a condition when the uterus does not contract following delivery.

25. Sudden shortness of breath, followed by cyanosis, immediately following delivery is suggestive of _____ _____ _____.

CHAPTER **38**

CARE OF THE NORMAL NEWBORN

Case Study

Chief Concern

A couple lives in a remote wooded area in the southwest corner of the county. Preferring a more natural lifestyle, they elect to have a home delivery. A nurse–midwife plans to attend the delivery, but her car breaks down. Therefore, the couple calls EMS.

As the Paramedic enters the house, he hears elation in the other room and the clearly audible cry of a newborn. "It's a boy!" yells Mack.

Critical Thinking Questions

1. What are the issues that a normal newborn must overcome?

_____

_____

2. What are the newborn's first two challenges?

_____

_____

History

"Hi, I am Barbara, I see I have come just in time." The mother is sitting at the edge of the bed, while Mack cradles the newborn below the mother.

As Barbara performs her physical examination, she asks the new mother a few questions such as her expected due date, her level of prenatal care, and if there is a chance of multiple gestations.

Critical Thinking Questions

1. What are the important elements of the history that a Paramedic should obtain?

_____

_____

2. What are the risks associated with prematurity?

_____

_____

Examination

After placing the newborn on the mother's abdomen and starting to dry the newborn, Barbara checks the infant for petechiae, swelling of the scalp, and softness of the skull. As she does so, she avoids applying pressure on the fontanels. Satisfied there is no birth trauma, she proceeds with the rest of her examination, looking for congenital anomalies.

Critical Thinking Questions

1. What are the elements of the physical examination of a newborn?

_____

_____

2. Why is a head-to-toe examination a critical element in this evaluation?

_____

_____

Assessment

Throughout the examination, the mother is anxious to hold her baby. Therefore, Barbara tries to complete the examination expeditiously. Barbara understands the importance of bonding and also understands the importance of the mother's first milk to the baby's future health.

Critical Thinking Questions

1. What is the significance of "bonding"?

_____

_____

2. What is the importance of the mother's first milk?

_____

_____

Treatment

With a bulb syringe in hand, Barbara stands by the newborn and his mother. Concerned about respiratory distress, Barbara is relieved when the newborn sneezes, indicating that he can maintain his own airway. Barbara relates that the newborn has a perfect APGAR score of 10.

Critical Thinking Questions

1. What is the APGAR score?

_____

_____

2. What is the treatment priority?

_____

_____

Evaluation

Barbara lets the newborn nurse. When it becomes apparent the newborn is either not ready or not capable of nursing, Barbara performs a heel stick to ascertain the newborn's blood glucose and ensure it is not the latter. The blood glucose is within normal limits, which is good news for the mother and father alike. As an added bonus, the stimulation of the heel stick stimulates the newborn to suckle.

Critical Thinking Questions

1. Why is a blood glucose reading important for a newborn?

   _____

   _____

2. What is the treatment for hypoglycemia in a newborn?

   _____

   _____

Disposition

As Barbara packs up her equipment, the nurse–midwife shows up. The two women have a conversation about the newborn as Barbara shares her findings. Together, the two women speak with medical control, who feels comfortable leaving the patient in the capable hands of the nurse–midwife.

Critical Thinking Questions

1. What is the most appropriate transport decision that will get the patient to definitive care?

   _____

   _____

2. Do all newborns need to be transported to the hospital?

   _____

   _____

Practice Questions
Multiple Choice

Select the best answer for each of the following questions.

1. Deoxygenated blood is passed to the umbilical arteries via which path?
   a. ductus venosus
   b. foramen ovale
   c. ductus arteriosus
   d. septal defect

2. Blood bypasses the lungs via which path?
   a. ductus venosus
   b. foramen ovale
   c. ductus arteriosus
   d. septal defect

3. The ligamentum arteriosum is the fetal remains of which path?
   a. ductus venosus
   b. foramen ovale
   c. ductus arteriosus
   d. septal defect

4. What is the direct cause of fetal distress?
   a. acidosis
   b. hypothermia
   c. hypoxia
   d. hypoglycemia

5. Which of the following is of the greatest concern to the Paramedic during neonatal resuscitation of the premature newborn?
   a. retinopathy of prematurity
   b. heart failure secondary to a patent ductus arteriosus
   c. respiratory distress from hyaline membrane disease
   d. thrombocytopenia

6. Prematurity is NOT associated with which of the following risk factors?
   a. cigarette smoking
   b. alcohol intoxication
   c. multiple gestations
   d. cocaine use

7. Which of the following is a risk for a postmature newborn with oligohydramnios?
   a. intrauterine infection
   b. placental abruption
   c. fetal distress
   d. all of the above

8. Which of the following is a sign of birth trauma?
   a. petechiae
   b. caput succedaneum
   c. cephalhematoma
   d. all of the above

9. The mother should be discouraged from breastfeeding if there is evidence of which condition?
   a. caput succedaneum
   b. laryngeal nerve injury
   c. omphalocele
   d. gastroschisis

10. What is the most dangerous abdominal wall defect?
    a. omphalocele
    b. gastroschisis
    c. diaphragmatic hernia
    d. umbilical hernia

11. Which infants are at risk for brachial plexus injury?
    a. newborns with shoulder dystocia
    b. breech deliveries
    c. macrosomic newborns
    d. all of the above

12. What is the most common birth defect?
    a. cleft palate
    b. spina bifida
    c. meningocele
    d. polydactyly

13. Which newborns are at risk for hypoglycemia?
    a. Newborns with low birth weight
    b. macrosomic newborns
    c. newborns with perinatal asphyxia
    d. all of the above

14. Which of the following is NOT a sign of neonatal hypoglycemia?
    a. jitteriness
    b. lethargy
    c. sweating
    d. tachycardia

15. Which condition may lead a Paramedic to suspect a risk of intrapartum infection?
    a. premature rupture of membranes
    b. foul-smelling amniotic fluid
    c. presence of fever
    d. all of the above

Short Answer

Write a brief answer to each of the following questions.

16. Explain the pathophysiology of hyaline membrane disease.

_____

_____

17. Explain how to care for a newborn with gastroschisis.

_____

_____

18. Explain how to care for a newborn with myelomeningocele.

_____

_____

19. Explain the process of preventing hypothermia.

_____

_____

20. List the complications common for premature infants.

_____

_____

Fill in the Blank

Complete each sentence by adding the appropriate word in the provided blanks.

21. Physical abnormalities of structure or function in the newborn are called _____ _____.

22. A birthweight over 4,000 grams is called _____.

23. Mothers with small hips and/or narrow pelvic outlets have _____ _____.

24. Sacral dimpling is suggestive of _____ _____ _____.

25. Premature newborns tend to be born in a _____ or breech position.

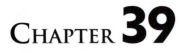

CHAPTER 39

SPECIAL CONSIDERATIONS IN NEONATOLOGY

Case Study

Chief Concern

Two words from the call remain stuck in Obie's mind: "Blue baby." As the ambulance pulls up to the brownstone, he sees another ambulance has already arrived, The crew already on-scene reports a "half-dead" teenage mother who has just given birth to a baby.

The attic scene Obie enters will stick in his mind for months to come. The "apartment" consists of a stained mattress on the floor, a single bare light bulb hanging from a cord for illumination, and urine-soaked newspapers, a product of the new puppy running around the apartment, barking up a storm.

"The baby, the baby!" Ernie yells, snapping Obie out of his daze. The baby is on the bathroom floor swaddled in a dirty bath rug. There is blood everywhere.

Critical Thinking Questions

1. What are some of the possible problems of prematurity?

   _____

   _____

2. What is the implication of the patient's statement that the baby is blue?

   _____

   _____

History

Ernie relates that the teenager is a runaway that has been living in the attic, courtesy of the landlord, who is also the baby's father. The girl has not seen a physician nor has there been any kind of prenatal care. The baby is almost 10 weeks premature according to his calculations, if the mother's estimate of the date of delivery is correct.

Critical Thinking Questions

1. What are the important elements of the history of the delivery that a Paramedic should obtain?

   _____

   _____

2. What are the important elements of the maternal history that a Paramedic should obtain?

   _____

   _____

Examination

The baby is tiny with red skin, sparse hair, and open eyes that confirm the baby is premature. Carefully picking the baby up from the floor, Obie places it on the mattress.

The tiny limbs stretch out, which is a good sign. Obie starts neonatal resuscitation, beginning with suctioning the airway with a bulb syringe. He is relieved to find the airway is clear.

"Clean towels, and get me a hot pack wrapped in another towel, plus cellophane!" Obie yells to his partner, who is already scampering down the stairs to the ambulance.

Critical Thinking Questions

1. What are the initial problems of transition that a newborn must overcome?

_____

_____

2. Why is wrapping the preterm newborn in plastic wrap important?

_____

_____

Assessment

Obie knows that the baby is a "premie," but at 30 weeks he should be viable. He also is unsure of the baby's sex, as the genitals are ambiguous. Obie reminds himself to stick to the discipline: A, then B, then C, then D.

Critical Thinking Questions

1. What is the most common "pathway" for newborn care?

_____

_____

2. What is the current thinking about meconium?

_____

_____

Treatment

After drying the neonate with the fresh towels, Obie reassesses the infant. Since the airway is patent, he decides to hold off on intubating. The neonate has good chest rise and is breathing rapidly. The baby's color has also improved, with the exception of the blue fingers and toes.

The infant's umbilical cord is still attached to the placenta that now is in a pile on the floor. Obie elects to cut the umbilical cord, obtaining venous access at the same time. Obie successfully cannulates the larger umbilical vein with a 3.5f catheter.

Critical Thinking Questions

1. What is the standard of care for neonatal resuscitation?

_____

_____

2. What are some of the patient-specific concerns of a Paramedic during a neonatal resuscitation?

_____

_____

Evaluation

Looking at the wraparound pulse oximeter, Obie notes that the pulse is starting to drop and the SpO_2 is still at 85%. Obie realizes he forgot to warm the little fellow.

Critical Thinking Questions

1. What are some of the predictable complications associated with neonatal resuscitation?

   _____

   _____

2. What is a simple mnemonic to remember the complications of newborn intubation?

   _____

   _____

Disposition

With the baby swaddled in fresh blankets and lying on a towel-wrapped hot pack, Obie makes his way down the stairs. Dispatch has already alerted University Hospital of an impending arrival of a neonate and a neonatal team is standing by in the emergency department anticipating their arrival.

Critical Thinking Questions

1. What is the most appropriate transport decision that will get the patient to definitive care?

   _____

   _____

2. Why must the heat pack be wrapped?

   _____

   _____

Practice Questions
Multiple Choice

Select the best answer for each of the following questions.

1. What is the first step in neonatal resuscitation?
   a. warming and drying
   b. suction
   c. blow-by oxygen
   d. compressions

2. Meconium aspiration can lead to all of the following EXCEPT _____.
   a. atelectasis
   b. increased peristalsis
   c. pneumothorax
   d. surfactant dysfunction

3. What is the therapeutic goal of ventilation of a neonate?
   a. 20 to 30 breaths per minute
   b. chest rise and fall
   c. 5 to 7 mL per kg
   d. 7 to 10 mL per kg

4. A congenitally small mandible, causing narrowing of the airway, is seen in children with which condition?
   a. Pierre Robin syndrome
   b. fetal alcohol syndrome
   c. Down syndrome
   d. prolonged QT syndrome

5. Which of the following is NOT necessarily an indication for intubation of a neonate?
   a. respiratory arrest
   b. prolonged bag ventilation
   c. ineffective mask seal
   d. meconium aspiration

6. What is the preferred laryngoscope blade for intubation of a neonate?
   a. Wis-Hipple
   b. Macintosh
   c. Grandview®
   d. Miller

7. The P in the DOPE mnemonic stands for _____.
   a. pulmonary atresia
   b. pulmonary embolism
   c. pulmonary edema
   d. pneumothorax

8. What is the preferred location for a needle decompression?
   a. second ICS at MCL
   b. fifth ICS at MCL
   c. second ICS at MAL
   d. fourth ICS at MAL

9. What is the preferred method of chest compression in the premature neonate?
   a. thumbs with fingers encircled
   b. first two fingers
   c. palm of one hand
   d. thumb of one hand

10. What is the preferred route of medication administration in the premature neonate?
    a. intraosseous
    b. intravenous
    c. umbilical
    d. subcutaneous

11. Naloxone should not be given for which condition?
    a. narcotic-induced respiratory depression
    b. maternal addiction
    c. field analgesia for labor
    d. all of the above

12. Which of the following will NOT make a neonate hypovolemic?
    a. placental abruption
    b. hypothermia
    c. placenta previa
    d. umbilical cord hemorrhage

13. Which of the following is NOT a life-threatening neonatal neurological disorder?
    a. intraventricular hemorrhage
    b. periventricular hemorrhage
    c. hydrocephalus
    d. all of the above

Case Studies & Practice Questions 215

14. Which of the following is suggestive of fetal hydrops?
    a. ascites
    b. pleural effusions
    c. pericardial effusions
    d. all of the above

15. Which of the following is NOT a physical sign displayed by the premature neonate?
    a. red, translucent skin
    b. bald head
    c. lids open
    d. scrotum empty

Short Answer

Write a brief answer to each of the following questions.

16. How do newborns make heat?

_____

_____

17. What are the three reasons that meconium aspiration leads to respiratory distress?

_____

_____

18. Describe the measurement and placement of an orogastric tube in a neonate.

_____

_____

19. Why is clear plastic wrap used for neonates?

_____

_____

20. What is kangaroo care?

_____

_____

Fill in the Blank

Complete each sentence by adding the appropriate word in the provided blanks.

21. The Paramedic's goal in caring for a newborn is to create a _____ _____ environment.

22. Increased respirations followed by bradypnea is an example of _____ _____.

23. Congenital narrowing of the nasal airway is called _____ _____.

24. The medical term for soft spots is _____.

25. Capillaries within the germinal layer matrix bleed in _____ _____ and _____ _____, thereby increasing intracranial pressure.

CHAPTER 40

ASSESSMENT OF THE STABLE CHILD

Case Study

Chief Concern

The school nurse, Meghan, meets the crew in the hallway outside the nurse's office. She explains that Jamie passed out in class while standing in line to go to gym.

The teacher, Mrs. Milkey, sent two students to the school's office and requested the nurse. When she arrived, Meghan found a very pale girl who was nevertheless awake and alert. Much relieved, she helped her to the nurse's office and called her parents, who wanted her transported to the emergency department immediately.

Critical Thinking Questions

1. What are the elements of the Pediatric Assessment Triangle?

   _____

   _____

2. What is the utility of the Pediatric Assessment Triangle?

   _____

   _____

History

From the doorway, Jamie looks fine. She is awake, alert, talkative, and has no trouble breathing. Although she appears to be naturally pale (she is blue-eyed and blond), her color now seems fine.

Josh approaches Jamie and, getting down on one knee in front of the 10-year-old, introduces himself. Jamie denies having a headache or that her neck hurts. She says she was just standing there when a black curtain fell over her eyes. The next thing she remembers is Mrs. Milkey kneeling next to her, holding her head up.

Critical Thinking Questions

1. What are the important elements of the history that a Paramedic should obtain?

   _____

   _____

2. How is obtaining a history different with children of different ages?

   _____

   _____

Examination

With her permission, Josh starts examining Jamie. Her scalp is intact, without deformity or tenderness. There is no drainage from her ears or nose and her facial bones are intact. Palpation of her neck confirms that Jamie does not have cervical tenderness or neck pain. In addition, a quick examination of her torso and extremities does not reveal any evidence of trauma.

The only finding that concerns Josh is Jamie's pants. They are ill-fitting and do not match, even though everything else Jamie is wearing does match. "Oh," the nurse whispers into Josh's ear, "She wet herself. We always keep extra clothes in the office just in case."

Critical Thinking Questions

1. What are the elements of the physical examination of a pediatric patient?

2. Is the pediatric patient's physical examination performed differently than an adult's?

Assessment

Josh's curiosity is piqued. Although no one mentioned any seizure activity, the incontinence suggests that Jamie might have had a seizure. Over Meghan's protestations, he elects to transport Jamie immediately to the emergency department, rather than wait for the parents. "Please tell the parents that we will be at Community Hospital when they get here," Josh notes.

Critical Thinking Questions

1. What is used to decide sick versus not sick?

2. What creates the urgency in this case?

Treatment

Once aboard the ambulance, Josh elects to reconfirm the pulse oximeter reading. The SpO_2 comes back normal. Electing to apply oxygen via nasal cannula to keep the SpO_2 stable, Josh explains to Jamie that he needs to start an IV. Jamie, who is a little frightened at first, agrees once Josh, in a calm and reassuring voice, explains that it is important for her safety.

Critical Thinking Questions

1. How is the treatment of pediatric patients different from treating other patients?

2. How is the treatment of pediatric patients similar to treating other patients?

Evaluation

With the ambulance less than five minutes away from the emergency department, Jamie suffers a seizure. Though the seizure does not last long (less than one minute), it confirms Josh's fear that she didn't pass out. Rather, it is more likely she seized and no one noticed or reported it.

Within minutes, Jamie is awake and asking what happened. "Jamie," Josh asks, "have you ever passed out before today?"

Critical Thinking Questions

1. What are some of the predictable complications associated with pediatric care?

_____

_____

2. What is the primary cause of decompensation in children?

_____

_____

Disposition

Forewarned by the school nurse by cellular telephone, Jamie's parents are waiting for her at the door. "Is she alright?" her mother implores of Josh. He reassures her that Jamie is alright but she needs to be seen in the emergency department.

Critical Thinking Questions

1. What is the most appropriate transport decision that will get the patient to definitive care?

_____

_____

2. Does the destination decision change if the child has special needs?

_____

_____

Practice Questions
Multiple Choice

Select the best answer for each of the following questions.

1. Which of the following is NOT part of the PAT assessment triangle?
   a. airway
   b. breathing
   c. appearance
   d. circulation

2. Which age group is known for "risk taking" behavior?
   a. toddlers
   b. preschool
   c. school-age
   d. adolescents

3. Which age group is known for its "literal thinkers"?
   a. toddlers
   b. preschool
   c. school-age
   d. adolescents

4. Which age group starts to be able to answer questions about their condition?
   a. toddlers
   b. preschool
   c. school-age
   d. adolescents

5. Which of the following groups does NOT tend to be modest?
   a. toddlers
   b. preschool
   c. school-age
   d. adolescents

6. At what age are both fontanels closed?
   a. 6 months
   b. 12 months
   c. 18 months
   d. 24 months

7. At what age should Paramedics introduce themselves by name to the patient?
   a. toddlers
   b. preschool
   c. school-age
   d. all of the above

8. Stranger anxiety is seen in children in which age group?
   a. toddlers
   b. preschool
   c. school-age
   d. adolescents

9. At which age group can the Paramedic revert to the standard head-to-toe assessment, as opposed to the toe-to-head assessment approach?
   a. toddlers
   b. preschool
   c. school-age
   d. adolescents

10. When should auscultation of lung sounds during a physical examination be done?
    a. immediately on arrival
    b. early in the exam
    c. before inspection
    d. toward the end of the exam

11. Which scale is used to assess pain in toddlers and preschoolers?
    a. Wong–Baker Faces scale
    b. Glasgow coma scale
    c. Anesthesiologist 0–10 scale
    d. no scale is used

12. At what age do respirations become "adult-like"?
    a. toddlers
    b. preschool
    c. school-age
    d. adolescents

13. A heart rate less than 80 is NOT a problem for which of the following age groups?
    a. newborns
    b. toddlers
    c. preschool
    d. school-age

14. What is the best thing on which to base medication dosing?
    a. weight at last pediatrician visit
    b. length-based tape
    c. rapid reference guides
    d. wheel guides

15. Which of the following is NOT acceptable for fluid administration?
    a. burette
    b. microdrip manually adjusted
    c. infusion pump
    d. three-way stopcock

Short Answer

Write a brief answer to each of the following questions.

16. What is the purpose of the PAT triangle?

_____

_____

17. What does the mnemonic TICLS stand for?

_____

_____

18. What does the mnemonic FLACC stand for?

_____

_____

19. Why don't some parents have their kids immunized against childhood diseases?

_____

_____

20. What are some examples of delivery complications?

_____

_____

Fill in the Blank

Complete each sentence by adding the appropriate word in the provided blanks.

21. Progressive improvement in physical, psychosocial, and intellectual skills is referred to as _____ _____.

22. A _____-_____ _____ is used to estimate medications, fluid resuscitation, venous catheters, endotracheal tubes, and so on.

23. A child's transition from compensated shock to decompensated shock is _____.

24. A depressed fontanel suggests _____.

25. A bulging fontanel suggests _____ _____ _____.

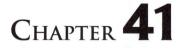

CHAPTER **41**

THE CRITICALLY ILL CHILD

Case Study

Chief Concern

Everyone in the station stops and turns to listen for the address after they hear, "Child in cardiac arrest." A flurry of activity then begins as crew members pull on their bunker pants, people yell, sirens scream, and the sole Paramedic, Joe, climbs into the rig. Slowly, the ambulance exits the bay and nudges into traffic behind the pumper.

Looking out the window at the sunny spring day, Joe starts to think of the causes of pediatric cardiac arrest. With reassurance that his crew members know their jobs, he can concentrate on the advanced life support.

Critical Thinking Questions

1. What are some of the possible causes of pediatric cardiac arrest?

2. What is the most common cause of pediatric cardiac arrest?

History

The call comes from a ball field, where a knot of people has formed around the child, a 10-year-old boy dressed in his baseball team's uniform. The coach and his assistant are busy performing CPR while another coach has the automated external defibrillator from the trainer's shed.

Dropping his gear near the child's head, Joe overhears the lieutenant asking what happened. The coach reports that the boy, who was playing middle field, just collapsed. Many thought he had just fainted until one of his teammates cried for help. The witnesses verify he has not been hit in the chest by a line drive.

Critical Thinking Questions

1. What are the important elements of the history that a Paramedic should obtain?

2. What may be the significance of being hit in the chest by a line drive?

Examination

Someone has already applied the automated external defibrillator pads and the machine advises them to shock, but to no effect. The child remains pulseless and apneic.

Firefighters replace the coach and restart CPR, minimizing the delay as much as possible, while Joe puts on the monitor. The data perplexes him, as it looks like torsades de pointes with the alternating waves undulating around the isoelectric line.

Critical Thinking Questions

1. What are the elements of the physical examination of a child in cardiac arrest?

2. If time permits, what other physical examination should be performed?

Assessment

Just as the team is about to load the boy onto the stretcher, his mother pulls up in her car, nearly hitting some oblivious bystanders in the process. With the engine still running, she leaps from the car and runs to the side of her son. "What happened?" she implores the firefighters who are doing CPR. "Ma'am, your son collapsed in the field. What can you tell us about him?"

Critical Thinking Questions

1. What diagnosis did the Paramedic announce to the patient's mother?

2. Should the mother be allowed to accompany her son?

Treatment

Joe elects to move the resuscitation to the back of the ambulance because of the crush of people crowded around to see the arrest. Once in the back of the ambulance, he reassesses the airway, breathing, and circulation. Satisfied that good CPR is in progress, he starts an intraosseous access. At first, the mother balks at the idea. However, Joe explains the importance of access and to giving drugs as quickly as possible.

Critical Thinking Questions

1. What is the standard of care for tachydysrhythmia in pediatric patients?

2. Should the child be cardioverted?

Evaluation

"Hold it" the lieutenant orders. The ECG monitor shows a narrow complex rhythm. "Check a pulse!" he orders. Seemingly every pulse point on the body is checked. "I've got one," one firefighter cries. "Me, too" cries another.

"OK," Joe says. "Let's keep CPR going, his heart's still weak. And let's get him in the rig. I want to intubate once we get inside." He further explains that he needs the EMT to get some ice packs going, since they were going to use the therapeutic hypothermia protocol.

"What's that?" the mother asks, the color in her face returning.

"Remember that Buffalo Bills player, Kevin Everett?" Joe asks the bewildered mother. She nods. "Well, cooling the body gives the brain more time to recover."

Critical Thinking Questions

1. What is the treatment for return of spontaneous circulation?

   _____

   _____

2. What is therapeutic hypothermia?

   _____

   _____

Disposition

Upon arriving at the hospital, and during a calmer moment, the mother explains that the boy's uncle had died from something called prolonged cutie syndrome, some kind of cardiac condition that can be passed from generation to generation. While the boy had seen a family pediatrician, he had never had a 12-lead ECG.

Critical Thinking Questions

1. What is the most appropriate transport decision that will get the patient to definitive care?

   _____

   _____

2. Are any special considerations needed as a result of the use of therapeutic hypothermia?

   _____

   _____

Practice Questions

Multiple Choice

Select the best answer for each of the following questions.

1. What is the most common cause of pediatric respiratory failure?
   a. asthma
   b. dehydration
   c. infection
   d. trauma

2. What is the most common cause of pediatric shock?
   a. hypovolemia
   b. anaphylaxis
   c. sepsis
   d. metabolic issues

3. The initial rhythm in pediatric cardiac arrest is most frequently what type of rhythm?
   a. ventricular tachycardia
   b. ventricular fibrillation
   c. asystole
   d. pulseless electrical activity

4. Symptomatic bradycardia is most often the result of _____ in children.
   a. hypoxemia
   b. hypoglycemia
   c. heart blocks
   d. hyperkalemia

5. What is the "break point" between sinus tachycardia and supraventricular tachycardia in children?
   a. 120
   b. 150
   c. 180
   d. 220

6. What is the "break point" between sinus tachycardia and supraventricular tachycardia in infants?
   a. 120
   b. 150
   c. 180
   d. 220

7. Torsades de pointes is most common in children with which condition?
   a. renal failure causing hypomagnesemia
   b. prolonged QT syndrome
   c. medication toxicology
   d. chest wall trauma

8. Which of the following represents a lower airway problem?
   a. gurgling
   b. stridor
   c. wheezes
   d. snoring

9. Which sign of respiratory distress is unique to children?
   a. pursed lip breathing
   b. intracostal muscle use
   c. nasal flaring
   d. sternal retraction

10. Which sign of inadequate perfusion is unique to children?
    a. pale skin
    b. dusky skin
    c. cyanotic skin
    d. mottled skin

11. What is the first line for fluid resuscitation in a newborn?
    a. 20 mL/kg of 0.9% NaCl solution
    b. 20 mL/kg of lactated Ringer's
    c. 10 mL/kg of 0.9% NaCl solution
    d. 10 mL/kg of lactated Ringer's

12. What is the vasopressor of choice for a child who is unresponsive to fluid resuscitation?
    a. epinephrine
    b. dopamine
    c. dobutamine
    d. phenylephrine

13. Adult defibrillation paddles/pads may NOT be used in which of the following?
    a. 1-year-old or older
    b. 30 inches or taller
    c. 10 kilograms or heavier
    d. never used on children

Case Studies & Practice Questions   **225**

14. Which dose of epinephrine is NOT the same as the others?
    a. 0.01 mg/kg of 1:10,000
    b. 0.1 mL/kg of 1:10,000
    c. 0.01 mg/kg of 1:1,000
    d. 0.1 mL/kg of 1:1,000

15. What is the correct amount of fluid resuscitation during a successful reversal of cardiac arrest with return of spontaneous circulation?
    a. 20 to 40 mL/kg
    b. 10 to 20 mL/kg
    c. 5 to 10 mL/kg
    d. no fluid resuscitation

Short Answer

Write a brief answer to each of the following questions.

16. What is the definition of a fever in a child?

    _____

    _____

17. What are the three additional elements of the history of present illness for a child?

    _____

    _____

18. What is the formula for roughly calculating the normal low systolic blood pressure of a child?

    _____

    _____

19. What is the first indicator of an altered mental status in a child?

    _____

    _____

20. Describe the anterior–posterior approach to defibrillation of a child.

    _____

    _____

Fill in the Blank

Complete each sentence by adding the appropriate word in the provided blanks.

21. The primary cause of cardiac arrest in the pediatric population is _____ _____.

22. Sudden cardiac death from a blow to the chest is called _____ _____.

23. Cyanosis of the nail beds, palms of the hands, and soles of the feet only is called _____.

24. Unexpected death of an infant may be the result of _____ _____ _____ _____.

25. A common cause of torsades de pointes in children is _____ _____ _____.

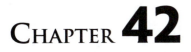

CHAPTER 42

PEDIATRIC MEDICAL EMERGENCIES

Case Study

Chief Concern

The mother is visibly distraught, as her infant son has just seized. She calls 9-1-1 and sits on the stoop, waiting for the ambulance. Although it only takes a few minutes to arrive, the time feels like hours to her. Even before Raylynn, the Paramedic on the rig, steps out of the ambulance, the mother is at the passenger's side door yelling, "We have to go the hospital RIGHT NOW!"

Critical Thinking Questions

1. What are some of the possible causes of the child's fever?

_____

_____

2. How can the fever and the seizure be related?

_____

_____

History

Once aboard the ambulance, the mother seems calmer. She reports that her son, who will be one year old in another month, was fine this morning. Right after lunch, however, he spiked a fever of 100.4°F. She immediately gave him a sponge bath and his temperature fluctuated until he seized.

Critical Thinking Questions

1. What are the important elements of the history that a Paramedic should obtain?

_____

_____

2. Why are immunizations an important part of the fever history?

_____

_____

Examination

While listening to the infant's mother, Raylynn puts on a mask and examines the child. He seems warm to the touch, but not abnormally so, and is flushed. He has a minor rash on the insides of his thighs, but Raylynn doesn't note any other rashes. Although the infant does not like the penlight, he does not reflexively withdraw his legs when she lifts his head and neck.

Case Studies & Practice Questions   227

Critical Thinking Questions

1. What are the elements of the physical examination of a patient with suspected febrile seizure?

_____

_____

2. Why is a blood glucose a critical element in this examination?

_____

_____

Assessment

The mother barrages Raylynn with questions: "What's happening to my baby? Will he have another seizure? Will he become an epileptic?" Raylynn tries to calm the mother by slowly answering her questions in a quiet manner.

Critical Thinking Questions

1. What diagnosis did the Paramedic announce to the patient's mother?

_____

_____

2. How does the Paramedic answer the mother's question about epilepsy?

_____

_____

Treatment

The infant seems to be brightening and is more interactive with the mother, much to her relief. Raylynn takes a pulse oximeter reading that reveals the infant's oxygen saturation is above 95%. Per protocol, she elects to watch the child's SpO_2 saturation. She is concerned that an oxygen mask might upset mother and child alike.

Next, Raylynn takes a blood sample by heel stick and checks the blood glucose, which is normal. As per routine, Raylynn attaches the ECG monitor and prepares to call the hospital.

Critical Thinking Questions

1. What is the standard of care of patients with suspected febrile seizure?

_____

_____

2. What is the danger of cooling the child too quickly?

_____

_____

Evaluation

While Raylynn is on the radio giving report, the monitor alarms go off. Raylynn instinctively checks the patient first. The baby is having another convulsion. Carefully noting the time, and understanding that most febrile convulsions are self-limited, Raylynn gets out the narcotics kit, removes the diazepam, and considers her best route of administration, in case the seizure doesn't stop.

Critical Thinking Questions

1. What are some of the predictable complications associated with febrile seizures?

_____

_____

2. What are some medication administration routes for benzodiazepines in children?

_____

_____

Disposition

Fortunately, the seizure stops just as the ambulance pulls into the ambulance bay. Carefully placing the oxygen mask over the infant's tiny face, Raylynn helps unload the patient. With the mother holding the infant's tiny hands, the team enters the emergency department.

Critical Thinking Questions

1. What is the most appropriate transport decision that will get the patient to definitive care?

_____

_____

2. What are some medication administration routes for benzodiazepines in children?

_____

_____

Practice Questions
Multiple Choice

Select the best answer for each of the following questions.

1. Which of the following is NOT an element of tetralogy of Fallot?
   a. pulmonary stenosis
   b. mitral regurgitation
   c. overriding aorta
   d. ventricular septal defect

2. Aortic stenosis, an outflow obstruction of blood, is diverted by _____.
   a. patent ductus arteriosus
   b. ventricular septal defect
   c. pulmonary stenosis
   d. mitral regurgitation

3. What is an early sign of an asthma exacerbation?
   a. cough
   b. sneeze
   c. nasal drip
   d. stridor

4. Which of the following is NOT a cause of bronchiolitis?
   a. respiratory syncytial virus
   b. parainfluenza virus
   c. rhino virus
   d. influenza A virus

5. Which condition is often confused with asthma?
   a. bronchiolitis
   b. croup
   c. laryngotracheobronchitis
   d. bacterial tracheitis

6. Which condition is congenital?
   a. bronchiolitis
   b. cystic fibrosis
   c. laryngotracheobronchitis
   d. bacterial tracheitis

7. Paramedics do NOT have an impact on which of the following causes of pediatric seizures in the field?
   a. hypoglycemia
   b. hypoxia
   c. poisoning
   d. infections

8. Which of the following is NOT included in the definition of status epilepticus?
   a. continuous seizure activity
   b. first time seizure
   c. two or more seizures
   d. prolonged post-ictal phase

9. What is the most frequent cause of an apparent life-threatening event in an infant?
   a. digestive problems
   b. neurological disorders
   c. cardiac anomalies
   d. respiratory compromise

10. What is the cause of sudden infant death syndrome?
    a. alcohol use during pregnancy
    b. exposure to secondhand smoke
    c. improper positioning in crib
    d. unknown etiology

11. Which of the following causes of abdominal pain in infants is NOT a potential surgical emergency?
    a. colic
    b. congenital inguinal hernia
    c. intussusception
    d. volvulus

12. Which condition does NOT represent a potentially serious underlying condition?
    a. convulsion lasting longer than 15 minutes
    b. single generalized seizure
    c. second febrile seizure in 24 hours
    d. focal seizures

13. What is the cause of the most dangerous meningitis?
    a. adenovirus
    b. herpes simplex
    c. influenza virus
    d. neisseria meningitidis

14. What is thought to be the cause of epiglottis, a bacterial infection?
    a. Haemophilus influenzae
    b. Neisseria meningitidis
    c. Group B Streptococci
    d. Streptococcus pneumoniae

15. What distinguishes the "whoop" of pertussis?
    a. expiratory stridor
    b. inspiratory wheeze
    c. inspiratory stridor
    d. expiratory wheeze

Short Answer

Write a brief answer to each of the following questions.

16. Describe the normal fetal circulation.

    _____

    _____

17. Describe the pathophysiology of cystic fibrosis.

    _____

    _____

18. Describe the pathophysiology of status asthmaticus.

    _____

    _____

19. When is croup most often seen?

    _____

    _____

20. Define status epilepticus.

    _____

    _____

Fill in the Blank

Complete each sentence by adding the appropriate word in the provided blank.

21. Infants with tetralogy of Fallot who pass out are said to have _____ _____.

22. Congenital heart anomalies with left-to-right shunting are termed _____ _____ _____.

23. The lay term for laryngotracheobronchitis is _____.

24. A child with unexplained weight loss and decreased feeding is a _____ _____ _____ child.

25. The old name for neonatal respiratory distress syndrome was _____ _____ _____.

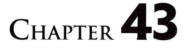

CHAPTER 43

CHILD ABUSE AND NEGLECT

Case Study

Chief Concern

The dispatch information calls out, "Respond to 1-year-old with fever of unknown origin." Rafael predicts, "Bet it's an ear infection." As a father of four children, Rafael is very experienced in these matters. Because of that, his junior partner, Jamila, has learned to defer to his judgment in these matters. Her thoughts are interrupted by the display on the mobile data terminal: "Police on-scene. Address with multiple reports of domestic violence."

Critical Thinking Questions

1. What is the implication of domestic violence and child abuse?

_____

_____

2. What connection does domestic violence have to a child with a fever of unknown origin?

_____

_____

History

Upon arrival, the Paramedics are greeted by the mother and ushered into a bedroom that is adorned with an abundance of toys and playthings. The infant, Liam, is lying in the crib. The Paramedics look at each other, as the child seems remarkably small for his age.

"He has been running a fever. I took it just five minutes ago and his rectal temperature was 102.5°F," his mother states as she waves the thermometer in front of Jamila's face. Although the thermometer does read 102.5°F, Liam is not warm to the touch.

Suddenly, and without apparent reason, the mother changes her mind, "I'll take him to his doctor," she says. Rafael looks over his shoulder, seeing a police officer standing in the doorway.

Critical Thinking Questions

1. What are the important elements of the history that a Paramedic should obtain?

_____

_____

2. What is the implication assumed when the mother changes her mind about EMS as soon as the police arrive?

_____

_____

Examination

Liam is clearly small for his age, yet he is reported to be a term baby. The mother denies smoking or drinking during the pregnancy as well. However, Liam looks emaciated, like those kids that appear on television from third world countries.

Critical Thinking Questions

1. What are the elements of the physical examination of a patient with suspected failure to thrive?

   _____

   _____

2. What is a good indicator of good nutrition?

   _____

   _____

Assessment

While Rafael speaks to the police officer, the two watch the mother walk around the room arranging stuffed animals and toys, oblivious to the infant in the crib. Jamila decides to make contact with the emergency department. The attending physician, who is familiar with the mother, orders the child to be transported.

Critical Thinking Questions

1. What diagnosis did the Paramedic announce to the patient's mother?

   _____

   _____

2. Should the Paramedic address the question of malnutrition on-scene?

   _____

   _____

Treatment

Rafael straps Liam's car seat onto the stretcher and Jamila goes back inside to escort the mother and child to the ambulance. Rafael returns, reporting that the officer has just left. He asks if he can be of any assistance.

Once again, the mother changes her mind, stating, "I think his fever broke. He's all better now."

Critical Thinking Questions

1. What is the standard of care of patients with suspected failure to thrive/neglect?

   _____

   _____

2. Should the Paramedic approach the mother with an accusation of child abuse?

   _____

   _____

Evaluation

Rafael does an about face and goes to the rig to ask the police officer to return while Jamila continues to press the case that the infant needs to be seen.

When the officer returns, the mother refuses to cooperate. Over her loud complaints, the infant is taken into police protective custody.

Critical Thinking Questions

1. Does the mother's second refusal raise the level of concern that the police need to be involved?

_____

_____

2. Could the Paramedic assume custody of the child?

_____

_____

Disposition

Both the on-duty police supervisor and the on-duty Paramedic supervisor meet the ambulance as it arrives at the hospital. Both Jamila and Rafael are taken "out of rotation" for calls so that they can complete their reports accurately.

In the interim, the physician gets a report from the mother regarding Liam's condition.

Critical Thinking Questions

1. Jamila has never reported child abuse and she is concerned about liability. What facts should the supervisor provide to Jamila?

_____

_____

2. Why is it important to get both the parent's report as well as the Paramedic's report?

_____

_____

Practice Questions
Multiple Choice

Select the best answer for each of the following questions.

1. What is the most common form of child abuse?
   a. sexual abuse
   b. physical abuse
   c. sexual exploitation
   d. neglect

2. Which group makes up the majority of child abusers?
   a. spouses
   b. paramours
   c. women
   d. strangers

3. Child abuse is more likely in which situation?
   a. poor families
   b. divorced families
   c. immigrant families
   d. single-parent families

4. Which of the following extraordinary circumstances can lead to child abuse?
   a. death in the family
   b. loss of employment
   c. loss of custodial support
   d. all of the above

5. Which of the following is NOT a parental indicator of child abuse?
   a. parental indifference
   b. cigarette smoking
   c. conflicting history
   d. alcohol use

6. What is the single greatest source of an abused child's behavior?
   a. fear
   b. love
   c. frustration
   d. confusion

7. What is the first stage in a pedophile's conditioning process?
   a. masturbation
   b. anal sex
   c. fondling
   d. oral sex

8. Which of the following would be considered atypical bruising?
   a. bruises of the shins
   b. bruises of the elbows
   c. bruises of the inner thigh
   d. bruises of the wrist

9. Which of the following burns may be accidental?
   a. cigarette burn to the palm of the hand
   b. hot water splash
   c. rope burns to the ankles
   d. radiator burns to the back

10. Which marks would be "marks of concern"?
    a. stocking burn
    b. pattern burn
    c. bruises in different stages of healing
    d. all of the above

11. Which fracture is associated with child abuse?
    a. greenstick
    b. spiral
    c. nondisplaced
    d. linear

12. Over 50% of deaths from child abuse are attributed to what cause?
    a. neglect
    b. sexual abuse
    c. shaken baby syndrome
    d. failure to thrive syndrome

13. What is the most common finding that suggests shaken baby syndrome?
    a. retinal hemorrhage
    b. inconsolability
    c. displaced skull fracture
    d. seizure

14. Who makes the majority of reports of child abuse?
    a. law enforcement
    b. family
    c. social workers
    d. healthcare professionals

15. The majority of cases of child abuse involve children in what age range?
    a. 0 to 1 year of age
    b. 1 to 4 years of age
    c. 5 to 10 years of age
    d. 10 to 15 years of age

Short Answer

Write a brief answer to each of the following questions.

16. What are the rights of a child in the United States?

    _____

    _____

17. How does the federal law define child abuse?

    _____

    _____

18. What are infanticide and abandoned infants acts?

    _____

    _____

19. Describe Munchausen by Proxy.

    _____

    _____

20. What is an "excited utterance"?

    _____

    _____

Fill in the Blank

Complete each sentence by adding the appropriate word in the provided blanks.

21. Statutory rape and juvenile sodomy are considered _____ _____.

22. Use of a child in a sexual performance, such as the production of pornography, is considered _____ _____.

23. The medical term for bedwetting is _____ and for self-soiling is _____.

24. A child with a subaverage growth for age may be identified as _____ _____ _____.

25. Nurses trained to care for victims of sexual abuse are called _____ _____ _____ _____.

CHAPTER **44**

GERIATRICS

Case Study
Chief Concern

"Squad ten, meet an elderly woman at the market corner of Quail and West Street. Complains of abdominal pain. The store manager will meet you." As the ambulance moves into the passing lane and the driver hit the lights, the medic student, Howard, talks to his Paramedic field training officer, Rich, about the possible causes of abdominal pain in the elderly.

Critical Thinking Questions

1. What are some of the serious causes of abdominal pain in the elderly?

   _____

   _____

2. What are some potentially life-threatening causes of abdominal pain in the elderly?

   _____

   _____

History

Mrs. Johnson, a pleasant elderly woman in her mid-eighties, is still independent and able to care for herself. She had gone to the corner market to pick up some more laxative medicine.

She complains that she frequently becomes "bound up" and needs a little help. She explains to Howard that she has been passing feces that "look like ribbon candy."

Critical Thinking Questions

1. What are the important elements of the history that a Paramedic should obtain?

   _____

   _____

2. What questions should the Paramedic ask about the medication history?

   _____

   _____

Examination

Mrs. Johnson is expected to have a lower than normal blood pressure, since she is slight of build. However, her blood pressure is abnormally low for anyone, even someone as small as Mrs. Johnson.

Rich suggests that Mrs. Johnson may be in shock, which leaves Howard with a quizzical look.

Critical Thinking Questions

1. How could Mrs. Johnson be in shock?

   _____

   _____

2. What is another danger of bowel obstructions?

   _____

   _____

Assessment

Rich convinces Howard that Mrs. Johnson may be in shock and that emergent treatment is necessary. Mrs. Johnson agrees to go to the hospital if the "boys" think it's necessary.

Critical Thinking Questions

1. What are some explanations for Mrs. Johnson's shock?

   _____

   _____

2. What are complicating factors that make ascertaining the source of the shock more difficult in the elderly?

   _____

   _____

Treatment

Mrs. Johnson is "vasculopathetic," meaning she has few acceptable veins for venous access. Howard cannot get an IV started even after two tries, so he elects to stop his attempts and instead keep her on high-flow, high-concentration oxygen while she is transported to the hospital with lights and siren.

Critical Thinking Questions

1. What are the concerns about using "standard care" for elderly patients?

   _____

   _____

2. How might treating the elderly be different from treating others?

   _____

   _____

Evaluation

While en route, Rich reminds Howard that "little old ladies" can surprise you with a heart attack and her hypotension may be cardiogenic. Howard immediately starts to obtain a 12-lead ECG.

Critical Thinking Questions

1. Why would the elderly be prone to an AMI?

   _____

   _____

2. Why would elderly female patients be prone to an acute myocardial infarction?

_____

_____

Disposition

When Howard and Rich return to the hospital later, the attending pulls them aside and says, "Good thing you guys rushed Mrs. Johnson in. She had a mesenteric infarction with peritonitis but she is stable now. Four or five more hours and she would have been dead."

1. What is the most appropriate transport decision that will get the patient to definitive care?

_____

_____

2. What happens if the patient is unstable?

_____

_____

Practice Questions
Multiple Choice

Select the best answer for each of the following questions.

1. A decubitus ulcer that is full thickness, with bone visible, would be in which stage?
   a. Stage IA
   b. Stage 3
   c. Stage IV
   d. Stage 6

2. What is another name for lentigines?
   a. sunspots
   b. liver spots
   c. age spots
   d. all of the above

3. What happens to total body water as a person gets older?
   a. remains the same
   b. increases with age
   c. decreases
   d. unknown

4. By age 70 approximately _____ of patients will have significant atherosclerosis.
   a. 40%
   b. 50%
   c. 60%
   d. 70%

5. Parkinson's disease is associated with which of the following?
   a. decreased dopamine
   b. increased serotonin
   c. decreased epinephrine
   d. increased monoamine oxidase

6. What is the most common cause of delirium?
   a. hypoxia
   b. hypoglycemia
   c. infection
   d. fever

7. What is the most lethal abdominal disease?
   a. appendicitis
   b. mesenteric infarction
   c. bowel obstruction
   d. abdominal aortic aneurysm

8. Lower back pain may be a kidney stone or it may be _____.
   a. appendicitis
   b. mesenteric infarction
   c. bowel obstruction
   d. abdominal aortic aneurysm

9. At what stage of renal failure is significant electrolyte imbalances, and cardiac dysrhythmias, seen?
   a. Stage 1
   b. Stage 2
   c. Stage 3
   d. Stage 4

10. Which of the following is NOT a sign of benign prostatic hypertrophy?
    a. urinary urgency
    b. nocturia
    c. urinary frequency
    d. foul-smelling urine

11. What is an abnormal forward curvature of the spine called?
    a. lordosis
    b. kyphosis
    c. scoliosis
    d. spina bifida

12. What is the gray-blue pigment around the iris called?
    a. presbycusis
    b. hyperopia
    c. presbyopia
    d. arcus senilis

13. Which of the following is potentially life-threatening?
    a. melanoma
    b. senile keratosis
    c. lentigines
    d. liver spots

14. Which of the following can lead to malnutrition in the elderly patient?
    a. gum atrophy
    b. decreased bowel motility
    c. decreased gastric acid secretion
    d. all of the above

15. Which of the following is NOT a cause of chronic constipation?
    a. volvulus
    b. malignancy
    c. laxative abuse
    d. intussusception

Short Answer

Write a brief answer to each of the following questions.

16. Define geriatrics.

_____

_____

17. Differentiate delirium from dementia.

_____

_____

18. What is kyphosis?

_____

_____

19. Why are the elderly prone to subdural hematomas?

_____

_____

20. What are the changes in pulmonary function associated with aging?

_____

_____

Fill in the Blank

Complete each sentence by adding the appropriate word in the provided blanks.

21. _____ differentiates chronic renal disease from end-stage renal disease.

22. Pain in the left colon is most likely due to _____.

23. Farsightedness, called _____, is one of the first changes associated with aging.

24. Use of a large number of prescribed medications that can potentially interact with one another is called _____.

25. Elderly patients with syncope should be assumed to have a _____ until proven otherwise.

CHAPTER **45**

PATIENTS WITH SPECIAL CHALLENGES

Case Study

Chief Concern

"NRN?" the rookie asks.

"Nine R Northgate," clarifies the caller. "It's a residence home for specially challenged patients." The call is for a person with difficulty breathing at a community residence for patients with developmental disabilities. The residence includes special rehabilitation services and a day respite program.

Critical Thinking Questions

1. What are some potential causes of shortness of breath for the ventilator-dependent patient?

   _____

   _____

2. What are some non-ventilator causes of shortness of breath?

   _____

   _____

History

The patient, Charlie, is ventilator-dependent and requires around the clock medical supervision. Charlie is 40 years old, but his parents still take care of him. However, the burden of care is enormous and the couple, now in their seventies and retired, are relieved to hear that NRN has respite services that allow them an occasional day to themselves.

When Charlie's ventilator alarms started to go off, the staff called 9-1-1, according to instructions. Meeting the crew at the door, the staff ushers them past rows of patients in wheelchairs with portable ventilators. Charlie is at the end of the row and is being manually ventilated by one of the staff.

The staff "ran the checklist," trying to isolate the problem. However, nothing has show up yet. They assume that Charlie must have a problem, which prompted the call to 9-1-1.

Critical Thinking Questions

1. What are some alarms on a home ventilator?

   _____

   _____

2. What should the Paramedic do when the ventilator alarm sounds?

_____

_____

Examination

Since he is ventilator-dependent, it is hard to tell if Charlie is having difficulty breathing. Although he does not appear to have central cyanosis, his pulse oximeter reading is in the mid-80s. Auscultation of his lungs reveals diffuse rales (crackles) proximal to the angle of Louis. Charlie has a G tube, but the feedings have been turned off and the pump is sitting in the corner. The rookie's field training officer leans in and whispers, "Aspiration."

Critical Thinking Questions

1. What are the elements of the physical examination of a ventilator-dependent patient?

_____

_____

2. What are the Paramedic's first assessment priorities?

_____

_____

Assessment

"Iatrogenic complications, medical complications, or both?" the rookie wonders. Since the hypoxia is real and Charlie needs immediate medical attention, the cause isn't the immediate concern.

Critical Thinking Questions

1. What diagnosis did the Paramedic announce to the patient?

_____

_____

2. What is different in the Paramedic's differential diagnosis of a technology-dependent patient?

_____

_____

Treatment

The rookie assists in ventilating Charlie while his field training officer prepares a new inner cannula to replace the one already there. When the inner cannula is removed, they see its inner lumen is coated with crud. "No wonder he was having trouble breathing."

After replacing the inner cannula, the rookie immediately notices Charlie's improved ventilation. "Problem solved," he triumphantly announces.

"Not so fast, rookie. Remember the rales!" his field training officer retorts.

Critical Thinking Questions

1. What is the standard of care of patients with suspected ventilator/tracheostomy-related difficulty breathing?

_____

_____

2. Should the Paramedic attempt to correct or reset the ventilator?

_____

_____

Evaluation

The Paramedics transfer Charlie from the wheelchair to the stretcher, which is no easy feat as Charlie is heavy and precautions have to be taken not to accidentally dislodge any of his "tubes": G tube, Foley catheter, PICC line.

While bagging Charlie, the rookie feels more resistance to the ventilation. Thinking his arm is tiring, he redoubles his effort, yet meets even more resistance. "Hey boss," he calls. "Charlie is really hard to bag and I think he may have gone unconscious."

Critical Thinking Questions

1. What are some of the predictable complications associated with a manual ventilation of the patient with a tracheotomy?

_____

_____

2. What would be the treatment for this patient?

_____

_____

Disposition

After turning Charlie over to the ED staff, the rookie goes outside for a breath of fresh air. "I almost killed that guy!" the rookie remarks. "Not likely," the field training officer assures him. He explains that ventilator-dependent patients have very thick mucus, owed to constant ventilation with air that dries the sputum. It is more likely that he just "coughed up" a mucous plug that blocked his bronchi. With one less lung, the rookie had unwittingly overventilated the remaining lung, causing a pneumothorax. "Hey," the field training officer suggests, "let's go back inside and talk to the doc about this case."

Critical Thinking Questions

1. What is the most appropriate transport decision that will get the patient to definitive care?

_____

_____

2. Does the destination decision change if the patient is unstable?

_____

_____

Practice Questions
Multiple Choice

Select the best answer for each of the following questions.

1. Patients who have been hearing impaired since birth most likely use _____ to communicate.
   a. speech reading
   b. American sign language
   c. visual language
   d. aided language

2. A sluggish ability to understand speech is a _____ disorder.
   a. language
   b. articulation
   c. voice production
   d. fluency

3. Inappropriate pitch, tone, volume, or quality indicates a _____ disorder.
   a. language
   b. articulation
   c. voice production
   d. fluency

4. Stuttering is a _____ disorder.
   a. language
   b. articulation
   c. voice production
   d. fluency

5. Inability to pronounce certain letters, such as R, is an example of a _____ disorder.
   a. language
   b. articulation
   c. voice production
   d. fluency

6. A feeding tube that enters the stomach is called a _____ tube.
   a. gastrostomy
   b. jejunostomy
   c. ileostomy
   d. colostomy

7. A feeding tube that decreases risk of aspiration is called a _____ tube.
   a. gastrostomy
   b. jejunostomy
   c. ileostomy
   d. colostomy

8. What is the most common complication of a feeding tube?
   a. dislodgement
   b. obstruction
   c. perforation
   d. equipment failure

9. Which of the following is a sign of an infection of a ventriculoperitoneal shunt?
   a. lethargy
   b. redness at the insertion
   c. abdominal pain
   d. all of the above

10. Which of the following is a sign of a malfunctioning ventriculoperitoneal shunt?
    a. Cushing's triad
    b. Beck's triad
    c. Murphy's triad
    d. Virchow's triad

11. What is the most common form of cerebral palsy?
    a. spastic
    b. dyskinetic
    c. ataxic
    d. athetoid

12. A large protruding tongue, abnormally shaped ears, and white spots in the iris of the eyes are characteristics of which condition?
    a. Down syndrome
    b. fragile X syndrome
    c. fetal alcohol syndrome
    d. Asperger syndrome

13. What is the most common form of inherited mental retardation?
    a. Down syndrome
    b. fragile X syndrome
    c. fetal alcohol syndrome
    d. Asperger syndrome

14. Gua sha involves the use of what object?
    a. coins
    b. spoons
    c. cups
    d. forks

15. Which culture never leaves the dying patient alone?
    a. Muslim
    b. Hispanic
    c. Jewish
    d. Buddhist

Short Answer

Write a brief answer to each of the following questions.

16. Explain the process that a Paramedic uses to troubleshoot ventilator problems.

    _____

    _____

17. What are nerve stimulators used for?

    _____

    _____

18. What is a vascular access device?

    _____

    _____

19. What is an analgesia pump?

    _____

    _____

20. What is an insulin pump?

_____

_____

Fill in the Blank

Complete each sentence by adding the appropriate word in the provided blanks.

21. Accommodations for the visually impaired are required under the _____ _____ _____
_____.

22. "Speaking trachs" are called _____ tubes.

23. A special noncoring needle used for implanted vascular access ports is called a _____ _____.

24. The other name for an indwelling urinary catheter is a _____ _____.

25. Patients with significant impairments in social interaction and communications are said to have _____
_____ _____.

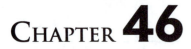

CHAPTER 46

CARE OF THE CHRONICALLY ILL PATIENT

Case Study

Chief Concern

"Medic 34, respond to 200 Looking Glass Lane. Assist the elderly patient who has fallen" the radio blares. The address is a new assisted living facility. Their management has a policy that staff cannot help lift a fallen client and that EMS has to be called instead.

The clientele at Looking Glass are varied, from elderly patients with early dementia to younger patients with cerebral palsy. All need some degree of assistance with their activities of daily living.

Critical Thinking Questions

1. What is the significance of the pre-existing medical condition to the fall?

2. Why might there be a "no-lift" policy in the facility?

History

Henrietta, an elderly 88-year-old woman, falls almost every week. She is seldom hurt and always insists she doesn't want to go to the hospital. She is dreadfully afraid of hospitals and is always quick to point out the MOLST form she has hanging on the back of the door in a clear plastic sleeve. The bright pink form clearly spells out her intentions. She would say, "Boys, respect my wishes."

Critical Thinking Questions

1. What are the different elements of the history that a Paramedic should obtain in the medically fragile patient?

2. What is the advantage of a MOLST?

Examination

Tonight Henrietta seems different. As usual, she had fallen, pressed her pendant alarm, and waited for personnel to respond. This time, however, when the Paramedic arrives, she doesn't mention the MOLST form, nor is she as sharp as usual.

A quick neurological examination reveals some weakness on the right side that was not there last week. A secondary examination reveals a small knot to the back of her head.

Critical Thinking Questions

1. Why is the comparison between the patient's present condition and baseline important?

_____

_____

2. Why is it important to ask why EMS was summoned?

_____

_____

Assessment

The patient care assistant relates, "She fell during the night but managed to get herself back to bed without assistance."

"Henrietta, I think you need to go to the hospital this time," the Paramedic states. "You may have hurt yourself." Unlike in the past, Henrietta agrees.

Critical Thinking Questions

1. Why is the staff members' input important?

_____

_____

2. What diagnosis will the Paramedic announce to the patient?

_____

_____

Treatment

Although a fall from a standing position to a carpeted floor is not normally a cause to take spinal precautions, it is in the case of the elderly. However, Henrietta is extremely kyphotic, to the point the Paramedic has to kneel down to look up into her eyes. Even a cervical collar is out of the question.

"I need blankets and pillows, as many as you can get me," the Paramedic requests from the patient care assistant.

Critical Thinking Questions

1. What is the standard of care for fluid resuscitation of an extremely elderly patient?

_____

_____

2. What are some of the patient-specific concerns for spinal immobilization of the extremely elderly patient?

_____

_____

Evaluation

Slowly Henrietta slips into unconsciousness. The Paramedic pulls out the MOLST form, taken from the back of the door when the crew left, and reviews the treatment options.

Oxygen and even ventilation is noted, but no intubation. Fluids via intravenous access is allowed, but no resuscitation medications. "Hmmm," the Paramedic murmurs, "all pretty straightforward." Then, he gets to work.

Critical Thinking Questions

1. What are some of the implications of the MOLST form?

_____

_____

2. What value does the MOSLT form have for the Paramedic?

_____

_____

Disposition

Arriving at the hospital, the Paramedic gives report. After report, he hands the MOLST form to the nurse. "Henrietta is very concerned about people following her wishes. Fortunately, she gave very clear instructions."

Critical Thinking Questions

1. What is the most appropriate transport decision that will get the patient to definitive care?

_____

_____

2. Why is a good patient report important?

_____

_____

Practice Questions
Multiple Choice

Select the best answer for each of the following questions.

1. Which of the following diseases does NOT tend to make patients who have them fall more frequently?
   a. cardiac disease
   b. muscular dystrophy
   c. lupus erythematosus
   d. multiple sclerosis

2. What is the lowest level of elderly group housing called?
   a. skilled nursing
   b. independent living
   c. assisted living
   d. facilitated living

3. What is a non-medical declaration of end-of-life wishes called?
   a. living will
   b. medical orders for life-sustaining treatment
   c. do not attempt resuscitation
   d. healthcare proxy

4. The Supreme Court decision in *Bartling v. Superior Court* affirmed the authority of this document.
   a. living will
   b. medical orders for life-sustaining treatment
   c. do not attempt resuscitation
   d. healthcare proxy

5. Which of the following is the most expansive advanced directive?
   a. living will
   b. medical orders for life-sustaining treatment
   c. do not attempt resuscitation
   d. healthcare proxy

6. Which of the following does NOT give a designated individual authority to make life or death decisions?
   a. healthcare proxy
   b. durable power of attorney for healthcare
   c. living will
   d. medical license

7. Which document can direct prehospital care?
   a. living will
   b. durable power of attorney for healthcare
   c. do not attempt resuscitation
   d. healthcare proxy

8. Which document can be revoked by the patient at any time?
   a. living will
   b. medical orders for life-sustaining treatment
   c. do not attempt resuscitation
   d. all of the above

9. Which constitutes a medical order?
   a. living will
   b. durable power of attorney for healthcare
   c. do not attempt resuscitation
   d. healthcare proxy

10. Which of the following must be signed by the patient, not a surrogate?
    a. living will
    b. do not resuscitate
    c. do not attempt resuscitation
    d. medical orders for life-sustaining treatment

11. Which document gives patient care directives before death?
    a. living will
    b. do not resuscitate
    c. do not attempt resuscitation
    d. medical orders for life-sustaining treatment

12. Which of the following potentially has authority over a Paramedic?
    a. healthcare proxy
    b. wife or closest kin
    c. durable power of attorney for heathcare
    d. hospice nurse

13. Once resuscitation begins, it cannot be terminated except for which situation?
    a. medical orders for termination
    b. rescuer exhaustion
    c. exposure to danger
    d. all of the above

14. Members of which of the following cultural groups may choose not to have advanced directives?
    a. Asian
    b. First American
    c. African American
    d. all of the above

15. A patient with which of the following disorders would most likely be eligible to donate organs?
    a. spinal cord injury
    b. diabetes
    c. severe cardiac disease
    d. septic

Short Answer

Write a brief answer to each of the following questions.

16. Define medically fragile.

    _____

    _____

17. Define hospice.

    _____

    _____

18. What is the Paramedic's liability if a DNAR is honored?

    _____

    _____

19. How is a durable power of attorney different than a power of attorney?

    _____

    _____

20. Why is good documentation of patient care important for the medically fragile patient?

    _____

    _____

Fill in the Blank

Complete each sentence by adding the appropriate word in the provided blanks.

21. Patients with a chronic medical condition are said to be _____ _____ because the balance that exists in their baseline status is easily tipped by relatively minor illnesses and trauma.

22. A durable power of attorney has the same effect as a _____ _____ .

23. The immediate step between independent living apartments and skilled nursing facilities is _____ _____ centers.

24. Psychiatric-related group homes are similar to _____ _____ centers.

25. A facility dedicated to end-of-life care is called a _____ .

CHAPTER 47

VIOLENCE IN THE COMMUNITY

Case Study

Chief Concern

It is five o'clock in the morning, and someone is apparently using her cell phone to call for help by repeatedly pressing 5. This sets off an alarm in the campus safety office, alerting them of violence on campus. The caller's name and photo appear on the dispatcher's computer monitor. Next to her physical description is a map of the campus with a flashing blue pin that identifies her exact location. University police are dispatched immediately.

Critical Thinking Questions

1. What are some of the reasons that a college co-ed might press the panic alarm?

_____

_____

2. What are the forms of nonconsensual sex?

_____

_____

History

Tabitha is a freshman at the university. Excited about her new possibilities, she plans to explore every opportunity. Therefore, she attends a frosh party held by one of the local fraternities. Once there, she meets a couple of "nice guys." The next thing she remembers is waking up mid-day with a splitting headache in the park. She cannot remember how she got there, and becomes alarmed when she realizes her pants are unbuttoned and she no longer has on any underwear.

Critical Thinking Questions

1. What are the important elements of the history that a Paramedic should obtain?

_____

_____

2. What resources could the Paramedic request to help on-scene?

_____

_____

Examination

With a little coaching from one of the female university police officers, Tabitha consents to being evaluated by EMS. Although a complete head-to-toe examination would be needed eventually, Tabitha has no apparent life-threatening injuries. Therefore, the Paramedic elects to limit the field examination.

Critical Thinking Questions

1. What additional responsibilities does the Paramedic have during the physical examination of a patient with suspected violence?

_____

_____

2. What responsibility does the Paramedic have in caring for the evidence?

_____

_____

Assessment

Tabitha repeatedly states she just wants to go home and shower, but the Paramedic explains the importance of gathering evidence immediately and the shorter timeline for drug-facilitated sexual assault evidence collection. After a few tearful moments, Tabitha agrees, saying, "I want to get those guys before they hurt anyone else."

Critical Thinking Questions

1. What is the common sequela of sexual assault and rape?

_____

_____

2. What psychological symptoms might the patient manifest following a sexual assault and rape?

_____

_____

Treatment

Tabitha is escorted to the back of the ambulance. On the Paramedic's insistence, the university officer accompanies her to the emergency department.

Tabitha repeatedly asks, "Why did this happen to me? I shouldn't have gone to that party. I should have stayed in my dorm room and studied." The Paramedic carefully explains that she is not responsible for the sexual assault and that their first priority is to make sure she is safe.

Critical Thinking Questions

1. What is the first priority of care of patients with suspected sexual assault?

_____

_____

2. What is the other patient care priority?

_____

_____

Evaluation

Suddenly Tabitha seems to become very "controlled." Her sudden change from sobbing to subdued concerns both the Paramedic and the police officer. They both know that she is trying to respond, reasonably, and trying to make sense out of an unreal situation. They also know her pain is real despite her outward appearance.

Critical Thinking Questions

1. What do the patient's behaviors represent?

   _____

   _____

2. What is the Paramedic's responsibility during care and transport of the patient?

   _____

   _____

Disposition

Tabitha is transported to a SAFE center where she is met at the door by a SANE nurse. She bypasses the main triage desk and is escorted to a private room away from the main emergency department. As the Paramedic and university police officer step out of the room to go write their reports Tabitha calls out quietly, "Thank you."

Critical Thinking Questions

1. What is the most appropriate transport decision that will get the patient to definitive care?

   _____

   _____

2. What are the documentation standards for wounds?

   _____

   _____

Practice Questions
Multiple Choice

Select the best answer for each of the following questions.

1. Violence in the community encompasses which of the following situations?
   a. intimate partner violence
   b. domestic violence
   c. sexual assault
   d. all of the above

2. What percentage of teenage girls and young women experience dating violence?
   a. 10%
   b. 20%
   c. 30%
   d. 50%

3. The number of battered pregnant women may be as high as what percentage?
   a. 5%
   b. 10%
   c. 25%
   d. 50%

4. Up to what percentage of women who seek emergency services or care are victims of intimate partner violence?
   a. 10%
   b. 20%
   c. 30%
   d. 50%

5. What percentage of men who batter their spouses also abuse their children?
   a. 10%
   b. 20%
   c. 30%
   d. 50%

6. Which of the following would be considered nonconsensual sex?
   a. patient mentally retarded
   b. patient is intoxicated
   c. patient is under age
   d. all of the above

7. Which of the following is a sign of drug-facilitated sexual assault?
   a. cameo recall
   b. euphoria and blackout
   c. amnesia
   d. all of the above

8. Rape can include which of the following acts?
   a. sodomy
   b. fellatio
   c. analingus
   d. all of the above

9. The majority of rapes are committed by which type of rapist?
   a. power reassurance rapists
   b. power assertive rapists
   c. anger-retaliatory rapists
   d. anger-excitation rapists

10. Which type of rapist is most likely to kill his victim?
    a. power reassurance rapist
    b. power assertive rapist
    c. anger-retaliatory rapist
    d. anger-excitation rapist

11. What is the most common form of elder abuse?
    a. sexual abuse
    b. physical abuse
    c. physical neglect
    d. emotional neglect

12. What factors make a person more prone to being a victim of elder abuse?
    a. female sex
    b. poverty
    c. social isolation
    d. all of the above

13. What are some warning signs of elder abuse?
    a. unexplained falls
    b. poor hygiene
    c. delays in seeking medical care
    d. all of the above

14. What is the maximum time frame for a sexual assault forensic examination?
    a. 24 hours
    b. 36 hours
    c. 72 hours
    d. 96 hours

15. What is the maximum time frame for emergency contraception medication?
    a. 24 hours
    b. 36 hours
    c. 72 hours
    d. 96 hours

Short Answer

Write a brief answer to each of the following questions.

16. Define youth violence.

_____

_____

17. Describe the cycle of abuse.

_____

_____

18. What is rape?

_____

_____

19. Define sexual elder abuse.

_____

_____

20. What are the Paramedic's responsibilities when caring for a victim of elder abuse?

_____

_____

Fill in the Blank

Complete each sentence by adding the appropriate word in the provided blanks.

21. The other name for domestic violence is _____ _____ _____.

22. A registered nurse who has undergone additional intensive training for treating victims of assault is called a _____ _____ _____ _____.

23. A temporary loss of ability to cope with life situations following sexual assault is called _____ _____ _____.

24. The governmental social service agency responsible for investigating elder abuse is _____ _____ _____.

25. The person who forces an elderly person to endure fondling and genital manipulation is guilty of _____ _____ _____.

SECTION **II**

NREMT SKILLS FOR PARAMEDIC CERTIFICATION

1. Patient Assessment—Medical

2. Patient Assessment—Trauma

3. Ventilatory Management
   - Adult
   - Dual Lumen Airway Device (Combitube® or PTL®)

4. Cardiac Management Skills
   - Dynamic Cardiology
   - Static Cardiology

5. IV and Medication Skills
   - Intravenous Therapy
   - Intravenous Bolus Medications

6. Oral Station

7. Pediatric Skills
   - Pediatric (<2 yrs.) Ventilatory Management
   - Pediatric Intraosseous Infusion

8. Random Basic Skills
   - Spinal Immobilization (Seated Patient)
   - Spinal Immobilization (Supine Patient)
   - Bleeding Control/Shock Management

National Registry of Emergency Medical Technicians
Advanced Level Practical Examination

PATIENT ASSESSMENT - MEDICAL

Candidate: _____   Examiner: _____

Date: _____   Signature: _____

Scenario: _____

Time Start: _____

	Possible Points	Points Awarded
Takes or verbalizes body substance isolation precautions	1	
SCENE SIZE-UP		
Determines the scene/situation is safe	1	
Determines the mechanism of injury/nature of illness	1	
Determines the number of patients	1	
Requests additional help if necessary	1	
Considers stabilization of spine	1	
INITIAL ASSESSMENT		
Verbalizes general impression of the patient	1	
Determines responsiveness/level of consciousness	1	
Determines chief complaint/apparent life-threats	1	
Assesses airway and breathing -Assessment (1 point) -Assures adequate ventilation (1 point) -Initiates appropriate oxygen therapy (1 point)	3	
Assesses circulation -Assesses/controls major bleeding (1 point) -Assesses skin [either skin color, temperature, or condition] (1 point) -Assesses pulse (1 point)	3	
Identifies priority patients/makes transport decision	1	
FOCUSED HISTORY AND PHYSICAL EXAMINATION/RAPID ASSESSMENT		
History of present illness -Onset (1 point) -Severity (1 point) -Provocation (1 point) -Time (1 point) -Quality (1 point) -Clarifying questions of associated signs and symptoms as related to OPQRST (2 points) -Radiation (1 point)	8	
Past medical history -Allergies (1 point) -Past pertinent history (1 point) -Events leading to present illness (1 point) -Medications (1 point) -Last oral intake (1 point)	5	
Performs focused physical examination [assess affected body part/system or, if indicated, completes rapid assessment] -Cardiovascular -Neurological -Integumentary -Reproductive -Pulmonary -Musculoskeletal -GI/GU -Psychological/Social	5	
Vital signs -Pulse (1 point) -Respiratory rate and quality (1 point each) -Blood pressure (1 point) -AVPU (1 point)	5	
Diagnostics [must include application of ECG monitor for dyspnea and chest pain]	2	
States field impression of patient	1	
Verbalizes treatment plan for patient and calls for appropriate intervention(s)	1	
Transport decision re-evaluated	1	
ON-GOING ASSESSMENT		
Repeats initial assessment	1	
Repeats vital signs	1	
Evaluates response to treatments	1	
Repeats focused assessment regarding patient complaint or injuries	1	

Time End: _____

CRITICAL CRITERIA	**TOTAL**	48	

_____ Failure to initiate or call for transport of the patient within 15 minute time limit

_____ Failure to take or verbalize body substance isolation precautions

_____ Failure to determine scene safety before approaching patient

_____ Failure to voice and ultimately provide appropriate oxygen therapy

_____ Failure to assess/provide adequate ventilation

_____ Failure to find or appropriately manage problems associated with airway, breathing, hemorrhage or shock [hypoperfusion]

_____ Failure to differentiate patient's need for immediate transportation versus continued assessment and treatment at the scene

_____ Does other detailed or focused history or physical examination before assessing and treating threats to airway, breathing, and circulation

_____ Failure to determine the patient's primary problem

_____ Orders a dangerous or inappropriate intervention

_____ Failure to provide for spinal protection when indicated

You must factually document your rationale for checking any of the above critical items on the reverse side of this form.

Candidate: _____ Examiner: _____

Date: _____ Signature: _____

Scenario # _____

Time Start: _____   NOTE: Areas denoted by "**" may be integrated within sequence of Initial Assessment

	Possible Points	Points Awarded
Takes or verbalizes body substance isolation precautions	1	
SCENE SIZE-UP		
Determines the scene/situation is safe	1	
Determines the mechanism of injury/nature of illness	1	
Determines the number of patients	1	
Requests additional help if necessary	1	
Considers stabilization of spine	1	
INITIAL ASSESSMENT/RESUSCITATION		
Verbalizes general impression of the patient	1	
Determines responsiveness/level of consciousness	1	
Determines chief complaint/apparent life-threats	1	
Airway -Opens and assesses airway (1 point) -Inserts adjunct as indicated (1 point)	2	

Breathing
  -Assess breathing (1 point)
  -Assures adequate ventilation (1 point)
  -Initiates appropriate oxygen therapy (1 point)
  -Manages any injury which may compromise breathing/ventilation (1 point)
	4	

Circulation
  -Checks pulse (1point)
  -Assess skin [either skin color, temperature, or condition] (1 point)
  -Assesses for and controls major bleeding if present (1 point)
  -Initiates shock management (1 point)
	4	

Identifies priority patients/makes transport decision	1	
FOCUSED HISTORY AND PHYSICAL EXAMINATION/RAPID TRAUMA ASSESSMENT		
Selects appropriate assessment	1	
Obtains, or directs assistant to obtain, baseline vital signs	1	
Obtains SAMPLE history	1	
DETAILED PHYSICAL EXAMINATION		

Head
  -Inspects mouth**, nose**, and assesses facial area (1 point)
  -Inspects and palpates scalp and ears (1 point)
  -Assesses eyes for PERRL** (1 point)
	3	

Neck**
  -Checks position of trachea (1 point)
  -Checks jugular veins (1 point)
  -Palpates cervical spine (1 point)
	3	

Chest**
  -Inspects chest (1 point)
  -Palpates chest (1 point)
  -Auscultates chest (1 point)
	3	

Abdomen/pelvis**
  -Inspects and palpates abdomen (1 point)
  -Assesses pelvis (1 point)
  -Verbalizes assessment of genitalia/perineum as needed (1 point)
	3	

Lower extremities** -Inspects, palpates, and assesses motor, sensory, and distal circulatory functions (1 point/leg)	2	
Upper extremities -Inspects, palpates, and assesses motor, sensory, and distal circulatory functions (1 point/arm)	2	

Posterior thorax, lumbar, and buttocks**
  -Inspects and palpates posterior thorax (1 point)
  -Inspects and palpates lumbar and buttocks area (1 point)
	2	

Manages secondary injuries and wounds appropriately	1	
Performs ongoing assessment	1	

Time End: _____   **TOTAL**   43

CRITICAL CRITERIA

____ Failure to initiate or call for transport of the patient within 10 minute time limit
____ Failure to take or verbalize body substance isolation precautions
____ Failure to determine scene safety
____ Failure to assess for and provide spinal protection when indicated
____ Failure to voice and ultimately provide high concentration of oxygen
____ Failure to assess/provide adequate ventilation
____ Failure to find or appropriately manage problems associated with airway, breathing, hemorrhage or shock [hypoperfusion]
____ Failure to differentiate patient's need for immediate transportation versus continued assessment/treatment at the scene
____ Does other detailed/focused history or physical exam before assessing/treating threats to airway, breathing, and circulation
____ Orders a dangerous or inappropriate intervention

You must factually document your rationale for checking any of the above critical items on the reverse side of this form.

National Registry of Emergency Medical Technicians
Advanced Level Practical Examination

VENTILATORY MANAGEMENT - ADULT

Candidate:_____ Examiner:_____

Date:_____ Signature:_____

NOTE: If candidate elects to ventilate initially with BVM attached to reservoir and oxygen, full credit must be awarded for steps denoted by "**" so long as first ventilation is delivered within 30 seconds.

	Possible Points	Points Awarded
Takes or verbalizes body substance isolation precautions	1	
Opens the airway manually	1	
Elevates tongue, inserts simple adjunct [oropharyngeal or nasopharyngeal airway]	1	
NOTE: Examiner now informs candidate no gag reflex is present and patient accepts adjunct		
**Ventilates patient immediately with bag-valve-mask device unattached to oxygen	1	
**Ventilates patient with room air	1	
NOTE: Examiner now informs candidate that ventilation is being performed without difficulty and that pulse oximetry indicates the patient's blood oxygen saturation is 85%		
Attaches oxygen reservoir to bag-valve-mask device and connects to high flow oxygen regulator [12-15 L/minute]	1	
Ventilates patient at a rate of 10-12/minute with appropriate volumes	1	
NOTE: After 30 seconds, examiner auscultates and reports breath sounds are present, equal bilaterally and medical direction has ordered intubation. The examiner must now take over ventilation.		
Directs assistant to pre-oxygenate patient	1	
Identifies/selects proper equipment for intubation	1	
Checks equipment for: -Cuff leaks (1 point) -Laryngoscope operational with bulb tight (1 point)	2	
NOTE: Examiner to remove OPA and move out of the way when candidate is prepared to intubate		
Positions head properly	1	
Inserts blade while displacing tongue	1	
Elevates mandible with laryngoscope	1	
Introduces ET tube and advances to proper depth	1	
Inflates cuff to proper pressure and disconnects syringe	1	
Directs ventilation of patient	1	
Confirms proper placement by auscultation bilaterally over each lung and over epigastrium	1	
NOTE: Examiner to ask, "If you had proper placement, what should you expect to hear?"		
Secures ET tube [may be verbalized]	1	
NOTE: Examiner now asks candidate, "Please demonstrate one additional method of verifying proper tube placement in this patient."		
Identifies/selects proper equipment	1	
Verbalizes findings and interpretations [compares indicator color to the colorimetric scale or EDD recoil and states findings]	1	
NOTE: Examiner now states, "You see secretions in the tube and hear gurgling sounds with the patient's exhalation."		
Identifies/selects a flexible suction catheter	1	
Pre-oxygenates patient	1	
Marks maximum insertion length with thumb and forefinger	1	
Inserts catheter into the ET tube leaving catheter port open	1	
At proper insertion depth, covers catheter port and applies suction while withdrawing catheter	1	
Ventilates/directs ventilation of patient as catheter is flushed with sterile water	1	
TOTAL	**27**	

CRITICAL CRITERIA

_____ Failure to initiate ventilations within 30 seconds after applying gloves or interrupts ventilations for greater than 30 seconds at any time
_____ Failure to take or verbalize body substance isolation precautions
_____ Failure to voice and ultimately provide high oxygen concentrations [at least 85%]
_____ Failure to ventilate patient at a rate of 10 - 12 / minute
_____ Failure to provide adequate volumes per breath [maximum 2 errors/minute permissible]
_____ Failure to pre-oxygenate patient prior to intubation and suctioning
_____ Failure to successfully intubate within 3 attempts
_____ Failure to disconnect syringe **immediately** after inflating cuff of ET tube
_____ Uses teeth as a fulcrum
_____ Failure to assure proper tube placement by auscultation bilaterally **and** over the epigastrium
_____ If used, stylette extends beyond end of ET tube
_____ Inserts any adjunct in a manner dangerous to the patient
_____ Suctions the patient for more than 10 seconds
_____ Does not suction the patient

You must factually document your rationale for checking any of the above critical items on the reverse side of this form.

p303/8-003k

DUAL LUMEN AIRWAY DEVICE (COMBITUBE® OR PTL®)

Candidate: _____   Examiner: _____

Date: _____   Signature: _____

NOTE: If candidate elects to initially ventilate with BVM attached to reservoir and oxygen, full credit must be awarded for steps denoted by "**" so long as first ventilation is delivered within 30 seconds.

	Possible Points	Points Awarded
Takes or verbalizes body substance isolation precautions	1	
Opens the airway manually	1	
Elevates tongue, inserts simple adjunct [oropharyngeal or nasopharyngeal airway]	1	
NOTE: Examiner now informs candidate no gag reflex is present and patient accepts adjunct		
**Ventilates patient immediately with bag-valve-mask device unattached to oxygen	1	
**Hyperventilates patient with room air	1	
NOTE: Examiner now informs candidate that ventilation is being performed without difficulty		
Attaches oxygen reservoir to bag-valve-mask device and connects to high flow oxygen regulator [12-15 L/minute]	1	
Ventilates patient at a rate of 10-12/minute with appropriate volumes	1	
NOTE: After 30 seconds, examiner auscultates and reports breath sounds are present and equal bilaterally and medical control has ordered insertion of a dual lumen airway. The examiner must now take over ventilation.		
Directs assistant to pre-oxygenate patient	1	
Checks/prepares airway device	1	
Lubricates distal tip of the device [may be verbalized]	1	
NOTE: Examiner to remove OPA and move out of the way when candidate is prepared to insert device		
Positions head properly	1	
Performs a tongue-jaw lift	1	

☐ USES COMBITUBE®	☐ USES PTL®		
Inserts device in mid-line and to depth so printed ring is at level of teeth	Inserts device in mid-line until bite block flange is at level of teeth	1	
Inflates pharyngeal cuff with proper volume and removes syringe	Secures strap	1	
Inflates distal cuff with proper volume and removes syringe	Blows into tube #1 to adequately inflate both cuffs	1	
Attaches/directs attachment of BVM to the first [esophageal placement] lumen and ventilates		1	
Confirms placement and ventilation through correct lumen by observing chest rise, auscultation over the epigastrium, and bilaterally over each lung		1	
NOTE: The examiner states, "You do not see rise and fall of the chest and you only hear sounds over the epigastrium."			
Attaches/directs attachment of BVM to the second [endotracheal placement] lumen and ventilates		1	
Confirms placement and ventilation through correct lumen by observing chest rise, auscultation over the epigastrium, and bilaterally over each lung		1	
NOTE: The examiner confirms adequate chest rise, absent sounds over the epigastrium, and equal bilateral breath sounds.			
Secures device or confirms that the device remains properly secured		1	
	TOTAL	20	

CRITICAL CRITERIA

_____ Failure to initiate ventilations within 30 seconds after taking body substance isolation precautions or interrupts ventilations for greater than 30 seconds at any time

_____ Failure to take or verbalize body substance isolation precautions

_____ Failure to voice and ultimately provide high oxygen concentrations [at least 85%]

_____ Failure to ventilate patient at a rate of 10-12/minute

_____ Failure to provide adequate volumes per breath [maximum 2 errors/minute permissible]

_____ Failure to pre-oxygenate patient prior to insertion of the dual lumen airway device

_____ Failure to insert the dual lumen airway device at a proper depth or at either proper place within 3 attempts

_____ Failure to inflate both cuffs properly

_____ **Combitube** - failure to remove the syringe immediately after inflation of each cuff

PTL - failure to secure the strap prior to cuff inflation

_____ Failure to confirm that the proper lumen of the device is being ventilated by observing chest rise, auscultation over the epigastrium, and bilaterally over each lung

_____ Inserts any adjunct in a manner dangerous to patient

You must factually document your rationale for checking any of the above critical items on the reverse side of this form.

p304/8-003k

DYNAMIC CARDIOLOGY

Candidate: _____   Examiner: _____

Date: _____   Signature: _____

SET #_____

Level of Testing: □ NREMT-Intermediate/99   □ NREMT-Paramedic

	Possible Points	Points Awarded
Time Start:_____		
Takes or verbalizes infection control precautions	1	
Checks level of responsiveness	1	
Checks ABCs	1	
Initiates CPR when appropriate [verbally]	1	
Attaches ECG monitor in a timely fashion [patches, pads or paddles]	1	
Correctly interprets initial rhythm	1	
Appropriately manages initial rhythm	2	
Notes change in rhythm	1	
Checks patient condition to include pulse and, if appropriate, BP	1	
Correctly interprets second rhythm	1	
Appropriately manages second rhythm	2	
Notes change in rhythm	1	
Checks patient condition to include pulse and, if appropriate, BP	1	
Correctly interprets third rhythm	1	
Appropriately manages third rhythm	2	
Notes change in rhythm	1	
Checks patient condition to include pulse and, if appropriate, BP	1	
Correctly interprets fourth rhythm	1	
Appropriately manages fourth rhythm	2	
Orders high percentages of supplemental oxygen at proper times	1	
Time End: _____ **TOTAL**	24	

CRITICAL CRITERIA

_____ Failure to deliver any shock in a timely manner

_____ Failure to verify rhythm before delivering each shock

_____ Failure to ensure the safety of self and others [verbalizes "All clear" and observes]

_____ Inability to deliver DC shock [does not use machine properly]

_____ Failure to demonstrate acceptable shock sequence

_____ Failure to immediately order initiation or resumption of CPR when appropriate

_____ Failure to order correct management of airway [ET when appropriate]

_____ Failure to order administration of appropriate oxygen at proper time

_____ Failure to diagnose or treat 2 or more rhythms correctly

_____ Orders administration of an inappropriate drug or lethal dosage

_____ Failure to correctly diagnose or adequately treat v-fib, v-tach, or asystole

You must factually document your rationale for checking any of the above critical items on the reverse side of this form.

p306/8-003k

National Registry of Emergency Medical Technicians
Advanced Level Practical Examination

STATIC CARDIOLOGY

Candidate: _____ **Examiner:** _____

Date: _____ **Signature:** _____

SET #_____

Level of Testing: ☐ NREMT-Intermediate/99 ☐ NREMT-Paramedic

Note: No points for treatment may be awarded if the diagnosis is incorrect.
Only document incorrect responses in spaces provided.

Time Start:_____

	Possible Points	Points Awarded
STRIP #1		
Diagnosis:	1	
Treatment:	2	
STRIP #2		
Diagnosis:	1	
Treatment:	2	
STRIP #3		
Diagnosis:	1	
Treatment:	2	
STRIP #4		
Diagnosis:	1	
Treatment:	2	
Time End: _____	**TOTAL** 12	

INTRAVENOUS THERAPY

Candidate: _____ Examiner: _____

Date: _____ Signature: _____

Level of Testing: ❑ NREMT-Intermediate/85 ❑ NREMT-Intermediate/99 ❑ NREMT-Paramedic

Time Start: _____

	Possible Points	Points Awarded
Checks selected IV fluid for: -Proper fluid (1 point) -Clarity (1 point)	2	
Selects appropriate catheter	1	
Selects proper administration set	1	
Connects IV tubing to the IV bag	1	
Prepares administration set [fills drip chamber and flushes tubing]	1	
Cuts or tears tape [at any time before venipuncture]	1	
Takes/verbalizes body substance isolation precautions [prior to venipuncture]	1	
Applies tourniquet	1	
Palpates suitable vein	1	
Cleanses site appropriately	1	
Performs venipuncture -Inserts stylette (1 point) -Notes or verbalizes flashback (1 point) -Occludes vein proximal to catheter (1 point) -Removes stylette (1 point) -Connects IV tubing to catheter (1 point)	5	
Disposes/verbalizes disposal of needle in proper container	1	
Releases tourniquet	1	
Runs IV for a brief period to assure patent line	1	
Secures catheter [tapes securely or verbalizes]	1	
Adjusts flow rate as appropriate	1	

Time End: _____ **TOTAL** 21

CRITICAL CRITERIA

_____ Failure to establish a patent and properly adjusted IV within 6 minute time limit
_____ Failure to take or verbalize body substance isolation precautions prior to performing venipuncture
_____ Contaminates equipment or site without appropriately correcting situation
_____ Performs any improper technique resulting in the potential for uncontrolled hemorrhage, catheter shear, or air embolism
_____ Failure to successfully establish IV within 3 attempts during 6 minute time limit
_____ Failure to dispose/verbalize disposal of needle in proper container

NOTE: Check here (_____) if candidate did not establish a patent IV and do not evaluate IV Bolus Medications.

INTRAVENOUS BOLUS MEDICATIONS

Time Start: _____

	Possible Points	Points Awarded
Asks patient for known allergies	1	
Selects correct medication	1	
Assures correct concentration of drug	1	
Assembles prefilled syringe correctly and dispels air	1	
Continues body substance isolation precautions	1	
Cleanses injection site [Y-port or hub]	1	
Reaffirms medication	1	
Stops IV flow [pinches tubing or shuts off]	1	
Administers correct dose at proper push rate	1	
Disposes/verbalizes proper disposal of syringe and needle in proper container	1	
Flushes tubing [runs wide open for a brief period]	1	
Adjusts drip rate to TKO/KVO	1	
Verbalizes need to observe patient for desired effect/adverse side effects	1	

Time End: _____ **TOTAL** 13

CRITICAL CRITERIA

_____ Failure to begin administration of medication within 3 minute time limit
_____ Contaminates equipment or site without appropriately correcting situation
_____ Failure to adequately dispel air resulting in potential for air embolism
_____ Injects improper drug or dosage [wrong drug, incorrect amount, or pushes at inappropriate rate]
_____ Failure to flush IV tubing after injecting medication
_____ Recaps needle or failure to dispose/verbalize disposal of syringe and needle in proper container

You must factually document your rationale for checking any of the above critical items on the reverse side of this form.

p309/8-003k

National Registry of Emergency Medical Technicians
Advanced Level Practical Examination
ORAL STATION

Candidate: _____   Examiner: _____

Date: _____   Signature: _____

Scenario: _____

Time Start: _____

	Possible Points	Points Awarded
Scene Management		
Thoroughly assessed and took deliberate actions to control the scene	3	
Assessed the scene, identified potential hazards, did not put anyone in danger	2	
Incompletely assessed or managed the scene	1	
Did not assess or manage the scene	0	
Patient Assessment		
Completed an organized assessment and integrated findings to expand further assessment	3	
Completed initial, focused, and ongoing assessments	2	
Performed an incomplete or disorganized assessment	1	
Did not complete an initial assessment	0	
Patient Management		
Managed all aspects of the patient's condition and anticipated further needs	3	
Appropriately managed the patient's presenting condition	2	
Performed an incomplete or disorganized management	1	
Did not manage life-threatening conditions	0	
Interpersonal relations		
Established rapport and interacted in an organized, therapeutic manner	3	
Interacted and responded appropriately with patient, crew, and bystanders	2	
Used inappropriate communication techniques	1	
Demonstrated intolerance for patient, bystanders, and crew	0	
Integration (verbal report, field impression, and transport decision)		
Stated correct field impression and pathophysiological basis, provided succinct and accurate verbal report including social/psychological concerns, and considered alternate transport destinations	3	
Stated correct field impression, provided succinct and accurate verbal report, and appropriately stated transport decision	2	
Stated correct field impression, provided inappropriate verbal report or transport decision	1	
Stated incorrect field impression or did not provide verbal report	0	

Time End: _____   **TOTAL**   **15**

Critical Criteria

_____ Failure to appropriately address any of the scenario's "Mandatory Actions"

_____ Performs or orders any harmful or dangerous action or intervention

You must factually document your rationale for checking any of the above critical items on the reverse side of this form.

p308/8-003k

PEDIATRIC (<2 yrs.) VENTILATORY MANAGEMENT

Candidate: _____ Examiner _____

Date: _____ Signature: _____

NOTE: If candidate elects to ventilate initially with BVM attached to reservoir and oxygen, full credit must be awarded for steps denoted by "**" so long as first ventilation is delivered within 30 seconds.

	Possible Points	Points Awarded
Takes or verbalizes body substance isolation precautions	1	
Opens the airway manually	1	
Elevates tongue, inserts simple adjunct [oropharyngeal or nasopharyngeal airway]	1	
NOTE: Examiner now informs candidate no gag reflex is present and patient accepts adjunct		
**Ventilates patient immediately with bag-valve-mask device unattached to oxygen	1	
**Ventilates patient with room air	1	
NOTE: Examiner now informs candidate that ventilation is being performed without difficulty and that pulse oximetry indicates the patient's blood oxygen saturation is 85%		
Attaches oxygen reservoir to bag-valve-mask device and connects to high flow oxygen regulator [12-15 L/minute]	1	
Ventilates patient at a rate of 12-20/minute and assures visible chest rise	1	
NOTE: After 30 seconds, examiner auscultates and reports breath sounds are present, equal bilaterally and medical direction has ordered intubation. The examiner must now take over ventilation.		
Directs assistant to pre-oxygenate patient	1	
Identifies/selects proper equipment for intubation	1	
Checks laryngoscope to assure operational with bulb tight	1	
NOTE: Examiner to remove OPA and move out of the way when candidate is prepared to intubate		
Places patient in neutral or sniffing position	1	
Inserts blade while displacing tongue	1	
Elevates mandible with laryngoscope	1	
Introduces ET tube and advances to proper depth	1	
Directs ventilation of patient	1	
Confirms proper placement by auscultation bilaterally over each lung and over epigastrium	1	
NOTE: Examiner to ask, "If you had proper placement, what should you expect to hear?"		
Secures ET tube [may be verbalized]	1	
TOTAL	**17**	

CRITICAL CRITERIA

_____ Failure to initiate ventilations within 30 seconds after applying gloves or interrupts ventilations for greater than 30 seconds at any time

_____ Failure to take or verbalize body substance isolation precautions

_____ Failure to pad under the torso to allow neutral head position or sniffing position

_____ Failure to voice and ultimately provide high oxygen concentrations [at least 85%]

_____ Failure to ventilate patient at a rate of 12-20/minute

_____ Failure to provide adequate volumes per breath [maximum 2 errors/minute permissible]

_____ Failure to pre-oxygenate patient prior to intubation

_____ Failure to successfully intubate within 3 attempts

_____ Uses gums as a fulcrum

_____ Failure to assure proper tube placement by auscultation bilaterally **and** over the epigastrium

_____ Inserts any adjunct in a manner dangerous to the patient

_____ Attempts to use any equipment not appropriate for the pediatric patient

You must factually document your rationale for checking any of the above critical items on the reverse side of this form.

p305/8-003k

PEDIATRIC INTRAOSSEOUS INFUSION

Candidate: _____ Examiner: _____

Date: _____ Signature: _____

Time Start:_____

	Possible Points	Points Awarded

Checks selected IV fluid for:
   -Proper fluid (1 point)
   -Clarity (1 point)
	2	

Selects appropriate equipment to include:
   -IO needle (1 point)
   -Syringe (1 point)
   -Saline (1 point)
   -Extension set (1 point)
	4	

Selects proper administration set	1	
Connects administration set to bag	1	
Prepares administration set [fills drip chamber and flushes tubing]	1	
Prepares syringe and extension tubing	1	
Cuts or tears tape [at any time before IO puncture]	1	
Takes or verbalizes body substance isolation precautions [prior to IO puncture]	1	
Identifies proper anatomical site for IO puncture	1	
Cleanses site appropriately	1	

Performs IO puncture:
   -Stabilizes tibia (1 point)
   -Inserts needle at proper angle (1 point)
   -Advances needle with twisting motion until "pop" is felt (1 point)
   -Unscrews cap and removes stylette from needle (1 point)
	4	

Disposes of needle in proper container	1	
Attaches administration set to IO needle (with or without 3-way)	1	
Slowly injects saline to assure proper placement of needle	1	
Adjusts flow rate as appropriate	1	
Secures needle with tape and supports with bulky dressing	1	

Time End: _____   **TOTAL**   23

CRITICAL CRITERIA

_____ Failure to establish a patent and properly adjusted IO line within the 6 minute time limit
_____ Failure to take or verbalize body substance isolation precautions prior to performing IO puncture
_____ Contaminates equipment or site without appropriately correcting situation
_____ Performs any improper technique resulting in the potential for air embolism
_____ Failure to assure correct needle placement
_____ Failure to successfully establish IO infusion within 2 attempts during 6 minute time limit
_____ Performing IO puncture in an unacceptable manner [improper site, incorrect needle angle, etc.]
_____ Failure to dispose of needle in proper container
_____ Orders or performs any dangerous or potentially harmful procedure

You must factually document your rationale for checking any of the above critical items on the reverse side of this form.

p310/8-003k

SPINAL IMMOBILIZATION (SEATED PATIENT)

Candidate: _____ Examiner: _____

Date: _____ Signature: _____

Time Start: _____	Possible Points	Points Awarded
Takes or verbalizes body substance isolation precautions	1	
Directs assistant to place/maintain head in the neutral, in-line position	1	
Directs assistant to maintain manual immobilization of the head	1	
Reassesses motor, sensory, and circulatory function in each extremity	1	
Applies appropriately sized extrication collar	1	
Positions the immobilization device behind the patient	1	
Secures the device to the patient's torso	1	
Evaluates torso fixation and adjusts as necessary	1	
Evaluates and pads behind the patient's head as necessary	1	
Secures the patient's head to the device	1	
Verbalizes moving the patient to a long backboard	1	
Reassesses motor, sensory, and circulatory function in each extremity	1	

Time End: _____   **TOTAL**   12

CRITICAL CRITERIA

_____ Did not immediately direct or take manual immobilization of the head

_____ Did not properly apply appropriately sized cervical collar before ordering release of manual immobilization

_____ Released or ordered release of manual immobilization before it was maintained mechanically

_____ Manipulated or moved patient excessively causing potential spinal compromise

_____ Head immobilized to the device **before** device sufficiently secured to torso

_____ Device moves excessively up, down, left, or right on the patient's torso

_____ Head immobilization allows for excessive movement

_____ Torso fixation inhibits chest rise, resulting in respiratory compromise

_____ Upon completion of immobilization, head is not in a neutral, in-line position

_____ Did not reassess motor, sensory, and circulatory functions in each extremity after voicing immobilization to the long backboard

You must factually document your rationale for checking any of the above critical items on the reverse side of this form.

SPINAL IMMOBILIZATION (SUPINE PATIENT)

Candidate: _____ Examiner: _____

Date: _____ Signature: _____

Time Start: _____

	Possible Points	Points Awarded
Takes or verbalizes body substance isolation precautions	1	
Directs assistant to place/maintain head in the neutral, in-line position	1	
Directs assistant to maintain manual immobilization of the head	1	
Reassesses motor, sensory, and circulatory function in each extremity	1	
Applies appropriately sized extrication collar	1	
Positions the immobilization device appropriately	1	
Directs movement of the patient onto the device without compromising the integrity of the spine	1	
Applies padding to voids between the torso and the device as necessary	1	
Immobilizes the patient's torso to the device	1	
Evaluates and pads behind the patient's head as necessary	1	
Immobilizes the patient's head to the device	1	
Secures the patient's legs to the device	1	
Secures the patient's arms to the device	1	
Reassesses motor, sensory, and circulatory function in each extremity	1	

Time End: _____   **TOTAL**   14

CRITICAL CRITERIA

_____ Did not immediately direct or take manual immobilization of the head

_____ Did not properly apply appropriately sized cervical collar before ordering release of manual immobilization

_____ Released or ordered release of manual immobilization before it was maintained mechanically

_____ Manipulated or moved patient excessively causing potential spinal compromise

_____ Head immobilized to the device **before** device sufficiently secured to torso

_____ Patient moves excessively up, down, left, or right on the device

_____ Head immobilization allows for excessive movement

_____ Upon completion of immobilization, head is not in a neutral, in-line position

_____ Did not reassess motor, sensory, and circulatory functions in each extremity after voicing immobilization to the device

You must factually document your rationale for checking any of the above critical items on the reverse side of this form.

p312/8-003k

BLEEDING CONTROL/SHOCK MANAGEMENT

Candidate: _____ Examiner: _____

Date: _____ Signature: _____

Time Start:_____	Possible Points	Points Awarded
Takes or verbalizes body substance isolation precautions	1	
Applies direct pressure to the wound	1	
NOTE: The examiner must now inform the candidate that the wound continues to bleed.		
Applies tourniquet	1	
NOTE: The examiner must now inform the candidate that the patient is exhibiting signs and symptoms of hypoperfusion.		
Properly positions the patient	1	
Administers high concentration oxygen	1	
Initiates steps to prevent heat loss from the patient	1	
Indicates the need for immediate transportation	1	
Time End: _____ **TOTAL**	7	

CRITICAL CRITERIA

_____ Did not take or verbalize body substance isolation precautions

_____ Did not apply high concentration of oxygen

_____ Did not control hemorrhage using correct procedures in a timely manner

_____ Did not indicate the need for immediate transportation

You must factually document your rationale for checking any of the above critical items on the reverse side of this form.

Chapter 1

Case Study

Case Study Questions

1. *What indicators prompted the Paramedic to obtain a 12-lead ECG?*

   A chief concern of substernal chest pain is a sufficient indicator to prompt the Paramedic to obtain a 12-lead ECG. The adage goes, "Any pain from the nose to the navel is considered cardiac until proven otherwise." Additionally, the presence of Levine's sign is suggestive of a myocardial infarction in evolution.

2. *Based on the patient presentation, what type of myocardial infarction should be suspected and where would the ECG changes be seen?*

   The patient presentation is somewhat classic for an anterior wall myocardial infarction in evolution. The Paramedic should expect to see ST elevations in leads V3 and V4.

Case Conclusion

1. *Why would the 12-lead ECG not show ST elevations if the patient is experiencing a myocardial infarction in evolution?*

   Approximately 50% of initial 12-lead ECG readings do not show ST elevations indicating a myocardial infarction in evolution. Nevertheless, prehospital 12-lead ECG readings are important as they serve as a baseline for comparison of future 12-lead ECG readings that may show ST elevations.

2. *What other ECG changes may have alerted the Paramedic to the potential for a myocardial infarction in evolution?*

   Other changes that are suggestive of an anterior wall myocardial infarction in evolution are reverse R wave progression, widening QT intervals, ST segment depressions, hyperacute T waves, and new onset left bundle branch block.

Pratice Questions

Multiple Choice

1. b		9. d	
2. a		10. b	
3. a		11. b	
4. c		12. c	
5. b		13. b	
6. a		14. d	
7. a		15. b	
8. d			

Short Answer

16. The American Heart Association standardized electrode placement.

17. A common mistake causing V1 and V2 to be placed too high is counting the first space under the clavicle as the first intercostal space when it is actually the second intercostal space.

18. The fourth electrode is placed "out of order" midline between the third and fifth electrode.

19. Left dominance means the left anterior coronary artery, rather than the right coronary artery, supplies blood to the AV node.

20. Reciprocal changes are concomitant ST segment depressions in the wall opposite of the ST segment elevations.

Fill in the Blank

21. wrist, ankles, chest, hips

22. rhythm strip

23. RSr

24. anterior

25. 25%, wide

Chapter 2

Case Study

Chief Concern

1. *What are some of the possible causes of Sam's symptoms?*

   An obvious cause of Sam's symptoms is food poisoning; however, an atypical presentation of myocardial infarction has to be considered as well.

2. *How can the bradycardia be related?*

   Someone who is vomiting is expected to have tachycardia. While vagal stimulation during retching can cause bradycardia, this patient is lying on the ground and not vomiting. This bradycardia may be of a cardiac origin.

History

1. *What are the important elements of the history that a Paramedic should obtain?*

   Although the patient is not complaining of pain, the OPQRST mnemonic is still useful. Sam's differential includes distress of a gastrointestinal origin versus that of a cardiac origin. Therefore, an abdominal history including a history of GERD, as well as a cardiac history, should be obtained.

2. *What are the risk factors associated with coronary artery disease?*

   Sam appears to be the poster child for coronary artery diseases. He is middle-aged, is overweight, has elevated cholesterol levels, and has hypertension. Perhaps most troubling is Sam's extensive smoking history.

Examination

1. *What are the elements of the physical examination of a patient with suspected acute coronary syndrome?*

   After performing the primary assessment and obtaining a set of vital signs, the Paramedic should proceed in a head-to-toe fashion looking for jugular venous distention, assessing the chest for accessory muscle use, and auscultating the chest for adventitious breath sounds as well as murmurs and a ventricular gallop. The abdomen should be assessed for tenderness and the ability to reproduce a hepatic jugular reflex. Finally, the Paramedic should assess for peripheral edema in the dependent areas, either sacrum or ankles.

2. *Why is a 12-lead ECG a critical element in this examination?*

   The patient presentation should make the Paramedic suspect acute coronary syndrome. In any case, "pain from the nose to the navel is cardiac until proven otherwise" and warrants a 12-lead ECG.

Assessment

1. *Hemodynamically speaking, what is the significance of dizziness and the bradydysrhythmia?*

   For whatever reason, most likely due to the heart's inability to mount a reflexive tachycardia secondary to the ischemia in the AV node, the patient becomes dizzy when trying to stand. Continued exertion could put a strain on the already compromised heart.

2. *What diagnosis did the Paramedic announce to the patient?*

   The patient should be advised that the problem may be gastrointestinal. However, it is even more possible that the problem is an acute coronary syndrome. Of the two, the one with the greater risks is the acute coronary syndrome.

Treatment

1. *What is the standard of care of patients with suspected inferior wall myocardial infarction?*

   MONA–B is the standard treatment regime. However, in this case, the patient has a suspected inferior wall myocardial infarction (IWMI). This patient population is preload dependent in many cases and administration of nitrate can lead to a precipitous drop in blood pressure. Although beta blockers have been shown to prevent sudden cardiac death from tachydysrhythmia, this patient has bradycardia.

2. *Why did Reba want venous access prior to Roger's administration of nitrates?*

   Patients with suspected inferior wall myocardial infarction tend to become hypotensive with the administration of nitrates. Furthermore, the patient has a borderline blood pressure as well.

Evaluation

1. *What are some of the predictable complications associated with an inferior wall myocardial infarction?*

   Inferior wall myocardial infarctions, without iatrogenic complications, tend to worsen in two ways: (1) extension of the inferior wall myocardial infarction into the right ventricle, or (2) the rupture of the chordae tendineae that anchor the mitral valve, as suspected in this case.

2. *Why did Reba request V4R?*

   If the inferior wall myocardial infarction had extended into the right ventricle, patterns of ischemia might be seen, thus warranting a 15-lead or right precordial chest 12-lead ECG.

Disposition

1. *What is the most appropriate transport decision that will get the patient to definitive care?*

   As Reba and Roger suspect an inferior wall myocardial infarction with rupture of the mitral valve, this patient needs to be transported immediately to an open heart center capable of valve replacements.

2. *While en route, what treatments should be instituted?*

   Since patients with an inferior wall myocardial infarction with rupture of the mitral valve are extremely preload dependent, the Paramedics should open the first venous line "wide open" with a liter bolus while establishing a second venous access. It is also important to monitor the patient's respiratory status, including pulse oximetry, for signs of decompensation. Continuous positive airway pressure (CPAP) and even positive pressure ventilation with a bag–mask assembly may be necessary if the patient shows signs of increased carbon dioxide retention or decreased oxygen saturation.

Practice Questions
Multiple Choice

1. b	9. b
2. d	10. a
3. a	11. c
4. b	12. a
5. d	13. b
6. b	14. b
7. c	15. d
8. d	

Short Answer

16. During hyperventilation, the patient reduces the blood's acid (i.e., makes the blood more alkaline), which in turn leads to hypocalcemia. The hypocalcemia causes coronary artery vasospasm.

17. Coronary arteries can be revascularized mechanically via angioplasty, chemically using fibrinolytics, and surgically with a coronary artery bypass graft.

18. A myocardial infarction may not show ST changes on the ECG because the myocardial infarction is early in evolution, in which case the Paramedic should look for hyperacute T waves, QT prolongation, ST depressions, and so on. Another option is that the myocardial infarction has completed its evolution, the infarction is complete, and there may or may not be a Q wave. This is called a non ST-elevation myocardial infarction.

19. Unstable angina is chest pain that increases in frequency, duration, or intensity that is not relieved with rest, oxygen, or nitroglycerine.

20. Pericarditis is an inflammation of the pericardium and can be caused by infections, malignancy, medications, systemic inflammatory conditions, renal failure, or myocardial infarction.

Fill in the Blank

21. diastole, aortic
22. preinfarction angina
23. mitral, aortic

24. second ICS at right sternal border
25. gastroesophageal reflux, heartburn

Chapter 3
Case Study
Chief Concern

1. *What are some of the possible causes of sudden shortness of breath?*

   Potential causes of acute shortness of breath are numerous and include pulmonary embolus, COPD, asthma, pneumonia, aspiration secondary to GERD, and sleep apnea, to name a few.

2. *How can the history of cardiac disease be related to shortness of breath?*

   Although the Paramedic must keep an open mind regarding other potential causes of shortness of breath, the history of heart disease might suggest shortness of breath secondary to heart failure.

History

1. *What are the important elements of the history that a Paramedic should obtain?*

   As the patient presents with both a respiratory concern as well as a potential cardiac concern, the Paramedic should focus on obtaining a history using the HAPISOCS and OPQRST mnemonics.
      The past medical history is particularly telling. Kareem has multiple risk factors for heart failure including coronary artery disease, myocardial infarction, hypertension, and tobacco abuse.

2. *What is the symptom pattern associated with a backward failure?*

   The previous history of exertional dyspnea and nocturia suggests that Kareem was already suffering from backward heart failure. However, his current paroxysmal nocturnal dyspnea is highly suggestive of heart failure.

Examination

1. *What are the elements of the physical examination of a patient with suspected heart failure?*

   The physical examination of the patient with suspected heart failure, based on history, consists of the ABCs and a focused physical examination that assesses the six cardinal signs of heart failure.

2. *Why is a 12-lead ECG a critical element in this examination?*

   One of the more ominous and potentially life-threatening causes of acute heart failure is a myocardial infarction. An inferior wall myocardial infarction with extension into the papillary muscles that anchor the mitral valve, as well as a massive anterior wall myocardial infarction that would reduce the myocardium's effectiveness as a pump, could lead to either forward or backward failure.

Assessment

1. *What were the symptoms, in the symptom complex, that led the Paramedic to the diagnosis?*

   The paroxysmal nocturnal dyspnea (PND), history of nocturia, night cough, dyspnea on exertion (DOE), jugular venous distention (JVD), rales, ventricular gallop, and a positive hepatojugular reflex (HJR) led the Paramedic to the diagnosis.

2. *What diagnosis did the Paramedic announce to the patient?*

   Using the Farmingham criteria, the Paramedic can be fairly safe in stating that the patient has heart failure.

Treatment

1. *What is the standard of care of patients with suspected heart failure?*

   Beyond assuring adequate oxygenation and ventilation, by monitoring the end-tidal carbon dioxide and oxygen saturation, the Paramedic should focus on reducing preload as long as the cardiac output remains stable. This can be accomplished by use of diuretics and even morphine sulfate. However, a growing body of literature supports the aggressive use of nitrates.

2. *Why was aspirin administered?*

Although the 12-lead ECG is inconclusive in many cases, the initial 12-lead ECG does not show patterns of ischemia. Therefore, the possibility of acute coronary syndrome cannot be altogether eliminated. Fortunately, the treatment of heart failure, with the addition of aspirin, can be the same as the treatment of acute coronary syndrome.

Evaluation

1. *What are some of the predictable complications associated with heart failure?*

Owed to the central role that the heart plays in the body, heart failure can lead to syncope, respiratory distress secondary to pulmonary edema, and cardiogenic shock.

2. *What are some of the predictable complications associated with the treatments for heart failure?*

As nitrates are the mainstay of heart failure therapy, hypotension is a likely complication. In some instances, as in this case, it is prudent to establish venous access in case a bolus of solution is needed. However, the effects of nitroglycerine are self-limiting. Therefore, persistent hypotension must be treated aggressively, using vasopressors, in order to maintain an adequate cerebral perfusion pressure.

Disposition

1. *What is the most appropriate transport decision that will get the patient to definitive care?*

Cardiogenic shock in the face of heart failure is an ominous sign associated with a high mortality. It is imperative that the patient be transported to a tertiary care center capable of providing mechanical circulatory support as well as critical care.

2. *What are some of the transportation considerations?*

While each case is different, cardiogenic shock associated with heart failure is a time-sensitive emergency that may warrant the use of air medical services for timely transportation to a tertiary care center.

Practice Questions
Multiple Choice

1. d		9. a	
2. a		10. b	
3. d		11. a	
4. a		12. d	
5. c		13. a	
6. d		14. c	
7. d		15. a	
8. c			

Short Answer

16. The pathological progression of heart failure starts with the patient's dropping blood pressure. This creates neurohormonal activitation (RAAS–norepinephrine), leading to cardiac hypertrophy. As a result, the body undergoes ventricular remodeling and decompensation, leading to activation of the neurohormonal axis.

17. As blood backs into the pulmonary tree during backward failure, breath sounds are diminished, starting from the base as a rule. These are often associated with a nonproductive cough. Then, as the airways narrow, wheezing (i.e., cardiac asthma) occurs. This is followed by frank rales (fine crackles) appreciated at the base of the lungs and then absent breath sounds as alveolar space collapses. Typically, these changes "layer out" in a caudal-to-cephalic manner.

18. The patient with heart failure lies recumbent at night, causing the blood that is normally sequestered in the legs to flood the core. The increased blood volume results in increased urine production, leading to nocturia or, more acutely, backward heart failure and pulmonary edema as a result of the heart's inability to compensate for the increased preload.

The patient who becomes hypoxic awakens to feeling short of breath and experiences paroxysmal nocturnal dyspnea (shortness of breath that occurs at night).

19. The six cardinal signs of heart failure are, from head to toe, jugular venous distention, ventricular gallop, pulmonary rales, hepatic jugular reflex, abdominal tenderness, and pedal (peripheral dependent) edema.

20. The three abdominal signs suggestive of heart failure are (1) development of abdominal tenderness, secondary to distention; (2) a hepatic–jugular reflex; and (3) ascites, as a result of abdominal fluids third-spacing when fluid backs up into the mesentery circulation.

Fill in the Blank

21. forward heart failure

22. cerebral perfusion pressure

23. diastolic dysfunction

24. weak, rapid

25. bradypnea

Chapter 4

Case Study

Chief Concern

1. *What are some of the possible causes of Sofia's weakness?*

   The causes of sudden weakness are numerous. However, the more ominous causes are hypoxia induced by a pulmonary embolism, for example, or a cardiac disorder, such as a myocardial infarction.

2. *What is the implication of an irregularly irregular pulse?*

   An irregularly irregular pulse indicates some dysrhythmia.

History

1. *What are the important elements of the history that a Paramedic should obtain?*

   While the standard OPQRST/SAMPLE history is indicated, the Paramedic should focus on the systemic impact of atrial fibrillation. The Paramedic should ascertain the time of onset but also if the patient was seated or standing and if there was any associated syncope. Atrial fibrillation can cause a loss in blood pressure leading to syncope. Similarly, the Paramedic should ask if the patient has any chest pressure or tightness as these may be anginal symptoms associated with hypotension and insufficient coronary artery filling. Finally, the Paramedic should ask about shortness of breath. In some cases, particularly protracted and untreated atrial fibrillation, the patient will develop backward failure and pulmonary edema.

2. *What is the cause of the "fluttering" and why would it invoke anxiety?*

   The fluttering in the patient's heart, called palpitations (i.e., the patient's awareness of one's heartbeat), often accompanies dysrhythmias that reduce blood pressure. This loss of blood pressure can induce anxiety or fear in some patients.

Examination

1. *What are the elements of the physical examination of a patient with suspected new onset atrial fibrillation?*

   A baseline neurological examination is indicated. Atrial fibrillation, especially paroxysmal atrial fibrillation, can cause strokes as mural thrombus detach and circulate through the carotids to the brain.

   The patient should also receive a thorough pulmonary examination as well. The patient is at risk for pulmonary embolism arising from prolonged bedrest for the hip fracture.

2. *Why is a 12-lead ECG a critical element in this examination?*

   Elderly women often have atypical presentations for myocardial infarction including sudden unexplained weakness as well as new onset atrial fibrillation.

Assessment

1. *What were the symptoms, in the symptom complex, that led the Paramedic to the diagnosis?*

   The sudden onset of weakness in the elderly made the Paramedic suspect there may be a cardiac origin to the complaint as well as the irregularly irregular pulse.

2. *What diagnosis did the Paramedic announce to the patient?*

   A diagnosis of error of automaticity would most likely confuse the patient. However, a diagnosis of suspected atrial fibrillation would not, provided it was accompanied by an explanation that it is an irregular heart rhythm.

Treatment

1. *What is the standard of care of patients with suspected errors of automaticity?*

   Typically, it is beyond the means of the Paramedic to ascertain the exact etiology of the error of automaticity. Therefore, it is incumbent on the Paramedic to ensure adequate oxygenation and circulation as well as correct any hypoglycemia. If the patient is symptomatic, certain pharmacological measures may be necessary, each according to the dysrhythmia and supportive care.

2. *What are some of the patient-specific concerns and considerations that the Paramedic should consider when applying this plan of care that is intended to treat a broad patient population presenting with atrial fibrillation?*

   If the patient is unstable, it may be necessary to perform cardioversion. However, in this case cardioversion should be avoided if at all possible. Cardioversion can dislodge mural thrombi and lead to a "shower of strokes."

Evaluation

1. *What are some of the predictable complications associated with atrial fibrillation with rapid ventricular response?*

   Hypotension is often a consequence of new onset atrial fibrillation with a rapid ventricular response, secondary to loss of the atrial kick and 30% of the cardiac output. A simple intravenous fluid bolus increases preload, augments the end-diastolic volume, and improves cardiac output: $SV \times HR = CO$.

2. *What are some of the predictable complications associated with the treatments for sustained wide complex tachycardia?*

   Overly aggressive fluid resuscitation can strain an already compromised heart, leading to backward failure and pulmonary edema. The ensuing hypoxia can worsen cardiac function, resulting in a downward spiral of hypoxia and hypotension that can result in cardiac arrest.

Disposition

1. *What is the most appropriate transport decision that will get the patient to definitive care?*

   Atrial fibrillation is such a common dysrhythmia that most general hospitals are prepared to evaluate and stabilize any patient. Treatment in most cases is started with anticoagulation in the hospital, with a long-term goal of conversion to a normal sinus rhythm in the future.

2. *What are some of the transportation considerations?*

   If the patient in this case was unstable, the Paramedic might consider transportation to a cardiac center where the physicians are more experienced with these cases.

Practice Questions
Multiple Choice

1. a
2. c
3. a
4. d
5. c
6. d
7. a
8. b
9. a
10. b
11. a
12. a
13. a
14. c
15. d

Short Answer

16. The origin of dysrhythmia, or arrhythmogenesis, is either errors of automaticity or errors of conduction. ECG clues to either can help determine which treatments are most effective.

17. The three chemical factors influencing errors of automaticity are hypoxia, acidosis, and hyperkalemia.

18. The suspected causes of atrial fibrillation are thyrotoxicosis, electrolyte imbalances such as hypocalcemia, acute alcohol intoxication, acute myocardial infarction, pericarditis, and pulmonary embolism.

19. Digitalis produces a positive inotropic effect and a negative chronotropic effect, thereby increasing output while slowing the heart.

20. A minor illness, such as the flu, leads to nausea, vomiting, and/or diarrhea. This, in turn, leads to digitalis toxicity. Digitalis toxicity leads to nausea, vomiting, and diarrhea, and so the cycle continues.

Fill in the Blank

21. dominance

22. accelerated idioventricular rhythm

23. prematurity

24. coupling interval

25. syncope

Chapter 5
Case Study
Chief Concern

1. *What are some of the possible cardiac causes of Mrs. Beckerman's weakness?*

   Cardiac problems can be broken down into problems of the myocardium (i.e., myocardial infarction), problems of the valves (i.e., mitral regurgitation), and problems of the electrical system (i.e., conduction disorders). Conduction disorders can be further broken down into disorders of conduction or disorders of automaticity.

2. *How can the dizziness be related?*

   As the dispatch information contained a clue (her heart was racing), a tachydysrhythmia cannot be ruled out. Cardiac output is a function of heart rate times stroke volume. An increase in one and/or the other can increase the cardiac output. An excessive increase (e.g., tachydysrhythmia) can actually lead to a decrease in cardiac output. In this case, a tachycardia can lead to insufficient ventricular filling secondary to a shortened diastole.

History

1. *What are the important elements of the history that a Paramedic should obtain?*

   When confronted with a tachydysrhythmia, the Paramedic should ascertain the following, in order of probability, following a standard OPQRST/SAMPLE history. First, the Paramedic should ask about the presence of palpitations, then dizziness. Next, the Paramedic should ask about any difficulty breathing or chest/neck pressure/pain. Finally, the Paramedic should ask if the patient lost consciousness or has nausea.

2. *What history would explain the diaphoresis?*

   As diaphoresis is an autonomic system response, specifically the release of epinephrine, the stimulus for this response could be hypoxia, hypoglycemia, or hypotension. Therefore, the history should also include the presence or absence of pulmonary disease, including recent events that would lead to a suspicion of pulmonary embolism, diabetes, or internal bleeding, such as recent trauma.

Examination

1. *What are the elements of the physical examination of a patient with suspected tachydysrhythmia?*

   After performing a primary assessment, the Paramedic should take the time to perform a cardiovascular examination along with vital signs and an ECG.

2. *Why is a 12-lead ECG a critical element in this examination?*

The 12-lead ECG, combined with clinical information, may help the Paramedic determine the type and origin of the tachydysrhythmia.

Assessment

1. *What were the symptoms, in the symptom complex, that led the Paramedic to the diagnosis?*

A dysrhythmia must be considered in any case of near-syncope. Near-syncope, combined with dizziness, diaphoresis, and pallor, is suggestive of loss of blood pressure.

2. *What diagnosis did the Paramedic announce to the patient?*

Although ventricular tachycardia sounds ominous, and can rapidly deteriorate into ventricular fibrillation, the chance of successful conversion (either chemical or electrical) is very high. Therefore, treatment on-scene to stabilize the patient is warranted in this case and the Paramedic should explain that to the patient in terms of a risk–benefit scenario.

Treatment

1. *What is the standard of care of stable patients with suspected ventricular tachycardia?*

Stable patients with suspected ventricular tachycardia can be treated with one of three medications. The first, and most common, is amiodarone administered in 150 mg bolus over 10 minutes. While it is possible to administer as much as 2.2 grams in one day, most Paramedics stop after the third bolus or 450 mg of amiodarone.

The next drug of choice is lidocaine, a Vaughn–Williams class I sodium channel blocker. Administered in bolus according to weight, in 0.5 to 1 mg increments to total 3 mg per kg, caution must be exercised as lidocaine can induce hypotension, thereby making a stable patient unstable.

The last drug is procainamide. Procainamide is effective but difficult to administer in the field. Administration is lengthy and has multiple contraindications and precautions.

2. *What are some of the patient-specific concerns and considerations that the Paramedic should consider when applying this plan of care that is intended to treat a broad patient population presenting with stable ventricular tachycardia?*

Although each medication has its individual complications, the greatest risk is the deterioration from stable ventricular tachycardia to unstable ventricular tachycardia to cardiac arrest and ventricular fibrillation. As these changes can occur within minutes, the Paramedic must be prepared to electively cardiovert the patient at a moment's notice.

Evaluation

1. *What are some of the predictable complications associated with a synchronized elective cardioversion?*

The complication with the greatest risk is the patient's deterioration into ventricular fibrillation and sudden cardiac death. For this reason alone, an elective synchronized cardioversion should only be performed if complete ALS equipment is available including intubation equipment, venous access supplies, medications, and so on.

2. *What is the greatest risk in applying this plan of care?*

This risk is greatest if the Paramedic fails to press the synchronization button. Inadvertent misfires can cause the energy to be delivered during the vulnerable period of repolarization, the period of relative refractoriness in the second half of the T wave.

If deterioration into ventricular fibrillation should occur, with or without elective synchronized cardioversion, the Paramedic must remember to turn off the synchronization button on the ECG monitor before delivering another countershock.

Disposition

1. *What is the most appropriate transport decision that will get the patient to definitive care?*

The patient in this case is going to need close monitoring for further episodes of ventricular tachycardia, including antiarrhythmic infusions and perhaps electrophysiology studies. Transportation to a cardiac center is warranted in this case.

2. *What other concerns should the Paramedic have for this patient?*

The Paramedic should be concerned about the reoccurrence of the dysrhythmia and should prepare an antidysrhythmic medication infusion.

Practice Questions
Multiple Choice

1. b
2. c
3. d
4. c
5. d
6. b
7. a
8. d

9. b
10. b
11. a
12. d
13. a
14. d
15. c

Short Answer

16. The two types of errors of conduction are (1) re-entry, in which the impulse circles around conducting tissue, and (2) blocks, in which impulses stop along the conduction pathway.

17. The heart normally fills during diastole. During a normal cardiac cycle, the heart is diastole two-thirds of the time. With tachycardia above 100 beats per minute, the heart is in diastole one-half of the time. In rates above 150 beats per minute, the heart is in diastole only one-third of the time. This does not allow sufficient time for coronary artery filling at a time when the myocardium demand, the mVO_2, is highest.

18. Valsalva is performed by asking the patient to take a deep breath and hold it. This increases intrathoracic pressure, compresses great vessels, and reduces venous return (i.e., preload). When the pressure is released and blood rushes to the heart, baroreceptors signal the heart to slow to accept the additional blood volume via the parasympathetic nervous system.

19. Secondary to changes of aging, the bundle branches are dysfunctional during sustained tachycardia. This results in temporary blocks that resolve when the tachycardia resolves.

20. After determining that the patient is stable, the Paramedic should obtain a 12-lead ECG. Analyzing the 12-lead ECG, the Paramedic should look for concordance, extreme axis deviation, and signs of A/V dissociation.

Fill in the Blank

21. sinoatrial node re-entry tachycardia
22. orthodromic
23. A/V re-entry tachycardia

24. abruptly, gradually
25. amiodarone

Chapter 6
Case Study
Chief Concern

1. *What are some of the possible causes of cardiac-related syncope?*

   The three causes of cardiac-related syncope are (1) ventricular diastolic disorders, such as cardiac tamponade; (2) dysrhythmia, either tachycardia or bradycardia; and (3) outflow obstructions, such as pulmonary embolism.

2. *Why is the cause of the fall more important than the fall?*

   Syncope while standing can be related to a lethal dysrhythmia, such as ventricular tachycardia or a pulmonary embolism.

History

1. *What are the important elements of the history that a Paramedic should obtain?*

   As ischemia-induced heart block is high on the list of differentials, the Paramedic should illicit a history suggestive of an acute coronary syndrome.

Preceding past the history of present illness, the Paramedic should obtain a complete past medical history, focusing especially on the patient's medications. Many medications have cardiac effects and some, such as those in the Vaughn–Williams classifications, are implicated in bradycardia.

2. *What is the symptom pattern associated with a bradydysrhythmia?*

In many cases, patients with bradycardia are asymptomatic or complain of mild symptoms such as dizziness, lightheadedness, or near-syncope. These complaints are all worthy of investigation and a cardiac monitor.

Examination

1. *What are the elements of the physical examination of a patient with suspected bradydysrhythmia?*

Beyond the standard cardiovascular examination, the Paramedic needs to obtain an ECG and carefully examine that ECG.

2. *What is the advantage of a 12-lead ECG in this case?*

In some cases, a 12-lead ECG can offer additional information, such as QT interval, that is measured and recorded on the printout. This feature can be convenient in the field where calipers are rare.

Assessment

1. *What diagnosis did the Paramedic announce to the patient?*

Any irregularity of the heart rhythm is worthy of a diagnostic workup. A simple explanation of "dropped beats" should be sufficient to convince the patient that it would be prudent to go to the hospital and get it checked out.

2. *Why is a 12-lead ECG a critical element in this examination?*

It appears to be a high-degree sinus arrest that could be a function of fibrosis secondary to changes of aging. However, because of the acute nature of the event, the Paramedic suspected occlusion of either circumflex or the right coronary artery. ECG changes in the lateral leads suggest that the circumflex is involved while ECG changes in the inferior leads suggest the right coronary artery is involved.

Treatment

1. *What is the standard of care of patients with suspected bradydysrhythmia?*

As the patient is not grossly symptomatic, routine care for a patient with observed syncope consists of O_2, IV, and ECG. It might be prudent to have atropine available if needed as well as a transcutaneous pacemaker.

2. *What are some of the patient-specific concerns that the Paramedic should consider when applying this plan of care that is intended to treat a broad patient population presenting with bradycardia?*

As bradycardia can be a precursor to potentially more lethal conditions, the Paramedic must remain vigilant for changes in the patient's condition. The Paramedic must always be prepared to initiate CPR as well as external pacing with the patient if needed.

Evaluation

1. *What are some of the predictable complications associated with an SA node infarction?*

As the SA node is the dominant pacemaker if the SA node is infarcted, a secondary pacemaker, such as the AV node, will likely create a junctional escape rhythm. This rhythm, while not ideal, is generally well tolerated unless (like this patient) there are other medical factors complicating care.

2. *What are some of the predictable complications associated with the treatments for sustained wide complex tachycardia?*

While the use of atropine in this case is acceptable practice, it must be understood that atropine will stress the already compromised SA node, perhaps hastening the onset of infarction. However, the therapeutic goal (increased heart rate to support a minimal cerebral perfusion) makes the risk acceptable provided the Paramedic has the tools (i.e., a transcutaneous pacemaker). This is applied if the patient should experience SA node infarction and symptomatic bradycardia from the junctional escape rhythm.

Disposition

1. *What is the most appropriate transport decision that will get the patient to definitive care?*

   This patient needs transportation to an interventional cardiology center, provided the patient can be transported to the cardiac center in reasonable time.

2. *Why would an interventional cardiology center be helpful?*

   The patient appears to need an emergent cardiac catheterization to restore blood flow to the SA node. It is also predictable that, even with reperfusion of the SA node, the cardiologist might suggest a pacemaker in the future.

Practice Questions

Multiple Choice

1. d
2. a
3. a
4. a
5. c
6. a
7. b
8. c
9. d
10. b
11. a
12. a
13. b
14. c
15. c

Short Answer

16. The formula for cardiac output is heart rate times stroke volume. While the body has mechanisms that increase the heart rate to compensate for decreased stroke volume, the body's mechanisms have a limited ability to increase the stroke volume to compensate for a low heart rate. Therefore, bradycardia has a tendency, below approximately 50 beats per minute, to compensate.

17. First, vasovagal syncope is an increase in parasympathetic tone, via vagal stimulation, causing a cardioinhibitory effect and bradycardia. Simultaneously, there is sympathetic suppression which causes vasodilation, resulting in decreased venous return (i.e., preload) and therefore decreased stroke volume. The combination of decreased heart rate and decreased stroke volume leads to decreased cardiac output and diminished cerebral perfusion. Diminished cerebral perfusion leads to syncope.

18. A third degree heart block implies infarction of the conductive tissue and a complete heart block. As a result, there is no connection between the atria and ventricles (i.e., A/V dissociation).

19. The two pacemaker pad placements are anterior–anterior and anterior–posterior. While anterior–anterior is more common among Paramedics that use dual service defib/pacer pads, the anterior–posterior placement may be more effective, causing less pectoral muscle contraction.

20. The triad of symptoms associated with pacemaker failure is syncope, palpitations, and bradycardia.

Fill in the Blank

21. Type II
22. sinus arrest
23. Wenckebach's
24. burst suppression
25. twiddler

Chapter 7
Case Study
Chief Concern

1. *What is the importance of early bystander CPR?*

   With the majority of cardiac arrest occurring in a prehospital setting, early bystander CPR can, in some instances, reverse a lethal rhythm. In the majority of cases, it is a holding action until the arrival of a defibrillator. In short, CPR increases the window of opportunity for a successful defibrillation. CPR may also indicate that an emergency response has been activated and that emergency medical services are on the way.

2. *What is the importance of early citizen defibrillation?*

   Early defibrillation provides the greatest chance of reversal of ventricular fibrillation.

History

1. *What is the importance of having an AED on-scene?*

   Cardiac arrest of a cardiac origin (i.e., sudden cardiac death) is amenable to immediate defibrillation. The AED is pervasive in the United States and can be found at most sporting venues, gyms, schools, and even airports.

2. *What is the implication of a "do not shock" warning from the AED?*

   The fact that the AED was at the patient's side almost immediately implies that the arrest may not be of cardiac origin, or that the cause of the arrest was so devastating that survival is unlikely.

Examination

1. *What are the causes of pulseless electrical activity?*

   There are several mnemonics to help the Paramedic remember the possible etiologies of pulseless electrical activity (PEA) such as ITCH PAD, THE HAT, and five H's and five T's.

2. *Which of the causes of pulseless electrical activity can a Paramedic have an impact on while in the field?*

   Although the American Heart Association advocates for the five H's and five T's, ITCH PAD may be more useful for Paramedics. The causes listed in ITCH PAD are amenable to prehospital treatment by Paramedics. The mnemonic ITCH PAD stands for infarction, tension pneumothorax, cardiac tamponade, five H's—hypoxia, hypovolemia, hypothermia, hyperkalemia, hypomagnesemia—pulmonary embolism, acidosis, and drugs.

Assessment

1. *What are the next priorities for the patient with a return of spontaneous circulation (ROSC)?*

   The key to survival is stabilizing the patient hemodynamically, as well as preparing the patient for therapeutic hypothermia, if indicated. The twin dangers for the patient with ROSC are acidosis and hypoxia, though it is prudent to check a blood glucose level as well.

2. *What is "reverse CPR"?*

   Many Paramedics do what is called reverse CPR. After confirming pulses at the carotid, there is a call for a pulse at the radial and a blood pressure. Provided the blood pressure is adequate, many medical authorities call for an antidysrhythmic medication to prevent relapse.

   Next, the Paramedic checks the patient's respiratory status, breathing, and airway. If the patient is breathing adequately, he or she should remain on high-flow, high-concentration oxygen. However, in many cases the patient is either ventilated manually or placed on a transport ventilator.

   Even if the patient is breathing, many medical authorities advocate that the patient be sedated, intubated, and ventilated to maintain a normal end-tidal carbon dioxide level.

Treatment

1. *What are the indications for therapeutic hypothermia?*

   The indications for therapeutic hypothermia include, in many jurisdictions, a pubescent patient with a ROSC GCS of eight or less and whose airway is controlled. Airway control is often accomplished by use of sedatives and/or paralytics.

2. *What is the standard of care for therapeutic hypothermia status post-return of spontaneous circulation?*

While procedures may vary, most start with the application of chemical ice packs at the neck, axilla, and groin after removal of clothing, then changing the ice packs every 10 to 15 minutes or as often as vital signs are obtained. Two large needles are then used to obtain venous access and 2 liters of chilled, 32°F to 34°F saline are infused. In some cases, either 20 mL/kg or 2 liters is infused, whichever is the smaller amount. The therapeutic goal is to lower the patient's core temperature to between 32°C and 34°C (90°F to 93°F), though in most cases only a 2°C to 4°C drop in temperature can be anticipated in the short time that the patient is with the Paramedic in the field.

Evaluation

1. *What are the hemodynamic parameters that the Paramedic should maintain?*

The Paramedic should maintain a mean arterial pressure (MAP) of greater than 65 mmHg. This helps assure minimal blood pressure for cerebral perfusion pressure.

2. *How does the Paramedic maintain these hemodynamic parameters?*

This can be accomplished by means of fluid bolus (2 liters should already be infusing) and/or use of dopamine. Likewise, hypertension should be controlled. Systolic blood pressures above 200 mmHg are treated with either nitroglycerin 400 mcg (0.4 mg) or a beta blocker such as metoprolol. A typical dose is 5 mg over 5 minutes every 5 minutes until either the blood pressure systolic is less than 200 mmHg or a maximum of 15 mg is used.

Disposition

1. *What is the most appropriate transport decision that will get the patient to definitive care?*

It is imperative that therapeutic hypothermia be continued for 12 to 24 hours. Therefore, only those hospitals that can sustain the field-induced hypothermia should receive the ROSC patients. These hospitals should, preferably have interventional cardiology capabilities in case an emergent angioplasty is needed.

2. *Why was a 12-lead ECG indicated following the return of spontaneous circulation?*

In many instances, the origin of sudden cardiac death is an underlying acute myocardial infarction.

Practice Questions
Multiple Choice

1. a
2. c
3. c
4. a
5. d
6. d
7. d
8. a
9. c
10. d
11. c
12. b
13. d
14. d
15. a

Short Answer

16. The four identifiable causes of cardiac arrest, from a mechanistic perspective, are (1) decreased preload, (2) decreased contractility, (3) errors of automaticity, and (4) increased afterload.

17. A tricyclic overdose is initially treated with sodium bicarbonate. If the QRS or QT interval remains prolonged, then it may be necessary to administer magnesium sulfate.

18. Although exhaled air contains sufficient oxygen to sustain life (i.e., 17%), it also contains carbon dioxide (approximately 4%). This carbon dioxide increases the acid load in the patient. Ambient air contains less than 1% carbon dioxide and does not contribute to the acid load.

19. The Paramedic's therapeutic goals during resuscitation of the patient in pulseless electrical activity (PEA) are reversal of acidosis through controlled ventilation and reversal of hypoxemia.

20. Overly aggressive hyperventilation, leading to air stacking and air trapping, decreases respiration of carbon dioxide. This leads to worsening acidosis, as well as increased intrathoracic pressures, that compress great vessels, reduce venous return, and decrease cardiac output and blood pressure.

Fill in the Blank

21. asystole

22. alkalosis

23. cricoid pressure

24. thoracic pump

25. conductive/cardiac pathway

Chapter 8

Case Study

Chief Concern

1. *What are some of the possible causes of shortness of breath for a trucker?*

   Possible etiologies could include carbon monoxide poisoning from truck fumes, emphysema from smoking, pulmonary edema secondary to heart failure or myocardial infarction, or pulmonary embolism.

2. *Which of the possible causes of shortness of breath could be directly related to the patient being a truck driver?*

   A truck driver may be exposed to carbon monoxide poisoning from exhaust fumes.

History

1. *What are the important elements of the history that a Paramedic should obtain?*

   Considering both the shortness of breath and the swelling in the legs, the Paramedic must consider pulmonary embolism along with cardiac etiologies such as atrial fibrillation. Truckers are prone to deep vein thrombus. The combination of venous stasis from bent knees, hypercoagulability, and inflammation (together referred to as Virchow's triad) creates the likelihood of pulmonary embolism.

2. *What is the symptom pattern associated with pulmonary embolism?*

   The traditional triad of symptoms that indicate PE in a patient is unexplained dyspnea, pleuritic-type chest pain, and hemoptysis. Together, these three signs are strongly suggestive of PE, although individually they are less supportive of the disorder.

Examination

1. *What are the elements of the physical examination of a patient with suspected deep vein thrombus?*

   The affected limb tends to be swollen, reddened, and painful to the touch. Although measuring the mid-calf in the prehospital setting is impractical, a manual comparison of the two limbs can help the Paramedic estimate the increased girth as well as warmth. Careful palpation will tend to illicit point tenderness as well.

2. *Why is a Homans' sign a critical element in this examination?*

   Although the Homans' sign is only 50% reliable, it is still considered a cardinal sign in the examination. The Homans' sign is elicited by asking the patient to dorsiflex the extended foot on the affected side.

Assessment

1. *What diagnosis did the Paramedic announce to the patient?*

   Hypoxia in the face of high-flow, high-concentration oxygen is, by definition, Type I respiratory failure.

2. *Why is a 12-lead ECG a critical element in this examination?*

   The possibility of myocardial infarction may exist. However, in this case the history is leading the Paramedic to suspect pulmonary embolism. If a PE occurred, then the 12-lead ECG may show a classic S1Q3T3 pattern and/or right heart strain/cor pulmonale, secondary to pulmonary hypertension.

Treatment

1. *What is the standard of care of patients with suspected pulmonary embolism?*

   A cardinal sign of PE is persistent hypoxia (Type I respiratory failure) despite the administration of high-flow, high-concentration oxygen. Little else can be done in the prehospital setting.

2. *What additional treatment might be considered in this case?*

   CPAP is a consideration, as increasing the partial pressure of oxygen may increase the $SaPO_2$.

Evaluation

1. *What are some of the predictable complications associated with a pulmonary embolism?*

   Another pulmonary embolism is always a risk. The triad of sudden unexplained hypotension, syncope, and refractory hypoxia suggests a saddle embolism.

2. *What are some of the predictable complications associated with a saddle embolism?*

   The longer the patient remains hypoxic, the greater the developing acid load and the greater the possibility of cardiac arrest. The loss of venous return in a saddle embolism leads to loss of preload and cardiac output. Often, these patients display pulseless electrical activity on the monitor.

Disposition

1. *What is the most appropriate transport decision that will get the patient to definitive care?*

   Transportation to the closest emergency department is probably acceptable. The survival of the patient in these cases is very low.

2. *What are some of the transportation considerations?*

   In consideration of the low survivability of a massive pulmonary embolism, prudence should be exercised to ensure that no other fatalities occur. The lights and siren response markedly increases the chance of an ambulance accident.

Practice Questions
Multiple Choice

1. a		9. a	
2. a		10. d	
3. d		11. b	
4. d		12. d	
5. c		13. c	
6. c		14. d	
7. d		15. b	
8. d			

Short Answer

16. Type I respiratory failure is the inability of the lungs to diffuse adequate oxygen into the blood.

17. The triad of symptoms associated with pulmonary embolism is made up of unexplained dyspnea, pleuritic chest pain, and hemoptysis.

18. The classic 12-lead ECG changes with pulmonary embolism are S1Q3T3—or a large S wave in Lead I, Q wave in Lead III, and an inverted T wave in Lead III.

19. The Fick equation calculates the amount of oxygen delivered to the tissues. It equals the cardiac output times the arterial oxygen amount minus the venous oxygen amount.

20. Both CPAP and PEEP work by providing positive pressure that stents the airway open and permits longer diffusion times for respiration.

Fill in the Blank

21. deep vein thrombus

22. Homans'

23. pulmonary embolism

24. AIDS

25. rigors

Chapter 9

Case Study

Chief Concern

1. *What are some of the possible respirator-related causes of shortness of breath?*

   The case suggests that the boss is a cigarette smoker with pulmonary disease. He could have asthma, chronic bronchitis (which is likely since he had a smoker's cough), and/or emphysema.

2. *How is the patient's shortness of breath possibly related to the early morning?*

   Often smokers who sleep lying prone build up congestion during the night. Coupled with open mouth breathing due to air hunger, which leads to dried secretions, mucous plugs can develop that block air passages.

History

1. *What are the important elements of the history that a Paramedic should obtain?*

   In the S portion of the SAMPLE history, the Paramedic should consider the use of HAPISOCS. The information obtained can help narrow down the possible etiologies of the shortness of breath. It is also important to get the list of medications, focusing on the use of beta/agonists (frequency) as well as steroids.

2. *What is the symptom pattern for Type II respiratory failure?*

   Patients with Type II respiratory failure have trouble exhaling carbon dioxide. Although the body has a capacity to compensate for the acidosis that results from carbon dioxide retention, that capacity is limited. When it is exceeded, the body decompensates.

Examination

1. *What are the elements of the physical examination of a patient with suspected Type II respiratory failure?*

   After ensuring the patient has a patent airway that can be maintained, and that oxygen or ventilation is being provided as needed, the Paramedic should proceed, in a head-to-toe fashion, with a pulmonary examination. Starting with the patient's mental status, since hypercarbia causes somnolence, the Paramedic should assess for nasal flaring, open mouth breathing, pursed-lip breathing, accessory muscle use, and central/peripheral cyanosis. Next, the Paramedic should listen for breath sounds and palpate the chest wall for fremitus and fractures.

2. *What assessment tools are critical elements in this examination?*

   The three tools that should be used are the ECG (used to look for ectopy, a sign of hypoxia), pulse oximeter, and an end-tidal capnography. These three tools can help the Paramedic determine the patient's cardiopulmonary status.

Assessment

1. *What is the significance of the elevated end-tidal carbon dioxide level?*

   The level is significant because the body is no longer able to compensate for the elevated carbon dioxide level. The somnolence confirms that the boss is decompensating.

2. *What does the use of a rescue inhaler suggest?*

   Unresponsiveness to a rescue inhaler suggests that the airway is constricted and the medication cannot get to the airway to open it.

Treatment

1. *What is the standard of care of patients with suspected Type II respiratory failure?*

   Ventilation is key. Although the patient retains carbon dioxide, the blood is acidotic and the oxyhemoglobin curve shifts to the right. The result is inefficient use of oxygen and hypoxia.

Traditionally, a two-fold attack is made to open the airway. First, a nebulizer is used to get a beta/agonist into the lungs through inhalation. Then, subcutaneous epinephrine is used to get a beta/agonist to the lungs via the capillary–alveolar interface.

2. *What are some of the patient-specific concerns and considerations that the Paramedic should consider when applying this plan of care that is intended to treat a broad patient population presenting with acute respiratory failure?*

Epinephrine—and beta/agonists in general—stimulate the heart, causing tachycardia. Stressing an already stressed heart (i.e., a hypoxic heart filled with acidotic blood) is a formula for cardiac irritability, ventricular fibrillation, and sudden cardiac death.

Evaluation

1. *What are some of the predictable complications associated with ventilation of the emphysemic patient in Type II respiratory failure?*

Blebs (or bullae) form on the surface of the emphysema patient's lungs. Positive pressure ventilation can lead to rupture of these blebs, creating a pneumothorax that can quickly progress to a tension pneumothorax with continued positive pressure ventilation.

2. *What are some of the predictable complications associated with the treatments for acute respiratory distress?*

The sudden loss of both oxygenation and ventilation can cause this patient to decompensate into cardiac arrest. Relief of the pneumothorax, by needle decompression, and the resumption of careful positive pressure ventilation, is needed to prevent the effects of hypoxia and hypercarbia.

Disposition

1. *What is the most appropriate transport decision that will get the patient to definitive care?*

This patient has high acuity and needs to be transported emergently to a tertiary care center with critical care capabilities.

2. *Why choose this hospital even if it means bypassing other hospitals?*

In this case, expert pulmonary management will be necessary, including chest tube insertion as well as ventilator support.

Practice Questions
Multiple Choice

1. a
2. d
3. b
4. c
5. b
6. c
7. a
8. c
9. a
10. b
11. b
12. b
13. d
14. b
15. c

Short Answer

16. Type II respiratory failure is the result of carbon dioxide retention.

17. The causes of wheezing are asthma, stasis (PE), toxins, heart issues (APE), mechanical issues (FBAO), allergies, trauma (pneumothorax), infection, and chronic obstructive pulmonary disease (COPD).

18. Aspirin can induce asthma and beta blockers can lead to bronchospasm.

19. Bronchospasm leads to retention of carbon dioxide. In turn, this increases blood acid and shifts the oxyhemoglobin curve, leading to hypoxia. Increased breath and increased work of breathing leads to increased acid load until the patient's acid load causes massive vasodilation, shock, and death.

20. With pulmonary disease, carbon dioxide (the normal stimulus to breathe) is elevated. However, the body compensates by retaining bicarbonate in the kidneys, buffering the acid created by the carbon dioxide. The resulting compensated respiratory acidosis is neutral (i.e., pH 7.35 to 7.45), and there is no stimulus to breathe. The body then depends on the secondary drive to breathe (hypoxia). When oxygen is administered to patients with hypoxic drive, breathing stops altogether.

Fill in the Blank

21. 10

22. sodium bisulfite

23. ibuprofen

24. PEEP

25. 55

Chapter 10

Case Study

Chief Concern

1. *What are some of the possible causes of convulsions in an infant?*

   Initial concern has to be for causes of hypoxia, such as FBAO, hypoglycemia (secondary to toxic ingestion), and hyperthermia. The last cause, hyperthermia, may be most common. Any infant with a fever should suggest to the Paramedic the possibility of a febrile seizure and/or meningitis.

2. *What immediate actions should the Paramedics take to safeguard this patient?*

   A primary assessment should help resolve any issues of the airway, ventilation, and so on. As the child is apparently post-ictal, supportive care (i.e., airway management, oxygen, etc.) at a basic level is all that may be needed.

History

1. *What are the important elements of the history that a Paramedic should obtain?*

   Since this is a first-time seizure, it eliminates the possibility of noncompliance and a breakthrough seizure. The obvious course of action is to ask the mother about the fever (i.e., onset, duration, etc.). The OPQRST SAMPLE may be useful in this case. However, the Paramedic should keep an open mind to other etiologies of a new onset convulsion such as alcohol (isopropyl alcohol is used to "rub down" the fever), stroke (infants can have strokes), and accidental ingestions of medications (one pill can kill). However, that is not likely in this case because of the child's developmental age.

2. *What is the symptom pattern associated with a seizure?*

   Most seizures start with an aura, which would be difficult to ascertain in this case, and then a clonic–tonic phase, followed by a post-ictal phase. The description makes it sound like the child is post-ictal. However, it would be important to get a full description of the seizure. Was it generalized or a partial complex seizure with secondary generalization? If it was the latter, then where did the Jacksonian march originate?

Examination

1. *What are the elements of the physical examination of a patient with suspected seizure disorder?*

   Following a careful primary assessment, the Paramedic should proceed with a head-to-toe examination starting with the fontanels. Bulging fontanels are a sign of increased intracranial pressure. The Paramedic should examine the eyes for reactivity and the presence or absence of doll's eyes, then end by examining the extremities for signs of injury.

2. *Why is an examination for meningeal signs a critical element in the neurological examination?*

   As high fever and seizures are consistent with meningitis as well as otitis media-induced febrile seizures, the Paramedic should assess for photophobia, nuchal rigidity, and Brudzinski's sign.

Assessment

1. *What diagnosis did the Paramedic announce to the patient's mother?*

   Although the obvious explanation of febrile seizure is introduced, the possibility of other etiologies is also entertained.

2. *Why should the Paramedic insist that the child be seen in the emergency department?*

Patients with a first-time seizure, even a pediatric febrile seizure, should be seen in the emergency department.

Treatment

1. *What is the standard of care of patients with suspected febrile seizure?*

While providing a supportive and protective environment during the post-ictal period, the Paramedic's care should focus on the primary assessment. If possible, and as the seizure subsides, the patient should be rolled into a lateral recumbent position (the recovery position) to allow passive drainage of secretions and to prevent aspiration. The Paramedic should suction as needed with a Yankauer suction tip to clear secretions collecting in the buccal pocket.

2. *Why is the use of an oropharyngeal airway discouraged?*

Use of the oropharyngeal airway is generally discouraged as it can stimulate retching and vomiting, potentially leading to aspiration. Use of the nasopharyngeal airway could be considered, especially if the patient's recovery seems slow or there is a concern about a repeated seizure. The application of oxygen in the immediate post-ictal period may reverse hypoxia associated with the seizure or other unknown etiologies, such as carbon monoxide poisoning.

Evaluation

1. *What are some of the predictable complications associated with a seizure?*

The most concerning complication is status epilepticus, which occurred in this case. Status epilepticus can be one prolonged seizure (greater than five minutes), two or more seizures without an intervening period of lucidity, or a prolonged twilight.

2. *What are the treatments if this complication occurs?*

Following airway management and administration of oxygen, the Paramedic should stop the seizure activity. The drug of choice is a benzodiazepine, administered either via venous access or rectally if need be. Midazolam is an alternative medication for status epilepticus. However, diazepam is preferred because midazolam takes three times longer to reach peak therapeutic effect (or two to three minutes) when compared with diazepam. Nonetheless, midazolam can be given nasally if venous access cannot be obtained.

Disposition

1. *What is the most appropriate transport decision that will get the patient to definitive care?*

The emergency department is appropriate. Most cases of status epilepticus can be managed with the medications available in the emergency department.

2. *Why should the Paramedic choose to go to a hospital with an available operating room?*

Benzodiazepines are thought to have only 70% effectiveness in stopping status epilepticus, so it is necessary to go to a hospital where anesthesia is available. Anesthesia is used to break persistent seizures that are unresponsive to benzodiazepines.

Practice Questions
Multiple Choice

1. a
2. c
3. b
4. c
5. b
6. b
7. b
8. c

9. a
10. c
11. a
12. d
13. c
14. b
15. b

Short Answer

16. Administration of naxolone to the newborn of an addicted mother may precipitate a seizure. Stimulation and assistance with a bag–mask assembly is usually sufficient to restore breathing. However, if the Paramedic administers the narcotic, and the newborn subsequently hypoventilates, it is safe to administer the naxolone.

17. An electrical storm is an imbalance of excitatory and inhibitory neurotransmitters that cascades across the brain's neural pathways, creating chaos. It is similar to a disruption in the sodium–potassium balance in the heart that leads to ventricular fibrillation.

18. Often starting with an automatism, such as a twitching finger or fluttering eyelid, a partial complex seizure spreads by secondary generalization across the entire body. This activity, which can be witnessed by a Paramedic, is called a Jacksonian march.

19. Brudzinski's sign is seen when the patient's head is lifted off the pillow and the legs lift involuntarily. Kernig's sign is pain with extension of the knee when the hip is flexed.

20. During status epilepticus, there is ineffective ventilation, hypercarbia (leading to acidosis), and continuous muscle activity (leading to hyperthermia). Coupled together, acidosis and hyperthermia shift the oxyhemoglobin curve to the right, leading to hypoxia and cerebral anoxia. Eventually, the acid load leads to massive vasodilation, hypotension, and pancerebral ischemia.

Fill in the Blank

21. reticular activating system

22. unconsciousness

23. atonic

24. automatism, absence

25. aura

Chapter 11
Case Study
Chief Concern

1. *What are some of the possible causes of sudden headache?*

   A sudden headache, as opposed to a headache that steadily builds to a crescendo, is suspicious for a rapid event such as meningitis secondary to an infection, subdural hematoma secondary to trauma, rupture of a congenital A/V malformation, or a subarachnoid hemorrhage.

2. *How could the sudden headache be related to the patient's photophobia?*

   The presence of the photophobia should immediately alert the Paramedic to the possibility of meningitis/encephalitis. Photophobia is also present in subarachnoid hemorrhage.

History

1. *What are the important elements of the history that a Paramedic should obtain?*

   Following the OPQRST should provide the Paramedic with a sufficient history, although more detail may be needed about the time immediately preceding the headache. A comprehensive past medical history should also be obtained.

2. *What is the importance of the previous headache?*

   Approximately 30% to 50% of subarachnoid bleeds have what is called a sentinel leak. These warning leaks are a precursor to a much larger event in the future.

Examination

1. *What are the elements of the physical examination of a patient with suspected disorder of cerebral circulation?*

   The Paramedic should perform a vectored neurological examination that includes elements of a rapid trauma examination, to rule out head trauma, as well as a cardiovascular exam, since atrial fibrillation can lead to stroke. As the patient has a meningeal sign (i.e., photophobia), the Paramedic should assess for other meningeal signs including the presence of fever.

2. *Why is a blood glucose test a critical element in this examination?*

Hypoglycemia, along with hypoperfusion and hypotension, can create symptoms that mimic a stroke. Cerebral function depends on a constant supply of glucose, oxygen, and blood for circulation.

Assessment

1. *What diagnosis did the Paramedic announce to the patient?*

Although the patient presentation is consistent with a rupture of the middle cerebral artery that is presently a grade II on the SAH severity scale, it is probably fair if the Paramedic only states that the patient has a medically dangerous headache that needs immediate medical attention.

2. *What symptoms led the Paramedic to the diagnosis?*

The severe "worst headache of my life" coupled with associated nausea and vomiting is suggestive of a medically dangerous headache.

Treatment

1. *What is the standard of care of patients with suspected subarachnoid hemorrhage?*

In the prehospital setting, medical treatment consists of monitoring the patient and providing supportive care. If the patient's mean blood pressure gets above 130 mmHg, then use of beta blockers or low dose loop diuretics might be indicated. However, use of nitrates is discouraged as it raises the intracranial pressure. In some cases, the use of mannitol may also be called on.

2. *What are some of the patient-specific concerns that the Paramedic should consider when administering mannitol?*

Although mannitol is an osmotic diuretic that is efficient in lowering intracranial pressure, rebound swelling can occur later.

Evaluation

1. *What are some of the predictable complications associated with a subarachnoid hemorrhage?*

The greatest risk with a subarachnoid hemorrhage is rebleeding and/or seizures.

2. *What is the problem with rebleeding?*

Rebleeding can lead to seizures, which can lead to additional rebleeding.

Disposition

1. *What is the most appropriate transport decision that will get the patient to definitive care?*

This patient needs high level neurological care that can typically only be found at a tertiary center, one capable of doing brain surgery.

2. *What are some of the transportation considerations?*

In some cases, patients with a subarachnoid hemorrhage will not tolerate either bright lights (photophobia) or loud sounds (such as the siren). In many cases, those patients with a mild case (i.e., low grade) subarachnoid hemorrhage are purposely kept in a dark, quiet room so as to prevent rebleeds until surgery is ready.

Practice Questions
Multiple Choice

1. d
2. b
3. a
4. c
5. d
6. d
7. b
8. d

9. b
10. d
11. b
12. a
13. b
14. a
15. a

Short Answer

16. The Cincinnati Stroke Scale (CSS) starts with a smile, for facial symmetry, followed by pronator drift for extremity weakness and speech.

17. Loss of the same half of a visual field in both eyes (e.g., both right sides of the two visual fields) is called homonymous hemianopia and is a typical sign of an occipital lobe stroke. Patients with homonymous hemianopia often have a gaze preference, and they tend to look toward the side with the stroke. Patients with homonymous hemianopia may be startled as the Paramedic approaches because they have lost the ability to distinguish objects, or people, approaching them.

18. The stroke symptom pattern may include monoparesis (a weakness in just one limb), quadriparesis (a weakness in all four extremities), or hemiparesis (weakness in one side of the body).

19. Patients who have experienced a cerebellar stroke may exhibit slurred speech, a loss of balance, and a staggering gait similar to drunken staggers when walking (this condition is called ataxia). The patient may also have nystagmus, a flickering extraocular eye movement (EOM) observed when assessing the cardinal gazes. Some patients may even experience hiccups.

20. The Romberg test checks the patient's ability to stand in a steady, upright position with the eyes closed. To have the patient perform the Romberg test, the Paramedic should ask the patient to stand with her feet together and eyes closed. It is important that the patient close her eyes tightly to prevent sensory feedback that will help her compensate. A positive Romberg test occurs when the patient starts to sway, demonstrating truncal instability. This may be indicative of a cerebellar stroke.

Fill in the Blank

21. sentinel
22. thunderclap
23. basilar
24. humming
25. glucose testing

Chapter 12

Case Study

Chief Concern

1. *What are some of the possible causes of unexplained weakness?*

   Although the symptom pattern is peculiar (bilateral weakness without trauma), the Paramedic should consider trauma (occult) as a possibility. Other possibilities include electrolyte disorders (particularly potassium abnormalities), central nervous system disorders (such as meningitis/encephalitis), and peripheral nervous system disorders such as multiple sclerosis, myasthenia gravis, and Guillain–Barré syndrome.

2. *How is trouble breathing related to the weakness?*

   The description sounds like an ascending paralysis. If it continues, the patient may hypoventilate and go into Type II respiratory failure.

History

1. *What are the elements of the physical examination of a patient with suspected neuromuscular disease?*

   Following the OPQRST AMPLE format should be sufficient. The Paramedic should focus on the symptom complex, trying to create a timeline of events and symptoms to create a symptom pattern. The history should include an extensive past medical history such as stroke, hypertension, diabetes, and so on.

2. *What are the symptoms associated with peripheral nervous systems disorders?*

   Symptoms associated with peripheral nervous system disorders include patterns of paralysis and paresthesia. The Paramedic should ask about unusual peripheral pain not associated with trauma (e.g., pain in the toes without stubbing the toe, flaccidity of muscle tone as manifested by difficulty performing activities of daily living, and paresthesia, the "pins and needles" feeling).

Examination

1. *What are the elements of the physical examination of a patient with suspected peripheral nervous system disorder?*

   After completing a primary assessment, and a system's examination according to the patient's chief concern, the Paramedic should perform a detailed neurovascular assessment of the extremities, starting distal and working proximal.

2. *Why perform the physical examination by starting distal and working proximal?*

   The nature of the weakness is better determined in this manner (i.e., peripheral nervous system disorder versus central nervous system disorder).

Assessment

1. *What diagnosis did the Paramedic announce to the patient?*

   The Paramedic might suspect a peripheral nervous system disorder—probably Guillain–Barré syndrome (GBS). However, at present the Paramedic should only tell the patient that, without further diagnostics, paralysis is abnormal.

2. *Is it possible to have unilateral weakness from a spinal cord injury?*

   A limited number of spinal cord injuries, such as Brown–Sequard syndrome as well as spinal tumor, can present with unilateral weakness.

Treatment

1. *What is the standard of care of patients with suspected peripheral nervous system disorder?*

   Care for the patient with suspected peripheral nervous system disorder includes supportive care (i.e., oxygen), venous access, and so on. Symptomatic care may be needed according to the patient's presentation.

2. *Would it be inappropriate to stabilize the patient's spinal column?*

   As the etiology of the paralysis is yet to be determined, it would not be inappropriate to stabilize the spinal column.

Evaluation

1. *What are some of the predictable complications associated with peripheral nervous system disorders?*

   This case is highly suggestive of Guillain–Barré syndrome (GBS). GBS presents with an ascending paralysis that can cause a number of autonomic derangements including hypo- and hypertension, bradycardia, and heart blocks.

2. *What is the greatest danger in Guillain–Barré syndrome?*

   Guillain–Barré syndrome (GBS) can progress to diaphragmatic paralysis and respiratory failure/arrest. One-third of GBS patients will need intubation and mechanical ventilation.

Disposition

1. *What is the most appropriate transport decision that will get the patient to definitive care?*

   In this case, the patient with suspected GBS may be a candidate for plasmapheresis (i.e., plasma exchange). Hospitals capable of plasmapheresis or immunoglobulin therapy should be considered.

2. *Is it acceptable to transport the patient to a community hospital?*

   Most patients with peripheral nervous system disorders do not present emergently (i.e., they are not in need of immediate special services). In most cases, the patient is transported to a community hospital for stabilization and then transferred for further diagnostic evaluation later.

Practice Questions

Multiple Choice

1. c
2. a
3. c
4. b
5. c
6. a
7. b
8. d

9. c
10. c
11. b
12. c
13. d
14. b
15. c

Short Answer

16. Post-polio syndrome can occur up to 30 years after the initial infection and involves a loss of the patient's surviving motor neurons. Patients with this condition often complain of muscle fatigue, weakness, joint pain, and sometimes new respiratory or speech difficulties. These new symptoms occur in muscles that were initially spared or recovered. Post-polio syndrome may progress to the point where the patient requires long-term respiratory support.

17. Peripheral neuropathies most commonly develop secondary to poorly controlled diabetes, renal disease, alcoholism, or liver disease.

18. Complex regional pain syndrome is a condition that produces severe and intense burning pain.

19. The patient should be examined for sensation in all extremities as well as the trunk if extremity sensory deficits are found. Muscle strength and equality are examined both distally and proximally, comparing both left and right upper and lower extremities to each other. A brief cranial nerve exam may indicate a more central problem involving the cranial nerves as well as issues with airway protection and gag reflex.

20. The patient may develop ptosis (drooping of the eyelid) and diplopia (double vision from ocular muscle weakness).

Fill in the Blank

21. Guillain–Barré
22. amyotrophic lateral sclerosis
23. Parkinson's disease

24. poliomyelitis
25. glove, stocking

Chapter 13

Case Study

Chief Concern

1. *What are some of the possible diabetic-related emergencies?*

   Altered mental status and diabetes suggest either hypoglycemia or hyperglycemia. While hyperglycemia is an urgent emergency, hypoglycemia is an emergency condition that needs immediate attention.

2. *What are other conditions that could mimic a diabetic-related emergency?*

   The conditions that could mimic a diabetic-related emergency include hypoxia and hypoperfusion. As the case provides scant information as to the etiology of the altered mental status, leaving the possibilities almost endless, the Paramedic should focus on hypoxia, hypoglycemia, and hypotension during the primary assessment.

History

1. *What are the important elements of the history that a Paramedic should obtain?*

   The Paramedic should determine the type of diabetes that the patient has (i.e., type 1 versus type 2), as well as associated medical conditions that would impact the patient, such as coronary artery disease, renal disease, and so on. A complete SAMPLE history also facilitates the history gathering.

2. *What is the symptom pattern associated with hyperosmolar nonketonic syndrome (HONKS)?*

The symptom pattern for HONKS includes altered mental status, up to and including coma, and extreme dehydration. Because of the insidious nature of HONKS, there are not many symptoms beyond confusion and declining mental status.

Examination

1. *What are the elements of the physical examination of a patient with suspected hyperglycemia?*

The key differential in hyperglycemia is DKA versus HONKS. Signs shared by both are altered mental status and dehydration. The patient should be examined for respiratory distress/compensation for acidosis. The patient's hemodynamic status should be assessed for signs of hypoperfusion secondary to hypovolemia.

2. *What is one key that helps differentiate HONKS from DKA?*

DKA takes days to occur whereas HONKS can take weeks to manifest.

Assessment

1. *What diagnosis did the Paramedic announce to his partner?*

In the case of hyperglycemia, the differential diagnosis is narrowed down to diabetic ketoacidosis (DKA) and hyperosmolar nonketotic syndrome (HONKS).

2. *How does the Paramedic differentiate between HONKS and DKA?*

The diagnosis of HONKS is almost a diagnosis of exclusion. If the patient does not have the signs of DKA (i.e., acetone on the breath and Kussmaul respirations), then the suspicion of HONKS is supported.

Treatment

1. *What is the standard of care of patients with suspected hyperglycemia?*

In the case of both DKA and HONKS, the patient is going to be hypovolemic and in need of fluid resuscitation. After ensuring a patent airway and adequate ventilation, the Paramedic should obtain venous access and initiate a fluid bolus.

2. *What are some of the patient-specific concerns and considerations that the Paramedic should consider when applying this plan of care that is intended to treat a broad patient population presenting with hyperglycemia?*

Mr. O'Connor has a history of heart failure; therefore, the fluid resuscitation should be judicious but cautious. Furthermore, the exact etiology of the coma is, as of yet, undetermined. Therefore, overly aggressive fluid resuscitation could result in increased intracranial pressure (in the case of cerebral edema) and subsequent herniation.

Evaluation

1. *What are some of the predictable complications associated with hyperglycemia?*

As the coma may be secondary to cerebral edema, seizure and herniation syndrome are possible. If the patient has DKA, seizures may occur secondary to hypoxia, despite the administration of high-flow, high-concentration oxygen. This hypoxia is partially owed to the rightward shift of the oxyhemoglobin curve secondary to acidosis.

2. *What are some of the predictable complications associated with the treatments for seizures secondary to cerebral edema?*

While respiratory depression is possible, the patient in a coma (i.e., with a Glasgow coma scale of less than 8) should already be intubated.

Disposition

1. *What is the most appropriate transport decision that will get the patient to definitive care?*

In Mr. O'Connor's case, transportation to any emergency department capable of caring for his condition is acceptable. Diabetes and diabetic emergencies have become so widespread that every emergency department is capable of managing this patient population.

2. *What is key to report when turning the patient over to the emergency department staff?*

It is important to relate the elevated blood glucose level as well as the time of onset of symptoms (i.e., days versus weeks of illness), in addition to any ECG abnormalities suggestive of hyperkalemia.

Practice Questions

Multiple Choice

1. a
2. b
3. c
4. a
5. b
6. b
7. a
8. d
9. c
10. d
11. b
12. a
13. a
14. b
15. c

Short Answer

16. Insulin can be classified according to onset of action, peak time of action, and duration of action.

17. Insulin resistance is the cell's inability to accept insulin and, therefore, the use of glucose.

18. Diabetic ketoacidosis is a life-threatening hyperglycemia resulting from the body's breakdown of fats and proteins—alternative energy pathways—that causes ketosis and acidosis.

19. Hyperosmolar nonketotic sydrome is a life-threatening hyperglycemia that is the result of a gradual buildup of glucose. However, it avoids alternative energy pathways because of minimal insulin secretion. HONKS is thought to be due to elevated epinephrine.

20. DKA occurs over days whereas HONKS develops over weeks. DKA produces acidosis as well as ketones whereas HONKS does not. HONKS tends to have a much higher glucose level than DKA; therefore, HONKS is associated with a greater degree of dehydration than DKA.

Fill in the Blank

21. random
22. diabesity
23. glucometer
24. neuroglycopenic
25. glucagon

Chapter 14

Case Study

Chief Concern

1. *What are some of the electrolyte problems associated with nausea, vomiting, and diarrhea?*

   Excessive nausea, vomiting, and diarrhea (NVD) can lead to hypokalemia and hypomagnesemia.

2. *What complications can these electrolyte disturbances produce?*

   Hypokalemia can cause generalized weakness, muscle cramps, tachycardia, and orthostatic hypotension. Hypomagnesemia can lead to generalized weakness, muscle cramps, tachycardia, and altered mental status.

History

1. *What are the important elements of the history that a Paramedic should obtain?*

   In this patient's case, the sudden cessation of steroids is important. The Paramedic should ascertain the dose and frequency of the steroids as well as when he stopped taking them.

2. *What is the symptom pattern associated with acute adrenocortical insufficiency?*

   Patients with acute adrenocortical insufficiency will complain of weakness and unexplained weight loss. Many patients with acute adrenocortical insufficiency will have diarrhea and abdominal pain.

Examination

1. *What are the elements of the physical examination of a patient with suspected adrenocortical insufficiency?*

   The suspicion of acute adrenocortical insufficiency is based on history; however, the supporting physical examination is consistent with shock.

2. *Why are orthostatic vital signs a critical element in this examination?*

   Patients with acute adrenocortical insufficiency often have orthostatic hypotension.

Assessment

1. *What diagnosis did the Paramedic announce to the patient?*

   The sudden cessation of steroids, coupled with the symptoms, would lead the Paramedics to suspect acute adrenal insufficiency.

2. *What is Addison's disease?*

   Addison's disease is the old name for adrenal insufficiency.

Treatment

1. *What is the standard of care of patients with suspected acute adrenal insufficiency?*

   After helping to maintain airway, breathing and circulation (resuscitation) the Paramedic should treat hypoglycemia with dextrose 50% and consider administration of hydrocortisone intravenously.

2. *What electrolyte disturbances should the Paramedic suspect?*

   While nausea and vomiting may induce hyponatremia and hypomagnesemia, two electrolyte disturbances that often accompany one another, the peaked T waves suggest hyperkalemia.

Evaluation

1. *What are some of the predictable complications?*

   The combination of the acute adrenal crisis, vomiting, and diarrhea can all contribute to hypoglycemia.

2. *What are other potential complications that could result from vomiting and diarrhea?*

   Complications that could result from excessive vomiting and diarrhea include hypokalemia, dehydration, and a metabolic alkalosis.

Disposition

1. *What is the most appropriate transport decision that will get the patient to definitive care?*

   Patients with complex electrolyte disturbances and/or hormonal disorders are often cared for in the intensive care unit. These patients should be transported to a hospital capable of handling patients with this acuity.

2. *What key points about the patient's condition should be discussed with the emergency department staff?*

   The emergency department staff should be made aware of hypotension as well as hypoglycemia, in the event of rebound hypoglycemia.

Practice Questions
Multiple Choice

1. c
2. a
3. d
4. d
5. c
6. b
7. a
8. a
9. a
10. b
11. c
12. d
13. c
14. b
15. b

Short Answer

16. Patients with diabetes insipidus and diabetes mellitus produce large quantities of urine and drink large quantities of water. However, the blood sugar of the patient with diabetes insipidus will be within normal limits and the patient will not have the signs of diabetic ketoacidosis (i.e., acetone smell on the breath or Kussmaul respirations) associated with diabetes mellitus.

17. As the blood concentration of sodium decreases, the concentration of sodium in the brain tissue remains relatively constant. This difference in sodium concentration produces a gradient that encourages water to move from the blood into the cerebral cells. This causes the brain cells to swell which, in turn, causes the agitation, coma, seizure, and death associated with hyponatremia.

18. Hyperkalemia can produce symptoms of weakness, paresthesias, depressed or absent deep tendon reflexes, ascending paralysis, nausea, vomiting, and diarrhea. Hyperkalemia can also cause life-threatening ECG changes.

19. Hypocalcemia secondary to hyperventilation can cause paresthesia around the mouth and fingertips, muscle weakness, and fatigue. Hypocalcemia can also cause carpal spasms, in which the forearm muscles contract and put the patient's wrists into a spastic position.

20. A thyroid storm can be mistaken for a psychiatric disorder. In this state of significantly increased metabolism, the patient becomes hyperthermic, agitated, tremulous, and psychotic.

Fill in the Blank

21. diabetes insipidus
22. toxic
23. exophthalmos
24. Chvostek's
25. hypomagnesemia

Chapter 15
Case Study
Chief Concern

1. *What are some of the possible causes of the patient's convulsions?*

    There are multiple etiologies. The "HIT + 1" mnemonic lists the major causes (hypoxia, hypoglycemia, heat exhaustion, high fever, heart-related iatrogenic trauma, tumor, toxemia of pregnancy, toxicology, tremens, and epilepsy).

2. *How can intoxication be related to the seizure activity?*

    Alcohol can be the direct cause, such as through ingestion of alcohol other than ethyl alcohol (i.e., toxicological emergency) or an indirect cause, secondary to alcohol withdrawal (i.e., delirium tremens). Alcohol can also be a contributing factor, either in terms of falls, traumatic injury, and seizure or subtherapeutic levels of anticonvulsant medications secondary to the diuretic effects of alcohol.

History

1. *What are the important elements of the history that a Paramedic should obtain?*

    First, the Paramedic should try to obtain a history of the current event. Was the seizure witnessed? Did the patient strike his head when he collapsed? Was the seizure a "whole body" seizure (i.e., tonic–clonic) or just one part of the body? Did the seizure start at one part of the body and progress, suggesting a Jacksonian march? How long did the seizure last and was the patient cyanotic?

    Using SAMPLE, the Paramedic should try to obtain a general history of seizures. This includes a description of the type of seizures (i.e., tonic–clonic or generalized) and the date or time of the last seizure. After allergies, the Paramedic should ask about medications, particularly anticonvulsant medications, and specifically the patient's compliance with those medications. A list of medications should be obtained, particularly new medications that might be seizure-provoking such as aminophylline, INZ for tuberculosis, tricyclic antidepressants, phenothiazines, and beta–lactam antibiotics, for example. The past medical history should include questions about respiratory disease (hypoxia-induced seizure), diabetes (hypoglycemia), and trauma (traumatic brain injury), as well as a history of epilepsy.

The last, in SAMPLE, include the last seizure and, in this case, the last drink. If greater than 24 hours, that should lead the Paramedic to a suspicion of tremens. The history should conclude with what the patient was doing prior to the seizure.

2. *What is the symptom pattern associated with an epileptic seizure?*

Seizures typically start with an aura, proceed to the tonic–clonic phase, and end with the post-ictal phase. Often, the patient collapses. However, in some cases the patient lowers himself to the ground. In most cases, the seizure activity is self-limiting and the patient slowly regains consciousness. It is problematic, and suggestive of status epilepticus, if the patient does not spontaneously recover within 10 to 15 minutes in most cases.

As most seizures are spontaneous, with a fleeting aura, there is no real symptom pattern. Paramedics must rely on eyewitness accounts of the event.

Examination

1. *What are the elements of the physical examination of a patient with suspected seizure disorder?*

Overall, the patient appears grossly diaphoretic and his vital signs indicate that he is hyperdynamic. Following the primary assessment and treatment of any hypoxia and/or hypoglycemia, the Paramedic should perform a neurological examination. Starting at the eyes, the Paramedic should check the cranial nerves. Barring suspected cervical spine trauma, the Paramedic should check for neck stiffness and ask the patient to flex, then extend, the knees, looking for signs of pain during extension.

2. *Why is a rapid trauma exam a critical element in this examination?*

Often patients experiencing a seizure collapse and may have injured themselves during the fall. A quick head-to-toe trauma assessment, using DCAP BTLS, can help the Paramedic discover any injuries that may have been sustained in the fall.

Assessment

1. *What is the significance of the alcohol withdrawal?*

Depending on the time since the patient's last drink, and assuming a history of chronic alcoholism, the patient may be in alcohol withdrawal, which may be the cause of seizures.

2. *What diagnosis did the Paramedic announce to the patient?*

The patient should be advised that he had a seizure and that seizure could be because he is "off his meds" (i.e., his anticonvulsant medication level is low). The patient may also be told that the seizure may be the result of his alcohol withdrawal and that there are methods that can help him through the withdrawal, as well as prevent further seizures.

Treatment

1. *What is the standard of care of patients with suspected seizure disorder?*

As most seizures are self-limiting, patient care involves providing a supportive and protective environment. In many cases, the patient is laid on the stretcher in the left lateral recumbent position to allow any secretions that have accumulated to passively drain.

2. *Are there any special considerations that the Paramedic should take?*

On occasion, a Yankauer suction will be used to assist the patient. If the patient is hypoxic, as indicated by pulse oximeters, oxygen may be utilized. In many EMS systems, high-flow, high-concentration oxygen by mask is routinely administered to the patient. Other care consists of monitoring the patient's level of consciousness for improvement as well as vital signs.

Evaluation

1. *What are some of the predictable complications of alcohol withdrawal?*

Although alcohol withdrawal can lead to a hyperdynamic state, with elevated heart rate and blood pressure which can result in an acute myocardial infarction or stroke, this is not the greatest concern. The saying goes, "seizures beget seizures." Since the underlying cause of the seizures has not been addressed (i.e., the alcohol withdrawal), it is reasonable to assume that the patient will seize again.

2. *What are some of the predictable complications associated with the treatments for alcohol withdrawal?*

As the treatment for alcohol withdrawal involves the use of benzodiazepines, the complications of treating alcohol withdrawal are the side effects of benzodiazepines, such as respiratory depression.

Disposition

1. *What is the most appropriate transport decision that will get the patient to definitive care?*

If the patient becomes unresponsive, secondary to another seizure (hopefully forestalled by the benzodiazepine), or experiences respiratory depression, secondary to the benzodiazepine, then the patient should go to the most appropriate hospital.

What is unacceptable in this case is if the patient refuses further medical assistance and transportation. The complexity of epilepsy, compounded by the alcoholism, not to mention the potential for traumatic brain injury with even minor trauma, makes it important that a physician see the patient. If the patient refuses, then medical control should be contacted.

2. *What are some of the transportation considerations?*

This patient should be transported to a hospital with an alcohol treatment center. While any emergency department should be capable of caring for a patient with a seizure disorder, this patient's case is complicated by the alcohol withdrawal. Taking the patient to a "detox center" eliminates the need to transfer him at a later time.

Practice Questions
Multiple Choice

1. d
2. d
3. d
4. d
5. d
6. d
7. d
8. d
9. d
10. d
11. d
12. d
13. d
14. d
15. c

Short Answer

16. The transient delirium seen in alcoholic patients is called Wernicke's syndrome.

17. Esophageal varices are most closely related to hematemesis.

18. Alcohol impacts a pregnancy through the development of fetal alcohol syndrome, which could lead to birth defects.

19. Benzodiazepines are used to treat alcohol withdrawal.

20. The C in the Alcohol Assessment Tool represents the question, "Have you ever tried to CUT down your drinking?"

Fill in the Blank

21. delirium tremens
22. benzodiazepine
23. limbic system
24. gynecomastia
25. asterixis

Chapter 16

Case Study

Chief Concern

1. *What are some of the possible causes of delirium?*

   While the obvious cause of hallucinations is psychiatric, all delirium is medical until proven otherwise. Possible medical causes include infections, withdrawal, electrolyte disturbances, toxins, stroke, hypoxia, Wernicke's encephalopathy, thyroid storm, hypertensive crisis, head injury, and heavy metal exposure.

2. *Which cause of delirium should be considered last?*

   The saying goes "all delirium is medical until proven otherwise." Delirium, as a sign of psychiatric illness, should be considered last.

History

1. *What are the important elements of the history that a Paramedic should obtain?*

   After scene safety has been established, and the primary assessment completed, the Paramedic needs to ascertain the type and amount of potential toxins ingested/injected and the time that the poisoning took place. The latter, the time of poisoning, has implications for the use of activated charcoal and antidotes.

2. *What is the symptom pattern associated with delirium?*

   The symptom pattern associated with delirium includes a sudden onset of abnormal behavior.

Examination

1. *What are the elements of the physical examination of a patient with suspected overdose?*

   After assessing the patient for hypoxia, hypoglycemia, and hypotension, the Paramedic needs to assess the patient according to the suspected toxidrome. In this case, three toxidromes come to mind: sympathomimetics (cocaine ingestion), anticholinergics (Trofanil), and possible toxic alcohol ingestion.

2. *Why is blood glucose a critical element in this examination?*

   All three of these toxidromes can induce hypoglycemia, which can be a source of delirium.

Assessment

1. *What diagnosis did the Paramedic announce to the patient?*

   While this case appears to be a suspected anticholinergic overdose, a sympathomimetic ingestion or other cause cannot be ruled out. It is important for the Paramedic to keep an open mind. The Vowels over TIPS (AEIOUTIPS) mnemonic (alcoholism, epilepsy, insulin, overdose, uremia, trauma-occult, infection, psychogenic, and stroke) can be helpful in remembering the causes of altered mental status.

2. *What are the three causes of delirium that should be evaluated and treated first?*

   The Paramedic should evaluate and treat any hypoxia, hypoglycemia, and hypoperfusion before moving onto a more complex differential diagnosis.

Treatment

1. *What is the standard of care of patients with suspected overdose?*

   If the toxin is known, it is reasonable to try the antidote if one is available. In this case—a suspected mixed overdose of a sympathomimetic and anticholinergic that may be the cause of the agitation—it may be appropriate to give a benzodiazepine.

2. *What basic care should be provided first?*

   Patients with an overdose are first given supportive care (i.e., oxygen, glucose as needed, and fluid resuscitation). In this case, cooling measures, using ice packs, are part of the supportive care.

Evaluation

1. *What are some of the predictable complications associated with a suspected anticholinergic overdose?*

   Tricyclic antidepressants work like sodium channel blockers (i.e., lidocaine) to lengthen QT intervals. As the QT interval progresses, the patient may go into torsades de pointes.

2. *What are some of the predictable complications associated with a suspected sympathomimetic overdose?*

   As a stimulant, a sympathomimetic overdose can lead to a hyperdynamic state including acute hypertension, hypertensive crisis, and stroke, as well as acute myocardial infarction and ventricular tachycardia.

Disposition

1. *What is the most appropriate transport decision that will get the patient to definitive care?*

   Patients with an overdose need to be seen in hospitals capable of critical care. In many instances, these patients will need special drug screening as well as intensive care.

2. *Given the choice of hospitals, which one would be preferred?*

   In many cases, the overdose patient may need to undergo hemodialysis. Therefore, any hospital with hemodialysis capabilities would be preferred.

Practice Questions
Multiple Choice

1. c
2. c
3. d
4. a
5. c
6. a
7. d
8. b
9. a
10. a
11. d
12. b
13. b
14. c
15. d

Short Answer

16. Toxicology is the study of the harmful effects that different chemicals—both natural and man-made—have upon the body. Therefore, it encompasses a wide variety of potential toxins and an equally wide spectrum of clinical effects. A toxin is any substance that can cause harmful physical effects when a person is exposed to it. Toxins may (1) produce little to no clinical effect; (2) produce very serious effects, such as leukemia or liver carcinoma, but not until years after exposure; or (3) produce immediate and life-threatening effects.

17. A toxidrome is a symptom pattern that is associated with a specific poison.

18. Patients with carbon monoxide poisoning initially complain of headache, nausea, and other flu-like symptoms.

19. The telephone number for poison control is 1-800-222-1222.

20. The carbon monoxide-poisoned patient is put in a hyperbaric chamber that increases pressure from 1 atmosphere (standard atmospheric pressure) to 2.8 atmospheres. The Paramedic administers 100% oxygen to the patient within the chamber. Under the increased pressure, a higher concentration of oxygen can be achieved in the tissues than at normal atmosphere. This has the effect of decreasing the percentage of blood bound to carbon monoxide (carboxyhemoglobin).

Fill in the Blank

21. organophosphate
22. sodium bicarbonate
23. fasciculations
24. 2-PAM
25. barbiturates, benzodiazepines

Chapter 17

Case Study

Chief Concern

1. *What are some of the possible causes of the woman's apparent abnormal behavior?*

   While this could be a case of situational depression, other possibilities have to be considered including psychiatric disorders.

2. *What are some medical causes of abnormal behavior?*

   Hypoxia, hypoglycemia, and hypoperfusion are possible medical causes of the abnormal behavior.

History

1. *What are the important elements of the history that a Paramedic should obtain?*

   The Paramedic should try to obtain a description of abnormal behaviors, such as regressive behaviors, as well as negative symptoms, such as alogia, affective flattening, and avolition. The Paramedic should further inquire about any interference with ADL.

2. *What is the symptom pattern for acute psychotic reaction?*

   While the symptom pattern is different from one psychiatric illness to another, from a Paramedic's perspective, any behaviors that interfere with ADL could be construed as an acute psychotic reaction.

Examination

1. *What are the elements of the physical examination of a patient with suspected acute psychotic reaction?*

   The Paramedic's examination should attempt to rule out any obvious organic cause of the behavior, such as hypoxia, hypoglycemia, or hypotension. A neurological examination, as well as a mini-mental status examination, is also part of the secondary assessment.

2. *Why are pulse oximeter and blood glucose critical elements in this examination?*

   The pulse oximeter and blood glucose help to eliminate hypoxia and hypoglycemia as possible causes of the behavior.

Assessment

1. *What is the significance of the hallucinations?*

   Julianna may be having auditory hallucinations, a sure sign of an acute psychotic reaction. Hallucinations, coupled with the other behaviors, suggest that Julianna has either hebephrenic schizophrenia or clinical depression.

2. *What safety concerns, if any, should the Paramedic have?*

   An auditory hallucination can be a command hallucination, which may direct the patient to behave other than normal (e.g., become combative).

Treatment

1. *What is the standard of care of patients with suspected acute psychotic disorder?*

   *Provided the patient is not violent and doesn't represent a danger to hersel*f or others, then the patient should be transported while supportive care is offered.

2. *What other safety concerns should the Paramedic have for the patient?*

   It is appropriate to ascertain if the patient has any suicidal thoughts as well.

Evaluation

1. *What are some of the predictable complications associated with auditory hallucinations?*

   Auditory hallucinations can become command hallucinations, which may direct the patient to either harm herself (i.e., commit suicide) or harm others (i.e., commit homicide). Therefore, justification exists for medical restraint.

2. *What is medical restraint?*

   Medical restraint is the application of devices (i.e., cravats, etc.) to prevent the patient from harming himself or others.

Disposition

1. *What is the most appropriate transport decision that will get the patient to definitive care?*

   This child is going to need mental health services following a medical evaluation to rule out other etiologies for her behavior. It is preferable to transport her to a hospital with these services.

2. *What are the advantages of transporting a patient with suspected acute psychotic disorder to these hospitals, even if that means bypassing other hospitals in the process?*

   Hospitals with mental health units are familiar with treating patients with acute psychotic reactions. It has been recognized that the sooner that treatment can begin, the less damaging the reaction.

Practice Questions
Multiple Choice

1. a
2. d
3. a
4. d
5. a
6. a
7. d
8. c
9. b
10. d
11. a
12. c
13. c
14. d
15. b

Short Answer

16. Psychogenic theorists believe that mental illness is the result of conflict between inner desires and opposing external demands. Somatogenic theorists believe that mental illness is a malfunction of the central nervous system. Both theorists believe that mental illness is a departure from the normal patterns of behavior.

17. Post-traumatic stress disorder (PTSD) is an anxiety disorder that occurs following a life-threatening event, such as personal combat or violent sexual assault. Subsequently, the patient experiences persistent and repetitive memories of the event. The all-consuming nature of this anxiety can lead to trouble concentrating as memories of the event invade the patient's thoughts. These invasive thoughts of the traumatic event, called flashbacks, can also lead to sleep disturbances and nightmares.

18. The potentially reversible causes of delirium can be found using the mnemonic DELIRIUM: drugs, electrolyte imbalances, lack of drugs, infection, reduced sensory input, intracranial pressure, uremia, and myocardial issues.

19. Dementia is a gradual and irreversible decline in mental function generally owed to an organic cause such as senility or Alzheimer's disease. Dementia is evident in disturbances of thought, such as poor judgment, socially inappropriate behaviors, and loss of the ability to think abstractly. Delirium is an acute and potentially reversible decline in mental function often associated with illness. The patient with delirium will have periods of lucidity and clarity of thinking whereas the demented patient generally does not.

20. A simple Romberg test involves tasks such as walking from heel to toe or running the heel of one foot over the shin of the other leg.

Fill in the Blank

21. Huntington's chorea
22. somatizing
23. bipolar
24. panic attack
25. acute dystonic reactions

Chapter 18
Case Study
Chief Concern

1. *What are some of the possible causes of this behavior?*

    Triggers for behavioral emergencies, including suicide, are life-threatening illness; personal injury or illness that is image altering or causes a functional loss, family abuse, loss of a loved one, divorce, and so on.

2. *What safety measures should the Paramedics consider on approaching the emotionally disturbed patient?*

    Methods of suicide include firearms, carbon monoxide, fire, motor vehicle crash, and falls from heights. Each of these methods represents a potential danger to the Paramedic. Therefore, the Paramedic should approach every scene of a potential suicide with a global view of the scene and pay attention to hazards and potential life threats.

History

1. *What are the important elements of the history that a Paramedic should obtain?*

    While the situation may appear to be a behavioral emergency, the possibility of a medical emergency must be considered first. Potential medical etiologies of behavioral emergencies are included in the mnemonic Vowels over TIPS: alcoholism, epilepsy, insulin, overdose, uremia, trauma-occult, infection, psychogenic, and stroke.

2. *What factors could exacerbate the situation, making it more dangerous?*

    In some cases, before the patient attempts suicide, she becomes intoxicated or ingests illicit drugs such as cocaine. These drugs tend to amplify the danger in the situation.

Examination

1. *What are the elements of the physical examination of a patient with a suspected behavioral emergency?*

    During a behavioral emergency, the physical assessment is often limited to a primary assessment and a rapid secondary assessment focusing on trauma.

2. *Why is a rapid trauma assessment a critical element in this examination?*

    A rapid trauma assessment is needed to ensure the patient did not attempt suicide by self-inflicted wounds, suffer head trauma that may have occurred from syncope, or experience any other potential wounds.

Assessment

1. *What is the significance of the patient's statements?*

    The words "I just want to die" establish that the patient is suicidal. While she does not voice her plan, nor have an apparent means to execute the plan, she seems determined to commit suicide. Therefore, all reasonable means to prevent her from doing so must be taken.

2. *What are the elements of a suicide threat?*

    A suicide threat must be either verbal or written, must be specific to a plan, and must be a plan that is executable.

Treatment

1. *What is the standard of care of patients with a behavioral emergency?*

    The safety of the patient with a behavioral emergency is paramount, only superseded by the safety of the crew. To ensure the patient's safety, it may be necessary to perform a medical restraint. A medical restraint consists of verbal de-escalation, physical restraint, and chemical sedation, each according to the need.

2. *What are some of the patient-specific concerns and considerations that the Paramedic should consider when applying this plan of care that is intended to treat a broad patient population presenting with a behavioral emergency?*

    Inherent to physical restraint are risks of injuries to the patient, the crew, and even the public in some instances. Every reasonable measure must be taken to mitigate these hazards and reduce the risk.

Evaluation

1. *What is the standard of care of patients for the medical restraint of an emotionally disturbed person?*

   Once a patient is restrained, and by definition powerless to care for herself, the Paramedic is responsible for ensuring the patient's safety. This includes all forms of supportive care as needed.

2. *What are some of the patient-specific concerns and considerations that the Paramedic should consider when applying this plan of care to the emotionally disturbed person?*

   Whenever restraints are used it is imperative that the Paramedic regularly check distal circulation as well as motor and neurological function. Typically, these restraint checks are performed when vital signs are obtained.

Disposition

1. *What is the most appropriate transport decision that will get the patient to definitive care?*

   While the patient will need immediate medical attention for any medical conditions that may have caused or arisen because of this suicide attempt, she will eventually need mental health care. Facilities capable of meeting these dual purposes are most appropriate.

2. *If in an either/or situation (i.e., medical facility or psychiatric hospital), to which hospital should be the patient be transported?*

   If the choice is a community hospital without psychiatric facilities or a psychiatric facility with an emergency department, the patient should go to the emergency department. The saying goes "all psychiatric patients are medical emergencies until proven otherwise."

Practice Questions
Multiple Choice

1. d	9. d
2. a	10. d
3. c	11. d
4. b	12. c
5. a	13. b
6. d	14. a
7. b	15. d
8. c	

Short Answer

16. Abnormal behavior is maladaptive behavior that does not permit the activities of daily living by reason of mental defect.

17. A person who exhibits aggressive behavior toward others or acts in a manner harmful to oneself, especially potentially self-destructive behaviors, is said to have a behavioral emergency.

18. A medical restraint is a medically necessary restriction of the patient's freedom so that he cannot harm himself or others.

19. The three levels of medical restraint are verbal persuasion, physical restraint, and chemical restraint.

20. The use of physical force to restrain a patient is acceptable for managing behavioral emergencies "only when less restrictive measures have failed and unanticipated aggressive or destructive behavior places the patient or others in imminent danger of self-harm."

Fill in the Blank

21. excited delirium

22. proxemics

23. therapeutic communications

24. protective restraint

25. hog-tying

Chapter 19

Case Study

Chief Concern

1. *What are some of the possible causes of gastrointestinal bleeding?*

   Although the causes of gastrointestinal bleeding are numerous, the number is reduced for a 1-year-old infant. In this case, as blood is in the stool, it could be dysentery, irritable bowel syndrome, intussusception, volvulus, or rectal fissures.

2. *Why should the Paramedic be concerned about blood in the stool of a 1-year-old infant?*

   The Paramedic has to consider the possibility that the blood in the stool is secondary to objects placed in the rectum, resulting in rectal fissures. This scenario is consistent with child abuse.

History

1. *What are the important elements of the history that a Paramedic should obtain?*

   The history should not change for an infant with this complaint. Using OPQRST, as part of the S in SAMPLE, should help start the conversation. The focus should be on recent bowel movements and past episodes of bleeding as well.

2. *Does the patient's vomiting have any relationship to the gastrointestinal bleeding?*

   Vomiting could be specific to the gastrointestinal disease, such as an obstruction. More likely, however, this constitutional sign indicates a more systemic effect. Vomiting can be the result of hypoperfusion or pain.

Examination

1. *What are the elements of the physical examination of a patient with suspected acute GI bleed?*

   The focus of the abdominal examination is to ascertain if the patient is in shock. While this infant is compensating, it should be remembered that infants can decompensate quickly and often without warning. After assessing circulation and perfusion, the Paramedic should focus on assessing the abdomen. In this case, it should be fairly easy to lie the infant on her back, expose her belly, and palpate for tenderness.

2. *Why would a diaper count be important?*

   Again, as the focus of abdominal examination is on hypoperfusion and shock, the diaper count will help the Paramedic gauge the infant's volume status. The smaller the diaper count (i.e., the less urine produced), the more likely the infant is volume depleted.

Assessment

1. *What diagnosis did the Paramedic announce to the patient's grandmother?*

   The grandmother should be advised that the infant has a potentially life-threatening emergency that requires immediate medical attention.

2. *How does the Paramedic explain an intussusception or volvulus to the grandmother in lay terms?*

   The Paramedic would describe the intussusception as the bowel telescoping into itself, whereas a volvulus is the bowel twisting itself.

Treatment

1. *What is the standard of care of patients with suspected gastrointestinal bleeding?*

   Standard advanced life support should be provided including high-flow, high-concentration oxygen (as needed), venous access (if possible), and consideration of a nasogastric tube.

2. *What issues are different when caring for a child with suspected gastrointestinal bleeding versus an adult?*

   Although the same care is provided to a child as is provided to an adult with suspected gastrointestinal bleeding, when caring for a child the Paramedic must also care for the parent(s).

Evaluation

1. *What are some of the predictable complications associated with acute GI bleed?*

   Any acute abdominal process has the potential to cause internal hemorrhage and hypotension.

2. *What should the Paramedic do if these complications arise?*

   If these complications arise, the Paramedic must be prepared to administer fluid bolus as a part of the resuscitation.

Disposition

1. *What is the most appropriate transport decision that will get the patient to definitive care?*

   This infant needs to be transported to a hospital with pediatric capabilities and preferably a pediatric surgeon. Typically, these services are only available in a tertiary care center.

2. *Why would surgery be necessary?*

   While most cases of intussusception resolve with a contrast enema preceding medical imaging, such as ultrasonography, a significant number may need surgical intervention.

Practice Questions
Multiple Choice

1. a
2. d
3. c
4. a
5. a
6. a
7. c
8. d
9. d
10. a
11. a
12. c
13. a
14. b
15. d

Short Answer

16. As the liver becomes cirrhotic, blood backs up into the portal system, creating portal hypertension. Distended veins in the throat, distended secondary to portal hypertension, become esophageal varices that rupture and bleed.

17. Irritable bowel syndrome can be confused with lactose intolerance, gluten sensitivity, and celiac disease.

18. Intussusception is an abnormal inwards telescoping of the bowel. The triad of symptoms associated with intussusception are vomiting, intermittent abdominal pain, and rectal bleeding. Volvulus is an abnormal twisting of the intestines and its triad of symptoms includes sudden severe and unremitting abdominal pain associated with nausea and vomiting as well as blood in the stool.

19. To check for orthostatic vital signs, the Paramedic should place the patient in a supine position for approximately two minutes, then assess the patient's blood pressure and heart rate. After helping the patient to stand, the Paramedic should wait for two minutes. One provider should be dedicated to monitoring the patient while a second provider reassesses the patient's blood pressure and pulse.

    A patient with a volume deficit will experience a decrease in preload, stroke volume, and cardiac output. This will show as a decrease in systolic blood pressure and an increase in heart rate. If the systolic blood pressure decreases more than 20 mmHg or the heart rate increases by more than 20 mmHg per minute from the supine to standing vital signs, the patient is said to have orthostatic vital signs or postural hypotension. The increase in heart rate is the more sensitive indicator of volume depletion.

20. The patient should be supine, with a pillow under her head. This prevents the patient from trying to look up to observe the Paramedic performing the exam and consequently tightening her abdominal muscles. The patient should be encouraged to place her hands to her sides and out of the Paramedic's way. The patient may be encouraged to bend her knees and place the soles of her feet on the bed. This helps to relax her abdominal muscles further.

Fill in the Blank

21. ligament, Treitz
22. Hamman's crunch
23. portal hypertension
24. inflammation
25. melena

Chapter 20

Case Study

Chief Concern

1. *What are some of the possible causes of right lower quadrant abdominal pain?*

   Possible causes of right lower quadrant abdominal pain include appendicitis, ascending urinary tract infection, inflammatory bowel syndrome, ovarian torsion, ruptured ovarian cyst, and ectopic pregnancy.

2. *Which of these causes of right lower quadrant abdominal pain are specific to women?*

   Possible causes of right lower quadrant abdominal pain specific to women would be ovarian torsion (rare), ruptured ovarian cyst, and ectopic pregnancy.

History

1. *What are the important elements of the history that a Paramedic should obtain?*

   Using the list of potential diagnoses and the mnemonic OPQRST, the Paramedic should ascertain the time and speed of onset, as well as associated symptoms.

2. *What history beyond the standard OPQRST AS/PN should the Paramedic obtain?*

   With any woman of childbearing age, it is important to ascertain the patient's last period, whether she is sexually active, and what form of contraception she is using.

Examination

1. *What are the elements of the physical examination of a patient with acute abdominal pain?*

   The abdominal examination consists of inspecting all four quadrants, from rib cage to pelvis, for bruises, swelling, and any discoloration. Next, the Paramedic may elect to auscultate for bowel sounds and/or use the stethoscope to gently palpate the abdomen for peritoneal signs. Next, the Paramedic should perform a deeper palpation of solid organs as needed. Pain with bimanual palpation of the kidneys might suggest nephritis secondary to an ascending urinary tract infection. Palpation at McBurney's point with point tenderness is suggestive of appendicitis. Alternatively, the Paramedic may wish to test for the obturator sign.

2. *Why are orthostatic vital signs a critical element in the patient's examination?*

   Patients with intra-abdominal processes are prone to hypovolemia via third-spacing or abdominal hemorrhage. Orthostatic vital signs can help the Paramedic identify potentially hypovolemic patients.

Assessment

1. *What is the significance of the abdominal pain?*

   The sudden onset of lower quadrant abdominal pain in a woman of childbearing age potentially could be a sign of a ruptured ectopic pregnancy or ruptured ovarian cyst. Both are potentially life-threatening surgical emergencies.

2. *What diagnosis did the Paramedic give to the patient?*

   The Paramedic's diagnosis is that the patient could be bleeding internally.

Treatment

1. *What is the standard of care for treating patients with acute abdominal pain?*

   As this is a potential surgical emergency, the patient should receive supportive care—including oxygen (as needed) and venous access—and be monitored.

2. *What is the concern in this case?*

The main concern is the possibility of an ectopic pregnancy, which is a surgical emergency. Any woman of childbearing age with lower abdominal pain is assumed to have an ectopic pregnancy until proven otherwise.

Evaluation

1. *What are some of the predictable complications associated with acute abdominal emergencies?*

Ruptured ovarian cyst, ruptured appendix, or ruptured ectopic pregnancy can lead to significant intra-abdominal bleeding.

2. *What are some of the predictable complications associated with the treatments for abdominal emergencies?*

Like trauma, the Paramedic must keep the principle of permissive hypotension in mind (i.e., just enough fluids to keep the brain perfused). In other words, the Paramedic should maintain a mean arterial pressure of 60 to 70 mmHg, while not diluting blood clotting factors and/or disrupting established clots.

Disposition

1. *What is the most appropriate transport decision that will get the patient to definitive care?*

As an acute abdomen (i.e., hot belly) is potentially a surgical emergency, the Paramedic should choose the closest hospital with an available surgical suite and appropriate diagnostic equipment.

2. *What key information should the Paramedic pass along to the emergency department and why?*

As abdominal pain is a common complaint, and many times benign, it is important that the Paramedic inform the emergency department that the patient is a female of childbearing age with lower quadrant abdominal pain.

Practice Questions
Multiple Choice

1. a
2. a
3. d
4. a
5. c
6. c
7. d
8. a
9. c
10. a
11. d
12. b
13. c
14. d
15. d

Short Answer

16. Paralytic ileus can be due to loss of mesentery blood flow (due to shock or loss of strength of muscular contraction), due to electrolyte imbalances, or due to loss of nervous control (secondary to anticholinergic medications, for example).

17. To test for the obturator sign, the Paramedic lies the patient supine with the right knee bent and right hip flexed 90 degrees. The Paramedic then takes the right ankle and gently rotates the hip away from the body. If the obturator is inflamed, then the patient will experience pain.

18. The rapid onset of belly pain, suggesting a surgical emergency, can be due to ovarian torsion, ruptured ovarian cyst, ruptured ectopic pregnancy, and ruptured abdominal aortic aneurysm.

19. Visceral pain comes from the abdominal organs, or viscera, which are innervated by the autonomic nerve fibers. These autonomic nerve fibers respond to abdominal distention (e.g., secondary to a bowel obstruction) and the muscular contraction of peristalsis. This can give the patient a dull, achy, and nauseating pain.

20. The effects of a large bowel obstruction are threefold. First, the fluid above the obstruction does not get reabsorbed; subsequently, the body's water volume is diminished and shock may ensue. Second, the resulting bowel dilatation causes impairment of blood flow to the intestines, with secondary edema and ischemia. Finally, as a result of edema, the permeability of the bowel walls increases, leading to bacterial invasion and systemic sepsis.

Fill in the Blank

21. biliary colic
22. jaundice
23. McBurney's point
24. Rovsing's sign
25. volvulus

Chapter 21

Case Study

Chief Concern

1. *What are some of the possible causes of weakness and dizziness in the dialysis patient?*

   Kidney-related reasons for weakness and dizziness include urinary tract infection, anemia, and heart failure.

2. *How is the time of the call related to the weakness and dizziness?*

   If the call was made pre-dialysis, then the Paramedics should be concerned about hyperkalemia as well as congestive heart failure secondary to hypervolemia. If the call was made post-dialysis, then the Paramedics should be concerned about hypovolemia or hypokalemia (which are both highly unlikely in this case) or disequilibrium syndrome.

History

1. *What are the important elements of the history that a Paramedic should obtain?*

   The differential diagnosis in this case ranges from the flu to stroke. Starting with mental status, the Paramedic should ascertain if there is paralysis or paresthesia in the extremities. The Paramedic should reaffirm the dialysis history including recent difficulties at dialysis.

2. *What is the symptom pattern for disequilibrium syndrome?*

   The symptom pattern is similar to the flu (i.e., headache and nausea). The symptom pattern is also like a stroke, including blurred vision, headache, and nausea.

Examination

1. *What are the elements of the physical examination of a patient with suspected disequilibrium syndrome?*

   Beyond the primary assessment, the Paramedic should perform a neurological examination, focusing on increased intracranial pressure. Both intracranial hemorrhage and disequilibrium syndrome can cause increased intracranial pressure. Regardless of the etiology, the Paramedic should monitor for signs of transtentorial herniation secondary to increased intracranial pressure.

2. *Why is a Cincinnati Stroke Scale a critical element in this examination?*

   Not only does the CSS help to reveal a possible stroke, but the tremors in Mrs. Washington's hands may be asterixis (i.e., liver flap).

Assessment

1. *Why does Abdullah suspect disequilibrium syndrome?*

   Mrs. Washington's symptom complex (the weakness, blurred vision), coupled with the liver flap, is suggestive of disequilibrium syndrome.

2. *What would be some signs of increased intracranial pressure?*

   Signs of increased intracranial pressure include rising blood pressure, falling heart rate, and changes in respiratory pattern.

Treatment

1. *What is the standard of care of patients with suspected increased intracranial pressure?*

   The Paramedic should focus on continuous monitoring of vital signs with an eye toward Cushing's triad.

2. *Are there any concerns about fluid resuscitation?*

   Fluid resuscitation, in Mrs. Washington's case, should be limited in light of her kidney failure.

Evaluation

1. *What is the process of obtaining venous access via an AV graft?*

   First, the Paramedic should assess the health of the AV graft/fistula by feeling for a thrill and/or auscultating for a bruit. Next, the Paramedic must determine the need for a tourniquet, which generally is only needed if the patient is in a low-flow state. Next, the Paramedic should use aseptic technique to prepare the area, followed by an introduction of sterile venous catheter at a 30-degree angle. Once the Paramedic observes a blood flash, the needle should run parallel to the plane of the arm. Once venous access is obtained, fluids should be run continuously to ensure the continued patency of the AV graft/fistula.

2. *What are some of the predictable complications associated with fluid resuscitation?*

   As the end-stage renal dialysis patient has limited ability to handle fluid overload, it is imperative that the Paramedic assess the patient for signs of overhydration and congestive heart failure.

Disposition

1. *What is the most appropriate transport decision that will get the patient to definitive care?*

   Although any emergency department could technically handle this emergency, in consideration of the possibility of a stroke, a stroke center would be preferable.

2. *What are the advantages of transporting a patient with suspected uremia to a hospital with a dialysis center, even if that means bypassing other hospitals in the process?*

   In the event that another dialysis-related complication occurs, it may be necessary to send Mrs. Washington to dialysis. Although most hospitals have the capability of emergency dialysis. it might be more convenient in this instance, from a medical records standpoint, to transport Mrs. Washington to the hospital where her dialysis center is located.

Practice Questions
Multiple Choice

1. a
2. d
3. c
4. d
5. c
6. d
7. c
8. c
9. d
10. a
11. d
12. a
13. c
14. c
15. b

Short Answer

16. Kidney stones generally form as a result of one of two mechanisms. In the first mechanism, a super saturation of the urine encourages the formation of crystals. In the second, there is an infectious foci.

17. In hemodialysis, blood is removed from the body and run through a machine that contains a semi-permeable membrane, called a dialyzer, which filters the blood, adds minerals and water, and then returns the purified and fortified blood to the patient's body.

18. Disequilibrium syndrome is a central nervous system disorder that is thought to be due to cerebral edema. The edema may result from osmotic shifts in the brain, urea removal, or changes in the intracellular pH in the brain. DDS usually occurs in younger patients and those who are new to dialysis.

19. As the nitrogenous waste builds up in the blood (azotemia), the patient will develop yellowed skin. This yellowed skin is not jaundice but results from the buildup of carotene in the skin. With jaundice, the sclera of the eyes is also yellowed, whereas in kidney failure-induced carotenodermia the sclera is not yellowed.

20. The stimulus for red blood cell production is erythropoietin. Patients with kidney failure lack erythropoietin, resulting in diminished red blood cells (i.e., anemia). This anemia causes patients to appear pale.

Fill in the Blank

21. occult

22. bladder cancer

23. anasarca

24. asterixis

25. uremic frost

Chapter 22

Case Study

Chief Concern

1. *What are some of the possible causes of a swollen, painful deformity?*

   The first and most obvious cause is a fracture, secondary to a trauma. If it is atraumatic, then everything from brittle bone disease (osteogenesis imperfecta) to bone cancer are possible.

2. *How is the patient's age related to these causes?*

   Some causes of atraumatic fractures, such as those secondary to osteoporosis, are unlikely in an adolescent. Others, such as gout, also become less likely.

History

1. *What are the important elements of the history that a Paramedic should obtain?*

   First, the Paramedics need to definitively determine if there was any trauma. For example, is it possible that Velma tried to get out of bed on her own and fell? Once satisfied that there was no trauma, they should proceed with the rest of the history. Sudden pain suggests an acute origin, such as a vascular occlusion or trauma. Following the OPQRST mnemonic, the Paramedic should obtain the time of onset; events preceding the onset of pain; the location, quality, recurrence, radiation, and relieving factors; and severity of the pain

2. *What additional history would be helpful?*

   The Paramedic should inquire if the patient has a history of fever, night sweats, or chills, which is suggestive of an infectious cause of the patient's extremity pain.

Examination

1. *What are the elements of the physical examination of a patient with suspected deep vein thrombus?*

   Examination of the painful extremity involves inspection and palpation of the extremity. First, the Paramedic should inspect the extremity for any obvious injury, deformity, areas of edema or erythema, or other skin changes. The Paramedic should palpate the extremity for skin temperature compared with the opposite extremity; palpate the extremity for bony and soft tissue tenderness; and assess the distal pulses, sensation, and muscle strength on each affected extremity, comparing it with the opposite side.

2. *Why was a temperature important?*

   A fever might indicate an infectious process and/or inflammation. This determination helps to narrow down the list of potential diagnoses.

Assessment

1. *What potential diagnoses are considered in Velma's case?*

   The worst case scenario would be an acute arterial occlusion. Maud eliminated that possibility by reviewing the five "P's." Alternate diagnoses include cellulitis, venous occlusion, or deep vein thrombus.

2. *What diagnosis seems most likely based on the patient's presentation?*

   A deep vein thrombus, with a potential of pulmonary embolism, seems most likely based on the patient's presentation.

Treatment

1. *What is the standard of care of patients with suspected acute venous occlusion or deep vein thrombus?*

   Beyond supportive care (i.e., ECG, venous access, and oxygen therapy as needed), there is little that a Paramedic can do for the patient in the prehospital setting.

2. *What is a PICC line?*

   A PICC line is a peripherally inserted central venous catheter that allows access to the great veins in the body. It is often used for patients who are vasculopathetic or for infusions of caustic medications.

Evaluation

1. *What are some of the predictable complications associated with acute venous occlusion or deep vein thrombus?*

   The risk of DVT is embolization of a portion of the DVT that travels to the heart and into the lung, becoming a pulmonary embolus (PE). The overwhelming majority of PEs originate from a lower extremity DVT.

2. *What are some signs of a pulmonary embolism?*

   The classic signs of a pulmonary embolism include shortness of breath with clear lung sounds; hypoxia in the face of high-flow, high-concentration oxygen; and chest pain without cardiac origin.

Disposition

1. *What is the most appropriate transport decision that will get the patient to definitive care?*

   Patients with unstable vital signs should be transported to the nearest emergency department for stabilization. Most hospitals will not have a concern with handling all of these patients who present with a complaint of extremity pain.

2. *What happens if the Paramedic suspects that the patient will need surgical intervention?*

   If the Paramedic suspects the patient may require surgical intervention by an orthopedist, general surgeon, or vascular surgeon, she should make reasonable attempts to bring the patient directly to an appropriate emergency department. If there is any question, the Paramedic should not hesitate to consult on-line medical control to ensure the appropriateness of the destination.

Practice Questions
Multiple Choice

1. d
2. d
3. a
4. a
5. c
6. c
7. a
8. a
9. d
10. a
11. a
12. c
13. b
14. a
15. a

Short Answer

16. Absent distal pulses and a cold extremity tend to differentiate arterial occlusion from venous occlusion.

17. Rhabdomyolysis, the breakdown of muscle, is a condition that is most often associated with crush injury, electrical injury, or prolonged soft tissue compression, although it can occur from a variety of causes including excessive exercise.

18. Arthritis is an inflammation of a joint, which can occur due to many different causes. The three types of arthritis covered in this chapter are osteoarthritis, rheumatoid arthritis, and gout.

19. Gonococcal arthritis is an infectious (septic) type of arthritis that occurs with those patients infected with gonorrhea.

20. Fibromyalgia is a painful syndrome that includes muscular pain, digestive disorders, chronic headaches, and even sleep disorders that may affect 3% to 6% of the population. The cardinal symptom of fibromyalgia is exhaustion that is coupled with muscle pain.

Fill in the Blank

21. slipped capital femoral epiphysis

22. lymphangitis

23. paronychia

24. pulselessness

25. bursitis

Chapter 23

Case Study

Chief Concern

1. *What are some of the possible causes of nosebleeds?*

   Nosebleeds could be the result of trauma (e.g., a fall), hypertension (secondary to a stroke), or a bleeding disorder. However, the most likely causes of a nosebleed are localized trauma and digital manipulation.

2. *What potentially life-threatening conditions could cause a nosebleed?*

   Nosebleeds can be a result of a simple fall, which can represent sudden syncope secondary to a potentially lethal dysrhythmia, such as ventricular tachycardia. The nosebleed can be an obvious minor injury that occurred secondary to a stroke. The nosebleed can also occur simultaneously with a traumatic brain injury.

History

1. *What are the important elements of the history that a Paramedic should obtain?*

   Beyond the history related to the chief concern, using mnemonics such as OPQRST, the Paramedic who suspects a bleeding disorder should also inquire about recent blood transfusions, as well as any history of liver and/or kidney disease.

2. *What specific medication history should the Paramedic obtain?*

   The medication history should focus on those medications that cause increased bleeding (i.e., anticoagulants such as aspirin), those medications that treat conditions that impair coagulation (such as liver disease or kidney disease), or medications that treat hypertension (such as ACE inhibitors).

Examination

1. *What are the elements of the physical examination of a patient with suspected bleeding disorder?*

   The Paramedic should perform a head-to-toe, secondary examination, following the primary examination, looking for evidence of bleeding. The Paramedic should examine the patient's head for evidence of cranial nerve dysfunction including pupil size, equality, and reaction. The Paramedic should examine the patient's chest for abnormal lung sounds and murmurs. She should also examine the abdomen for signs of internal bleeding, including tenderness, firm distention, or bruising on the flanks. The Paramedic then examines for painful extremities to determine distal function, including pulses, sensation and motor function, and bony tenderness. She should examine swollen joints for tenderness and stability. Finally, the Paramedic should examine the patient's skin for color, temperature, moisture, petechiae, and bruising.

2. *Why is a neurological assessment a critical element in this examination?*

   Bleeding evident on the outside may mean that there is internal bleeding as well, which leads to increased intracranial pressure. The brain, within its cranial vault, cannot tolerate much bleeding. A neurological examination may reveal evidence of increased intracranial pressure and signs of transtentorial herniation.

Assessment

1. *What is the significance of the widespread bruising?*

   The widespread bruising that is described may be purpura fulminans, a coagulation disorder associated with disseminated intravascular coagulation. This purpura looks similar to lividity but is not dependent and occurs on any surface.

2. *If disseminated intravascular coagulation, secondary to sepsis, is suspected, what other workups are needed?*

Disseminated intravascular coagulation is seen in late-stage sepsis. Traditional sources of infection in the elderly follow the PUS triad: pulmonary infections, urinary tract infections, and skin breakdown.

Treatment

1. *What is the standard of care of patients with suspected DIC secondary to sepsis?*

The treatment of most bleeding disorders is usually supportive, focusing on optimizing oxygen delivery by maintaining an adequate airway, breathing, and circulation.

2. *Assuming the MOLST form did not prohibit administration of any medications, what medication would be given to support the blood pressure?*

Patients with sepsis experience distributive shock and need medications, such as dopamine or epinephrine, for vasoconstriction.

Evaluation

1. *What are some of the predictable complications associated with DIC?*

As a coagulopathy, Andrea can expect bleeding from any "instrumentation" (i.e., venous catheters, indwelling urinary catheters, and so on), as well as any mucous membrane, from the airway and lungs to the gastrointestinal tract. Bleeding in some cases can be significant and life-threatening.

2. *Beyond vasopressor support, what else can a Paramedic do to help the patient with end-stage sepsis?*

After treating the "pipes" with vasopressors and the "fluid" with fluid boluses of saline solution, the Paramedic can support the bradycardiac "heart" with cardiac compressions or external pacing.

Disposition

1. *What is the most appropriate transport decision that will get the patient to definitive care?*

This patient is critically ill and will need to be transported to a hospital with a critical care/intensive care unit for hemodynamic monitoring and vasopressor support.

2. *What special hospital services may the patient need beyond intensive care?*

Understanding the pathophysiology of DIC, the Paramedic should consider facilities with a blood bank, for transfusion of blood products, as well as one with critical care.

Practice Questions
Multiple Choice

1. b
2. b
3. c
4. a
5. a
6. c
7. a
8. d
9. d
10. b
11. d
12. d
13. a
14. d
15. b

Short Answer

16. Disseminated intravascular coagulation (DIC) is a condition in which there is an overactivation of both the coagulation and fibrinolytic systems. The overactivation of the coagulation system produces significant amounts of fibrin which clot the smaller blood vessels and capillaries, thereby consuming platelets and clotting factors. The overactivation of the fibrinolytic system causes breakdown of larger clots and promotes bleeding. Often the smaller clots that occlude the smaller blood vessels are not affected. DIC becomes a paradoxical condition in which the patient is both clotting and bleeding at the same time.

17. The problem with polycythemia is the viscosity, or thickness, of the blood is increased, becoming more like a jelly or syrup. The thicker blood does not flow as well through the smaller blood vessels. The slower the blood flows, the less the venous return, which in turn reduces stroke volume and therefore cardiac output. Furthermore, polycythemia causes the heart to work harder, pumping viscous blood, leading to further decline.

18. In autoimmune hemolytic anemia, the patient develops antibodies that work against the patient's own red blood cells. In other words, the immune system attacks and destroys the patient's own red blood cells.

19. Vitamin B_{12}, folate, and iron are needed for the production of red blood cells.

20. Von Willebrand disease is a hereditary coagulation disorder that results in a lack of von Willebrand factor (vWf) in the inner lining of the blood vessels.

Fill in the Blank

21. coagulopathy

22. anemia

23. alloimmune hemolytic anemia

24. hemolytic uremic syndrome

25. malaria

Chapter 24

Case Study

Chief Concern

1. *What are some of the possible musculoskeletal causes of back pain?*

   Sources of musculoskeletal back pain include muscle strain (common), disk herniation (often traumatic), infections including spinal osteomyelitis, diskitis, epidural hematoma, cancer (either bone cancer or metastasis), and osteoporosis.

2. *What are some nontraumatic, nonmusculoskeletal causes of back pain?*

   Sources of atraumatic, nonmusculoskeletal back pain include rupture of an abdominal aortic aneurysm, kidney stones, or kidney infection (pyelonephritis, for example).

History

1. *What are the important elements of the history that a Paramedic should obtain?*

   After eliminating trauma in the differential diagnosis, the Paramedic should ask about saddle anesthesia, changes in bowel and bladder control including stool incontinence and/or urinary incontinence, and factors such as night sweats, fever, or unintended weight loss.

2. *What are the important elements of the patient's past medical history?*

   First, the Paramedic should ascertain if the back pain is acute or chronic. If it is chronic, what is the diagnosis and what treatments, including surgery, have been undertaken for the back pain? Next, the Paramedic should determine any past medical history, looking for signs of hypertension, cancer, and aortic aneurysm. For the post-menopausal women and elderly males, the Paramedic should find out if the patient has osteoporosis.

Examination

1. *What are the elements of the physical examination of a patient with back pain?*

   After completing a primary assessment and a full set of vital signs, the Paramedic should inspect and palpate the spine for tenderness, swelling, and deformity along the midline. Muscle spasm adjacent to the spine should also be assessed.

2. *Why is a peripheral neurological examination a critical element in this examination?*

   Peripheral weakness may be an indication of spinal nerve involvement. Any difference in strength, sensation, or pulses should be noted.

Assessment

1. *What is the significance of the leg weakness?*

   The leg weakness is suggestive of spinal cord nerve impingement and potential problems with ambulation in the future.

2. *What diagnosis did the Paramedic announce to the patient?*

Pat probably already understands that her leg weakness represents the progression of a problem beyond a simple backache. As the specter of permanent disability is always present, the patient needs immediate medical attention.

Treatment

1. *What is the standard of care of patients with suspected acute cord compression?*

After establishing standard ALS care, such as venous access, the Paramedic should focus on analgesia as needed and other supportive measures.

2. *What analgesia might be used in this case?*

Any opiate, such as morphine sulfate or fentanyl, would be appropriate. Fentanyl may be preferable because it has a rapid onset and fewer hemodynamic effects. However, morphine may be preferable if a long transport time is expected.

Evaluation

1. *What are some of the predictable complications associated with acute cord compression?*

While the case may present as acute cord compression, the Paramedic should be watchful for an aortic aneurysm as both acute cord compression and aortic aneurysm present with a similar symptom pattern. The Paramedic should not rely solely on the presence or absence of a midline abdominal pulsation to differentiate the two pathologies. Some patients, particularly heavy patients, may not present with a pulsating midline mass.

2. *How would an aortic aneurysm present?*

An aortic aneurysm that dissects would cause a rapid loss of blood pressure as well as a loss of pulses in the legs. Therefore, the Paramedic should monitor pedal, popliteal, and femoral pulses.

Disposition

1. *What is the most appropriate transport decision that will get the patient to definitive care?*

Any hospital capable of providing neurosurgical services, including magnetic resonance imaging or computerized tomography scan, is capable of caring for patients like Pat.

2. *What special hospital services might be needed?*

Acute cord compression often requires surgery to decompress the spinal cord and support adjacent spinal vertebrae. Rehabilitation often follows back surgery. Many of these hospitals have a rehabilitation facility attached to the hospital.

Practice Questions
Multiple Choice

1. b
2. a
3. c
4. b
5. b
6. b
7. c
8. d
9. a
10. d
11. a
12. c
13. d
14. d
15. d

Short Answer

16. Infections can occur in the disk (diskitis) or within the spinal canal (epidural abscess) and produce pain or compression of the spinal cord. These infections are most often due to bacteria that have travelled in the bloodstream from another location in the body to the disk or around the spinal cord.

17. Saddle anesthesia is a numbness or "pins and needles" sensation located in the skin territory of the perineum between the legs, the external genitalia, and the anus. Sensation to this area of the skin is covered by the S4 and S5 nerves, which are the most distal nerves in the spinal cord.

18. Stool incontinence occurs as the control of the anal sphincter is lost and the sphincter relaxes, allowing stool to ooze from the anus.

19. If a patient has abdominal pain associated with back pain, the Paramedic should be concerned about the presence of an aortic aneurysm rupture.

20. Following a primary assessment with vital signs, the Paramedic should inspect the spine for deformities, contusions, or masses. Next, the Paramedic should palpate along the length of the spine for deformity, point tenderness, and muscular spasm. Next, the Paramedic should check for signs of incontinence, equality of femoral pulses, equality of leg strength, and the presence of pedal pulses. Finally, the Paramedic should assess for sensation along the medial and lateral surfaces of the lower legs, the dorsum of the foot, and the plantar surface.

Fill in the Blank

21. pyelonephritis

22. spinal stenosis

23. saddle anesthesia

24. analgesics/opiates

25. diskitis

Chapter 25
Case Study
Chief Concern

1. *What are some of the primary causes of Joe's headache?*

   Primary headaches include migraine, tension, and cluster headaches, but of more concern are secondary headaches.

2. *What are some of the secondary causes of a headache?*

   Secondary headaches are those headaches caused by another pathology such as hemorrhagic stroke, meningitis/encephalitis, and hypertensive crisis.

History

1. *What are the important elements of the history that a Paramedic should obtain?*

   The Paramedic should get a complete clinical picture of the headache using OPQRST and identify other associated symptoms including problems of vision, paresthesia, or weakness.

2. *What are some of the important elements of the past medical history that a Paramedic should obtain?*

   Past medical history should include risk factors such as hypertension, diabetes, cardiovascular disease, renal failure, and stroke.

Examination

1. *What are the elements of the physical examination of a patient with suspected hypertensive emergency?*

   After completing the primary assessment and treating any immediate life threats, the Paramedic should proceed to perform a neurological examination as well as a cardiovascular examination. The neurological examination should be repeated frequently, and following every medication, to trend changes as well as detect subtle findings that may indicate deterioration.

2. *Why is a cardiovascular examination, including a 12-lead ECG, a critical element in this examination?*

   Hypertensive emergencies have profound effects on the cardiovascular system and can lead to future ischemic events and even heart failure.

Assessment

1. *What diagnosis did the Paramedic announce to the patient?*

   The symptom complex presented is suggestive of a hypertensive emergency. The patient should be informed of the potential for stroke, seizures, or heart attack.

2. *Why would the patient not be aware of the seriousness of the illness?*

As the symptoms of an acute hypertensive crisis may be subtle (which explains why hypertension is called the "silent disease"), it may be necessary to enlist a physician's assistance to get the patient to seek medical attention.

Treatment

1. *What is the standard of care of patients with suspected hypertensive crisis?*

While in the past Paramedics aggressively lowered acute hypertension with beta blockers, resulting in hemorrhagic strokes in some cases, current wisdom suggests a more cautious approach using nitrates.

2. *Why are nitrates preferred in the prehospital treatment of suspected hypertensive crisis?*

Nitrates, either sublingual or topical, can be administered in the prehospital setting, with the therapeutic goal of lowering blood pressure gradually by titrate of the nitrates, if possible.

Evaluation

1. *What are some of the predictable complications associated with acute hypertensive crisis?*

Patients with acute hypertensive crisis are at risk for strokes, seizures, and acute myocardial infarction.

2. *What are some of the predictable complications associated with the treatments for acute hypertensive crisis?*

The patient, as in this case, may have had a hypertension-induced stroke or a hemorrhagic stroke. In either case, the Paramedic should treat the patient like any other patient with a stroke.

Disposition

1. *What is the most appropriate transport decision that will get the patient to definitive care?*

A patient with a hypertensive crisis will need to be transported to a hospital with a neurosurgical service (if possible) and to a facility with MRI or CT scanning capabilities.

2. *What specialty hospitals have these capabilities?*

Often stroke centers have a neurological service as well as advanced medical imaging such as CT scanners and/or MRI.

Practice Questions
Multiple Choice

1. c
2. d
3. b
4. a
5. d
6. b
7. d
8. a
9. d
10. d
11. c
12. d
13. d
14. d
15. d

Short Answer

16. Hypertension leads to increased cerebral perfusion pressures. The increased CPP leads to microscopic damage to the blood vessels. These vessels can either rupture, causing a hemorrhagic stroke, or the narrowed blood vessels can be blocked by a clot, leading to a thrombotic stroke.

17. Hypertension increases the work of the heart, leading to left ventricular hypertrophy and ventricular remodeling. The combined effect is a weakened heart that ejects less blood and results in heart failure.

18. The kidneys are the most likely organ to be affected by hypertension. Hypertension limits blood flow to the kidneys and impairs the kidney's ability to function as a filter. This sets into motion the renin–angiotensin–aldosterone mechanism that further increases the blood pressure, creating a cyclical decline in kidney function.

19. The Paramedic should ask the patient about headaches, nausea, visual disturbances, and any numbness or weakness.

20. The Paramedic should ask the patient about chest pain/pressure (or anginal equivalents) or shortness of breath that is suggestive of backward failure.

Fill in the Blank

21. hypertensive encephalopathy

22. hypertensive urgency

23. uremia

24. eclampsia

25. renin, angiotensin, aldosterone system

Chapter 26

Case Study

Chief Concern

1. *What are some potential causes of eye injury?*

   Foreign body presence, infection, glaucoma, retinal detachment, corneal abrasion

2. *What are some "secondary" or indirect causes of blurred or lost vision?*

   Strokes can be a cause of blurred or lost vision, as well as certain medications, such as amiodorane, and even psychiatric illness (hysterical blindness).

History

1. *What are the properties of cement dust?*

   Cement contains lime. Lime, as an alkali, can cause a severe burn that continues to burn beyond the surface, a process called liquefaction necrosis.

2. *Was Amanda's advice correct?*

   Copious irrigation is the key to neutralize and dilute the alkali. The sooner the irrigation, the less likely ocular damage will occur. Alkali substances can penetrate the anterior within five minutes.

Examination

1. *What are the elements of the physical examination of a patient with an ocular burn?*

   The priority should be a primary assessment. While ocular burns are very painful, it is possible that Mark also inhaled the cement dust. The Paramedic should start with a visual inspection of the oropharynx and auscultate the throat and apices of the lung, continuing with the remainder of the primary assessment.

2. *What are the elements of the eye exam?*

   To conduct an eye exam, the Paramedic should check each eye for visual acuity.

Assessment

1. *What diagnosis does the Paramedic tell the patient?*

   In this case, it is obvious that the patient has an eye injury.

2. *What is the prognosis for a burn to the eye?*

   Alkali burns to the eyes have led to cases of prolonged disability and even blindness.

Treatment

1. *What is the standard of care for patients with ocular burns?*

   Irrigation with copious quantities of water is the standard of care for patients with ocular burns. No attempt should be made to neutralize the alkali with a weak acid. While the alkali might be neutralized, the exothermic chemical reaction, producing heat, would further injure the already injured eye.

2. *What device might be helpful with irrigation?*

Commercial devices such as the Morgan® Lens are particularly useful as they contain a plastic shield that sits on the eye and permits a constant stream of sterile saline to irrigate the eye.

Evaluation

1. *Is the irrigation still needed?*

Irrigation of ocular burns, particularly burns from alkalis, should be continuous if possible and minimally last for 20 minutes.

2. *When should the irrigation stop?*

If after 20 minutes of continuous irrigation the eye is pain-free and vision has returned to normal, then the irrigation can be stopped.

Disposition

1. *What is the most appropriate transport decision that will get the patient to definitive care?*

Ocular emergencies are so common that any emergency department should be able to manage the patient.

2. *What specialty hospital may be preferred?*

Often a trauma center will have an on-duty ophthalmologist or ophthalmologist resident.

Practice Questions
Multiple Choice

1. a
2. b
3. c
4. a
5. a
6. b
7. a
8. a

9. d
10. a
11. b
12. d
13. a
14. c
15. b

Short Answer

16. The origins of dizziness are found in the vestibular system, which is part of cranial nerve VIII. It is responsible for providing information to the brain on one's location in space and orientation. Disruption of this system, either from mechanical forces (e.g., a spinning amusement park ride) or from physiological causes (e.g., dehydration, vertigo, or infection), can give the patient the feeling of spinning.

17. Peripheral vertigo is a disturbance of the vestibular organs whereas central vertigo is a central nervous system disorder.

18. Disequilibrium is a feeling of being off-balance or unsteady on the feet.

19. In acute angle–closure glaucoma, the pressure within the eye increases rapidly and dramatically and can cause dysfunction of the optic nerve, leading to permanent loss of vision.

20. Acidic irritants tend to cause less damage than alkaline agents. The reason for this is that the acidic irritants cause the proteins on the front of the eye to coagulate, or clump together, preventing further penetration into the eye. Alkaline agents, on the other hand, rapidly penetrate through the cornea, essentially melting the structures as it burns deeper.

Fill in the Blank

21. tinnitus
22. vertigo
23. disequilibrium

24. conjunctivitis
25. epistaxis

Chapter 27

Case Study

Chief Concern

1. *What are some of the possible pulmonary causes of hemoptysis?*

   Pulmonary causes of hemoptysis include cancer, tuberculosis, and even the plague.

2. *What are some of the extrapulmonary causes of hemoptysis?*

   Extrapulmonary causes of hemoptysis include epistaxis, strep throat, and esophageal reflux.

History

1. *What are the important elements of the history that a Paramedic should obtain?*

   The Paramedic should obtain a history of the present illness including a history of pulmonary disease, activity at onset, and so on (HAPISOCS). In this case, the patient's overseas travel should be explored in more depth.

2. *Why should the patient's overseas travel be explored in more depth?*

   Tuberculosis is still endemic to certain regions of the world, particularly third world countries.

Examination

1. *What are the elements of the physical examination of a patient with suspected tuberculosis?*

   A comprehensive pulmonary examination is in order. In both the anterior and posterior chest, the Paramedic should inspect the thorax, making some decisions about the work of breathing and the use of accessory muscles. Next, the Paramedic should auscultate each of the five lobes for signs of lung consolidation. Next, the Paramedic should use the diagnostic tools available. The Paramedic can expect the SpO_2 to be lower than normal and the $EtCO_2$ to be elevated.

2. *Why is a 12-lead ECG a critical element in this examination?*

   Pulmonary disease can put a strain on the heart. The patient may not note the chest pressure because of the pleuritic chest pain or the work of breathing.

Assessment

1. *What diagnosis did the Paramedic announce to the patient?*

   While the presumption is tuberculosis, owed to the symptom complex, the Paramedic can only be sure that Mr. Wentworth is infected and is experiencing respiratory distress.

2. *What other medical conditions could cause the symptom complex?*

   The patient may also have lung cancer with secondary metastasis to the lymph nodes and a secondary pulmonary infection.

Treatment

1. *What is the first priority of care for the Paramedic treating the patient with suspected tuberculosis?*

   The first priority of patient care is isolation and protection. The combination of weight loss, fever, and night sweats is highly suggestive of tuberculosis.

2. *What is the next priority of care for the Paramedic treating the patient with suspected tuberculosis?*

   The next order of business is respiratory support (i.e., oxygenation) and ventilation as needed.

Evaluation

1. *What are some of the predictable complications associated with suspected tuberculosis?*

   As tuberculosis is a pulmonary disease, it can be expected that these patients will need respiratory support, up to and including intubation, for the respiratory failure.

2. *What advanced complications can be expected for the patient with tuberculosis?*

   As tuberculosis is an infectious disease, it can be expected that these patients will eventually become septic and will need vasopressor support.

Disposition

1. *What is the most appropriate transport decision that will get the patient to definitive care?*

   Tuberculosis is an all too common disease and therapy can be started at any hospital.

2. *What specialty hospital might be preferred in this case?*

   The patient in this case is critically ill and will need the intensive care found at a tertiary care facility.

Practice Questions
Multiple Choice

1. a
2. a
3. b
4. c
5. c
6. a
7. c
8. b
9. a
10. d
11. d
12. a
13. d
14. d
15. a

Short Answer

16. A carrier is an asymptomatic (i.e., without signs of infection) conveyance for infection that is unaware of being the reservoir for the disease.

17. Turbidity in urine, a sign of urinary tract infection, is caused by bacteria suspended in the urine, making the urine cloudy or hazy.

18. Broadly defined, virulence speaks to several factors in pathogenesis, such as ease of entry, route of entry, dose, and host defense. More narrowly, virulence speaks to the fitness of the microbe to survive and thrive in the host.

19. The four stages of infection are incubation, prodromal phase, infectious period, and the recovery time.

20. A residual is a physical remnant of the infection whereas the sequela is a morbid condition as a result of the disease.

Fill in the Blank

21. competitive inhibition
22. contagious
23. fomites
24. attenuated
25. acme

Chapter 28
Case Study
Chief Concern

1. *What are some of the possible infectious causes of pediatric rashes?*

   Some possible causes are measles, mumps, rubella, roseola, and chickenpox.

2. *What infectious disease(s) would be a problem for the Paramedic if she were pregnant?*

   Rubella can cause serious birth defects.

History

1. *What are the important elements of the history that a Paramedic should obtain?*

   After ascertaining the patient's chief complaint, the Paramedic should inquire about symptoms that may have occurred during the prodrome/incubation period of the infection.

2. *What specific questions beyond the standard SAMPLE history should the Paramedic ask?*

The Paramedic may ask questions about headaches, meningeal signs, productive cough, gastrointestinal symptoms (nausea, vomiting, and diarrhea, as well as anorexia), and constitutional signs such as fever, myalgia, and pruritus.

Examination

1. *What are the elements of the physical examination of a patient with suspected infection?*

A head-to-toe examination looks for meningeal signs, respiratory embarrassment, and gastrointestinal disorders. It ends with an examination of the extremities for exanthema, vesicles, purpura, and petechiae.

2. *What would a limited number of vesicles around a wrist, for example, suggest?*

A limited distribution of lesions in a certain location, such as around the patient's wrist or waist, without the accompanying systemic signs (such as fever) is suggestive of contact dermatitis of a noninfectious origin.

Assessment

1. *What diagnosis did the Paramedic announce to the patient's father?*

A centrifugal rash, such as the one described, is suggestive of rubeola (measles), rubella (German measles), or chickenpox.

2. *Is the location of the rash important to the diagnosis?*

A rash starting on the trunk (i.e., a central rash) is suggestive of smallpox. A "centrifugal" rash (i.e., one starting in the periphery) is suggestive of chickenpox, and other "disseminated" rashes are suggestive of measles.

Treatment

1. *What is the standard of care of patients with a suspected communicable disease?*

The Paramedic should provide the patient with a chance to rest and should consider reducing the fever and relieving any discomfort, if possible. Antiemetics may be in order if the patient is nauseous. The Paramedic may also use venous access for a fluid bolus if the patient is dehydrated secondary to insensible losses such as sweat from fever.

2. *What are some of the patient-specific concerns and considerations that the Paramedic should consider when applying this plan of care that is intended to treat a broad patient population presenting with communicable disease?*

First and foremost, the Paramedic should be concerned about self-protection. Gloves and a mask may be used at a minimum in these cases. However, even prior to the call for EMS the Paramedic should have the proper vaccinations.

Evaluation

1. *What are some of the predictable complications associated with a suspected communicable disease?*

Most of the suspected communicable diseases are capable of producing meningitis.

2. *What symptom pattern would alert the Paramedic to this complication?*

The Paramedic should be alert to changes in mental status as well as the classic triad of meningeal signs: photophobia, nuchal rigidity, and headache.

Disposition

1. *What is the most appropriate transport decision that will get the patient to definitive care?*

As many of these childhood diseases are highly contagious but are self-limited infections, transportation to the emergency department may not be necessary as long as the child does not have secondary complications.

2. *What are some of the transportation considerations?*

If a child with suspected chickenpox (varicella zoster) is to be transported, then standard precautions are in order as well as advanced notification of the emergency department so that an isolation room may be prepared.

Practice Questions
Multiple Choice

1. c
2. b
3. d
4. a
5. b
6. a
7. a
8. c
9. c
10. d
11. a
12. a
13. b
14. c
15. b

Short Answer

16. Clusters are events such as multiple cases of diarrhea or flu-like symptoms. These events are compared against the expected incidence of those symptoms within a given population in order to identify variation.

17. Social distancing is a less noxious, but also less effective, method of movement restriction. Social distancing, while not a strict quarantine, prevents the spread of communicable disease by banning public gatherings (i.e., limiting access to places where groups of people congregate, such as theaters and schools).

18. In ring vaccination, the persons immediately at risk due to their proximity with the infected or ill people (the "ring" around the infected population), even if they haven't had direct contact with them, are vaccinated. This procedure works like a fire break. Like a fire break, it needs to be instituted early, during the disease's incubation period.

19. With the disease contained, the remaining population in the affected area receives a targeted vaccination. Targeted vaccinations are effective at preventing epidemics in some cases, but the effectiveness of these vaccination campaigns are limited by mobility and mass transit.

20. If the origin of the disease cannot be found, then mass vaccination of the potential population at risk is in order. The problem with mass vaccination is that it is expensive in terms of both human and medical resources.

Fill in the Blank

21. sexually transmitted disease
22. pruritus
23. contact tracing
24. erythema
25. chlamydia

Chapter 29
Case Study
Chief Concern

1. *What are some of the possible causes of nontraumatic joint pain?*

    Nontraumatic joint pain is usually caused by an autoimmune disease such as systemic lupus erythematosus (SLE or lupus), rheumatoid arthritis (RA), dermatomyositis, polymyositis, ankylosing spondylitis, and inclusion-body myositis. Although each of these syndromes is rare, systemic lupus erythematosus and rheumatoid arthritis are two of the more common diseases.

History

1. *What are the important elements of the history that a Paramedic should obtain?*

    As fever is a classic sign of inflammation, the Paramedic should try to discern the etiology of the fever and rule out infection, if possible. The nurse practitioner appears to have started that line of thinking already.

2. *Why should the Paramedic take a careful medication history?*

    Several medications have been implicated in autoimmune disorders including chlorpromazine, hydralazine, isoniazid, quinidine, procainamide, and methyldopa.

Examination

1. *What are the elements of the physical examination of a patient with suspected autoimmune disorder?*

   The physical examination should focus on potential etiologies of the fever (i.e., bronchitis, pneumonia, and urinary tract infection, three infections with a high probability in this patient population).

2. *What signs would suggest systemic lupus erythematous?*

   The malar rash, a fixed erythema in the shape of a butterfly on the face, is almost pathomimetic for systemic lupus erythematosus (SLE).

Assessment

1. *What diagnosis would be probable in this case?*

   Based on the triad of symptoms (i.e., fever, joint pain, and malar rash), the Paramedic is led to suspect systemic lupus erythematosus (SLE). However, a more extensive diagnostic workup will be needed to confirm the suspicion.

2. *What diagnosis did the Paramedic announce to the patient?*

   At this point, the Paramedic can only suspect an autoimmune disorder of unknown etiology.

Treatment

1. *What is the standard of care of patients with suspected autoimmune disorders?*

   In general, Paramedics can only offer supportive care for patient-specific complaints.

2. *Why would the Paramedic withhold the steroid?*

   If the patient is immunocompromised, steroids could further lower her immunity and leave her susceptible to infection.

Evaluation

1. *What are some predictable complications of systemic lupus erythematosus (SLE)?*

   Joint pain is a common complication of SLE. While ibuprofen is the drug of choice for SLE, many services do not routinely carry the medication.

2. *What is the cause of death for patients with SLE?*

   The cause of death for patients with SLE is often an infection.

Disposition

1. *What is the most appropriate transport decision that will get the patient to definitive care?*

   As autoimmune disorders can be complex, it is advisable to transport these patients to medical centers with advanced diagnostic capabilities and those facilities capable of providing long-term care and follow-up to these chronic diseases.

2. *What important assessment information should the Paramedic relay to the emergency department staff?*

   The Paramedic should relay any signs or symptoms that would suggest an infection, such as fever, chills, and so on.

Practice Questions
Multiple Choice

1. d		9. a	
2. d		10. d	
3. b		11. b	
4. d		12. d	
5. d		13. d	
6. d		14. a	
7. d		15. d	
8. d			

Short Answer

16. Mast cells release a variety of granules and chemicals, including histamine, heparin, and other cytokines (immune chemicals) that are responsible for the body's reaction to immune stimulation.

17. The results of mast cell secretions include vascular leaking, smooth muscle stimulation, and increased secretions from nasal, bronchial, or gastric cells.

18. Among the autoimmune diseases are systemic lupus erythematosus (SLE or lupus), rheumatoid arthritis (RA), dermatomyositis, polymyositis, ankylosing spondylitis, and inclusion-body myositis. Although each of these syndromes is rare, systemic lupus erythematosus and rheumatoid arthritis are two of the more common diseases.

19. HIV is responsible for creating immune deficiency, and particularly targets the body's T cells. Since T cells are responsible for the initial stimulation of an immune response, a deficiency in the number of circulating T cells will ultimately result in a diminished immune response. People infected with HIV are susceptible to a wide variety of diseases, ranging from the simple colds that affect everyone else, to the opportunistic infections of Kaposi's sarcoma, thrush, cytomegalovirus, and various fungal infections.

20. Acute transplant rejection occurs as early as a week after transplant but can occur months to years after transplant as well. In acute rejection, the immune system attacks the transplanted organ and causes symptoms that are related to the failure of that organ.

Fill in the Blank

21. antigens
22. urticaria
23. neutropenic

24. angioedema
25. autoimmune

Chapter 30
Case Study
Chief Concern

1. *What are some of the possible causes of anaphylaxis caused by injection?*

   The typical causes of anaphylaxis are insect bites (especially from wasps and bees).

2. *What are some of the possible causes of anaphylaxis caused by ingestion?*

   Certain foods (such as peanuts and eggs) and certain medications (especially the penicillins) have a tendency to cause anaphylactic reactions.

History

1. *What are the important elements of the history that a Paramedic should obtain?*

   As time is often critical in these cases, the Paramedic needs an efficient history that minimizes unimportant information while getting to the heart of the matter. The use of the OPQRST/AMPLE format can help facilitate that process.

2. *What important additional information should a Paramedic try to obtain?*

   Anaphylactic reactions are caused by foreign proteins that are inhaled, injected, or ingested; therefore, the Paramedic should try to ascertain what offending substance was ingested, inhaled, or injected.

Examination

1. *What is the first priority in the physical examination of a patient with suspected anaphylaxis?*

   Anaphylaxis reactions affect the airway and breathing, potentially leading to suffocation and death. Therefore, the Paramedic should focus the examination on looking for signs of airway compromise and bronchoconstriction.

2. *What is the next priority in the physical examination of the patient with suspected anaphylaxis?*

   After ensuring an adequate airway and ventilation, the Paramedic should focus the examination on signs of hypoperfusion. Anaphylaxis can lead to widespread vasodilation with subsequent hypotension that leads to unconsciousness and cardiac failure.

Assessment

1. *What is the significance of stridor?*

   The audible stridor suggests that the airway is narrowly constricted and that the Paramedic may have to adjust airway management accordingly.

2. *What diagnosis did the Paramedic announce to the patient?*

   While the patient may appear to be experiencing anaphylaxis, the Paramedic was correct to break the problem down to the obvious and apparent issue.

Treatment

1. *What is the first priority in the care of the patient with suspected anaphylaxis?*

   The Paramedic must address any airway, breathing, or circulation issues as the first priority of treatment. In the case of a patient with severe anaphylaxis, the soft tissues of the patient's upper airway can become edematous and can rapidly result in occlusion of the airway. All patients with anaphylaxis should be placed on high-flow, high-concentration oxygen via a nonrebreather face mask. The Paramedic should consider endotracheal intubation if airway edema is present and progressing. In severe anaphylaxis, intubation can be very difficult due to the edema. If so, a surgical airway may be needed.

2. *What is the next priority in the care of the patient with suspected anaphylaxis?*

   After ensuring adequate ventilation (via a patent airway) and oxygenation, the Paramedic should address any issues of hypoperfusion. Hypoperfusion is first treated with supplemental epinephrine administered intramuscularly or subcutaneously followed by fluid resuscitation.

Evaluation

1. *What are some of the predictable complications associated with anaphylaxis?*

   If the patient is hemodynamically unstable, the Paramedic should rapidly establish IV access, administer IV fluid boluses, and position the patient supine with legs elevated.

   Epinephrine is the drug of choice for the treatment of anaphylaxis. Epinephrine is a sympathomimetic medication that causes bronchodilation and peripheral vasoconstriction, increasing blood pressure. The dose of epinephrine for moderate allergic reactions is 0.3 to 0.5 mg (0.3 to 0.5 mL) of a 1:1,000 solution administered intramuscularly.

2. *What are some of the predictable complications associated with the treatments for anaphylaxis?*

   Epinephrine, as a potent vasoconstrictor, can increase the workload of an already taxed heart, leading to ischemia and even acute myocardial infarction. Epinephrine should be cautiously administered to the patient with suspected coronary artery disease.

Disposition

1. *What is the most appropriate transport decision that will get the patient to definitive care?*

   Patients with a tentative airway that has the potential to deteriorate should be transported to the closest definitive care. In most cases, a community hospital is capable of caring for these emergent patients.

2. *What important patient information should be shared with the emergency department staff?*

   The emergency department staff will need to know what offending agent is suspected of inducing the anaphylaxis, the symptom pattern that led the Paramedic to suspect anaphylaxis, and the treatment provided to the patient for the anaphylaxis.

Practice Questions
Multiple Choice

1. c
2. d
3. a
4. a
5. b
6. d
7. a
8. c
9. c
10. a
11. a
12. c
13. a
14. a
15. a

Short Answer

16. Comparisons of epinephrine administered subcutaneously versus epinephrine administered intramuscularly show the time to therapeutic serum concentration is significantly shorter with intramuscular injection (5 minutes intramuscular versus 20 minutes subcutaneous).

17. The Paramedic should use caution when administering epinephrine to the elderly and those with heart disease due to the added stress that the resultant tachycardia can have on the patient's heart. This stress can lead to ischemia.

18. Signs of poor perfusion include altered mental status, diaphoresis (sweating), cool skin, and delayed capillary refill.

19. The Paramedic should exclude chronic obstructive airway disease. In addition to asthma, airway obstruction from foreign body aspiration is also possible.

20. Epinephrine is the drug of choice for the treatment of anaphylaxis. Epinephrine is a sympathomimetic medication that causes bronchodilation and peripheral vasoconstriction, increasing blood pressure.

Fill in the Blank

21. urticaria
22. anaphylactoid
23. pruritis
24. erythema
25. antigen

Chapter 31
Case Study
Chief Concern

1. *What are some of the possible medical conditions that would cause a fall?*

   The list of possible causes of syncope include dysrhythmia (number one on the list), seizure, stroke, hypoglycemia, hypoxia, and hypotension, to name a few.

2. *How is trouble breathing related to the patient's obesity?*

   Due to a functional restrictive lung disorder created by the panniculus, morbidly obese patients cannot tolerate lying flat.

History

1. *What past pulmonary history should the Paramedic obtain?*

   The Paramedic should try to obtain any history of dyspnea on exertion, paroxysmal nocturnal dyspnea, and signs of reactive airway diseases such as asthma.

2. *What past cardiac history should the Paramedic obtain?*

   The Paramedic should try to obtain any history of congestive heart failure and acute myocardial infarction, as well as any medical studies, such as echocardiograms, that indicate cardiomyopathy or cardiomegaly.

Examination

1. *What confounds the physical examination of the obese patient with suspected respiratory failure?*

   The large panniculus markedly reduces audible breath sounds, making any differentiation between normal and abnormal breath sounds difficult. The examination is further confounded by the presence of chronic atelectatic rales created by the compression of the base of the lungs by the panniculus.

2. *What confounds the physical examination of the obese patient with suspected heart failure?*

   The six cardinal signs typically seen in a patient with heart failure are jugular venous distention, ventricular gallop, pulmonary edema manifested by rales, hepatojugular reflex, dependent peripheral edema, and peripheral cyanosis. These signs are obscured in the obese patient.

Assessment

1. *What is the significance of the falling oxygen saturation?*

   The Paramedic's history for the morbidly obese patient with falling oxygen saturation should keep three etiologies in mind: backward heart failure, cor pulmonale, and restrictive lung defect.

2. *What is the significance of the syncope in the obese patient?*

   The syncope could be the result of Pickwickian syndrome (an obesity hypoventilation syndrome that occurs due to transient hypoxia) and hypercarbia. The syncope could also be the result of a transient lethal dysrhythmia, such as a run of ventricular tachycardia. This patient population has several risk factors for sudden cardiac death that are owed, in part, to their unique physiology.

Treatment

1. *What are some of the patient-specific cardiac concerns and considerations that the Paramedic should consider when applying a plan of care to a morbidly obese patient?*

   Stress on the already enlarged heart can lead to congestive heart failure as well as ischemia.

2. *What are some of the patient-specific respiratory concerns and considerations that the Paramedic should consider when applying a plan of care to a morbidly obese patient?*

   The combination of restrictive lung defect, leading to hypercarbia, and the obesity–hypoventilation syndrome can lead the patient to rapid respiratory embarrassment and respiratory failure.

Evaluation

1. *What are some of the predictable complications associated with having a bariatric patient lie flat?*

   Post-obstructive pulmonary edema (POPE) can occur when the patient breath-holds while being laid flat, after which the airway suddenly becomes occluded. The resulting increase in blood flowing back into the lungs causes an increase in pulmonary capillary pressures. The increased pulmonary capillary pressure causes fluids to leak into the alveolar space and pulmonary edema to form almost instantly.

2. *What are some treatments that could help prevent post-obstructive pulmonary edema?*

   The patient with POPE should immediately be raised to the seated position. The Paramedic should treat this type of flash pulmonary edema aggressively with high-flow, high-concentration oxygen and continuous positive airway pressure (CPAP).

Disposition

1. *What are the advantages of transporting a bariatric patient to these hospitals, even if that means bypassing other hospitals in the process?*

   Certain hospitals have invested in equipment capable of caring for a large patient, including bariatric wheelchairs, heavy-duty Hoyer® lifts, and open CAT scans. These technologies will prevent delays in patient care.

2. *What patient information should be shared with the emergency department staff while en route?*

   Beyond a routine report with the patient's chief concern and vital signs, the Paramedic should share information about the patient's weight. In many instances, special equipment has to be obtained from a warehouse or storage to treat these patients.

Practice Questions

Multiple Choice

1. b
2. a
3. d
4. c
5. b
6. d
7. b
8. a

9. b
10. d
11. a
12. b
13. a
14. c
15. c

Short Answer

16. The body mass index (BMI) is a calculation which starts with the patient's weight in kilograms and divides it by the patient's height, in meters, squared. The resulting number represents the BMI.

17. In cardiac remodeling, the heart of the patient who is obese has to overcome hypertension. To do so, it must beat harder and faster. As a result, the hyperdynamic, or forcefully beating, heart starts to hypertrophy, resulting in increased muscle mass. This hypertrophy changes the shape and volume of the ventricular chambers, a process called remodeling. The remodeled ventricle is no longer able to accept the same quantity of blood as a normal left ventricle. Therefore, there is a decreased cardiac output, which in turn leads to more tachycardia, ventricular remodeling, and so on. In other words, there is a positive feedback loop with negative consequences.

18. The obese patient is prone to transient hypoxia, particularly when lying flat. This hypoxia can be most pronounced at night when the patient is sleeping and can result in sleep apnea. Because of the recurrent hypoxia, the hormone erythropoietin (EPO) is secreted by the kidneys, which in turn stimulates the bone marrow to produce erythrocytes, or red blood cells. The resulting increase in red blood cells, as measured by hematocrit, creates a condition called polycythemia. Physiologic polycythemia is a condition of increased viscosity that makes it more difficult for the patient's heart to pump the blood, resulting in further deterioration of the patient's cardiac function.

19. A useful working definition of obesity may be excessive body fat that results in an impairment of health. This definition speaks to the consequences of obesity and not to the patient's actual weight.

20. Patient lift teams are called for when the patient is morbidly obese. These lift teams have trained together to prevent uncoordinated lifts, which lead to back injury. These lift teams are also fitted for back belts, which help stiffen the spine and decrease internal spinal forces.

Fill in the Blank

21. insulin resistance
22. Pickwickian syndrome
23. body habitus

24. panniculus
25. post-obstructive pulmonary edema

Chapter 32

Case Study

Chief Concern

1. *What are some of the possible causes of the patient's bleeding?*

   Patients with a terminal disease may have blood dyscrasia from their disease (such as leukemia), chemotherapy, radiation, or severe sepsis.

2. *Why did the patient request "no lights or siren"?*

   The patient understands that his condition is terminal and his end-of-life decision is to not have the Paramedic take heroic measures.

History

1. *What are the important elements of the history that a Paramedic should obtain?*

   The questions in the medical history of a patient with a terminal illness are less focused on rooting out the source of the disease and more on the quality of life and the activities of daily living. The Paramedic should ask questions about the fundamental human needs such as freedom from pain and adequate nutrition.

2. *Why isn't Mrs. Jancin eating?*

   Mrs. Jancin has anorexia. Anorexia is thought to be due to metabolic derangements caused by the cancer.

Examination

1. *What are the elements of the physical examination of a patient with suspected paraneoplastic syndrome?*

   The Paramedic should perform a neurological examination. Many of the signs of paraneoplastic syndrome mimic those of a stroke: slurred speech, difficulty swallowing, memory loss, and visual problems.

2. *Why is a blood glucose level a critical element in this examination?*

   While the patient's malaise may be related to the paraneoplastic syndrome, it could just as easily be related to malnutrition and hypoglycemia.

Assessment

1. *What is the Paramedic's primary concern for the terminally ill patient?*

   The first priority in palliative care is freedom from pain. The Paramedic should inquire about the pain plan and what has recently been done to relieve the patient's pain.

2. *What are some of the Paramedic's concerns about analgesia?*

   When analgesia is indicated, it can ease the pain of the disease. However, the side effects of analgesia, particularly opiates, can lead to respiratory depression and hasten death.

Treatment

1. *What is the standard of care of patients with suspected paraneoplastic syndrome?*

   Care for the patient with suspected paraneoplastic syndrome consists of comfort measures and palliative care.

2. *What is the nature of the special Paramedic–patient relationship for the patient with paraneoplastic syndrome?*

   The Paramedic's first responsibility is to ascertain if there are any advanced directives regarding care. Next, understanding that the patient's needs may be urgent but not an emergency, the Paramedic should consult with the patient regarding every treatment and obtain permission.

Evaluation

1. *What is the most predictable complication associated with paraneoplastic syndromes?*

   Nausea is the most common complaint, followed by concerns about pain and shortness of breath.

2. *What would be the preferred treatment for this complication?*

   In this case, the nausea is treated with intranasal ondansetron.

Disposition

1. *What is the most appropriate transport decision that will get the patient to definitive care?*

   Definitive care is not the issue for this patient. The appropriate transportation decision is to transport Mrs. Jancin to a place where she can get the care and comfort that she needs.

2. *What is the difference between hospice care and hospital care?*

   Hospital care focuses on the cure of the patient whereas hospice care focuses on the care of the patient. Hospitals have a diagnostic goal whereas hospice has a palliative goal.

Practice Questions
Multiple Choice

1. d
2. c
3. d
4. a
5. b
6. a
7. b
8. b

9. a
10. d
11. c
12. d
13. b
14. c
15. a

Short Answer

16. Hospice is a place of rest for terminally ill patients. Hospice care, whether provided at home or in the hospital, provides care for both the patient and the family through a multidisciplinary team of nurses, doctors, social workers, clergy, and counselors. Hospice care encompasses physical, mental, and spiritual care to manage the patient's distress and to decrease her suffering.

17. Anorexia is an eating disorder characterized by a lack of desire to eat. Unlike the psychiatric disorder anorexia nervosa, anorexia is the medical symptom for decreased appetite that owes its origins to a metabolic disturbance, such as cancer. One of the characteristics of anorexia is early satiation, a feeling of fullness after eating very little.

18. Cachexia is a wasting syndrome that is thought to be induced by inflammatory cytokines. Associated signs of cachexia include a swollen belly secondary to ascites (accumulation of fluid in the peritoneal cavity).

19. Pancytopenia is demonstrated by large ecchymotic areas or purpura. The purpura, caused by bleeding under the skin, is secondary to the anemia which often accompanies terminal cancer.

20. Although the HIV virus itself does not lead to the patient's death, the destruction of the patient's immune system permits opportunistic infections, like tuberculosis, to infect the patient in end-stage, or class IV, AIDS.

Fill in the Blank

21. jiroveci
22. chemotherapy
23. alternative

24. remission
25. palliative

Chapter 33
Case Study
Chief Concern

1. *What are some key concerns that a Paramedic should address when confronted with a critically ill patient?*

   Since cerebral resuscitation is the therapeutic goal, the key concerns are oxygen, ventilation, and circulation as well as provision of adequate glucose.

2. *What is the "order of resuscitation"?*

   The "primary survey" dictates the order of resuscitation. Starting with level of consciousness, the Paramedic focuses on airway, breathing, and circulation, in that order.

Disposition

1. *What is the most appropriate transport decision that will get the patient to definitive care?*

   Any patient with an altered mental status should be transported to an emergency department for further diagnostic workup. The therapeutic goal of resuscitation is to ensure adequate cerebral oxygenation, perfusion, and the provision of glucose.

2. *What is the minimum standard of care for an ALS-worthy patient?*

   Any patient with altered mental status is "ALS-worthy" and should minimally receive high-flow, high-concentration oxygen, assistance with ventilation, venous access, glucose determination, and ECG monitoring, as needed. In many cases, a 12-lead ECG is also appropriate.

Practice Questions
Multiple Choice

1. a
2. b
3. c
4. b
5. d
6. a
7. b
8. b

9. a
10. b
11. d
12. a
13. c
14. b
15. a

Short Answer

16. The brain needs oxygen, glucose, circulation, and the elimination of carbon dioxide to survive.

17. The adequate delivery of oxygen is based on four main components. The first key component is a clear and unobstructed airway. The second key component is adequate oxygenation of the patient. The third key component is adequate ventilation. The final key component is adequate tissue perfusion.

18. Paramedics often can determine if their patient is critically ill at the moment of initial patient contact (i.e., sick versus not sick). Sick patients (i.e., those in extremis) appear to be in distress. Patients in distress can look like they are fighting to remain conscious, have difficulty breathing, or are pale and diaphoretic.

19. Distraction from treatment priorities is a real concern in the limited resource environment during prehospital care. Multiple intubation attempts in effect put blinders on the Paramedic as he focuses all of his efforts at successfully intubating the patient. Critically ill patients often have multiple problems across multiple body systems requiring multiple interventions.

20. The three components to consider in the management of inadequate perfusion include the heart (pump), circulating blood volume, and vascular tone (pipes).

Fill in the Blank

21. acidosis
22. balloon pump
23. overresuscitation

24. goal-directed therapy
25. CPAP

Chapter 34
Case Study
Chief Concern

1. *What are some of the possible causes of vaginal bleeding in women of childbearing age?*

   Conditions that can cause vaginal bleeding are spontaneous abortion, threatened abortion, placenta previa, and placental abruption.

2. *What is the implication of the comment, "I think I'm losing the baby!"?*

   The most obvious implication is that Xian–Lun is having a miscarriage. However, that assumption is based on limited information.

History

1. *What are the important elements of the history that a Paramedic should obtain?*

   Utilizing the standard OPQRST/AMPLE mnemonic, the Paramedic should try to obtain as complete a prenatal history as possible.

2. *What additional history should the Paramedic obtain?*

   The three key historical points should be the last menstrual period (LMP), the expected date of delivery (EDD), and if the patient is receiving prenatal care.

Examination

1. *What are the elements of the physical examination of a patient with vaginal bleeding?*

   The abdominal examination for a patient with vaginal bleeding includes inspection (for contusions, abrasions, distention, and masses), auscultation (for bowel sounds), and palpation (for tenderness or pain).

2. *What is a "pad count"?*

   A pad count is the number of pads that the woman has soaked through and is used as a rough estimation of the severity of her bleeding.

Assessment

1. *What is the significance of the vaginal bleeding?*

   Vaginal bleeding could represent placenta previa, placenta abruptio, or possibly an aborted pregnancy.

2. *What is the risk with vaginal bleeding during pregnancy?*

   Patients with vaginal bleeding of an unknown etiology may be compensating for the blood loss. Even if there are no outward indications that the pregnancy is threatened, the Paramedics should take all precautions to protect the patient and the unborn baby.

Treatment

1. *What is the standard of care of patients with vaginal bleeding?*

   Care for a woman with heavy vaginal bleeding is largely supportive, and consists of providing oxygen and obtaining venous access.

2. *When is fluid resuscitation necessary?*

   Fluid resuscitation may be necessary if the patient is showing signs of hypoperfusion such as tachycardia. If the mother is in compensated shock, the fetus may be in decompensated shock as blood is shunted away from the placenta first.

Evaluation

1. *What are the implications of domestic violence in this case?*

   The Paramedic must more seriously entertain the possibility of placental abruption, a medical emergency for both mother and baby. The combination of trauma—from domestic violence, heavy vaginal bleeding, and abdominal pain—leads to that conclusion.

2. *What responsibilities does a Paramedic have to report domestic violence?*

   Although the Paramedic generally does not have a duty to report domestic violence, the Paramedic should support the patient if she chooses to report the domestic violence.

Disposition

1. *What is the most appropriate transport decision that will get the patient to definitive care?*

   As placental abruption may represent a surgical emergency, it is important to transport the patient with suspected placental abruption to a place capable of providing both obstetrical service and surgical service.

2. *What should the Paramedic report to the emergency department staff?*

   The Paramedic should report that the patient may be a victim of domestic violence. Many hospitals have special procedures, including private and secure rooms, for caring for victims of domestic violence.

Practice Questions

Multiple Choice

1. c
2. d
3. b
4. c
5. d
6. a
7. d
8. c

9. a
10. b
11. c
12. a
13. b
14. a
15. b

Short Answer

16. Patients with an ectopic pregnancy may complain of abdominal pain, vaginal bleeding, or both. Although some patients will know that they are pregnant, many will not know at the onset of symptoms. It is important for the Paramedic to consider ectopic pregnancy in any young woman of childbearing age who complains of lower abdominal pain and/or vaginal bleeding.

17. The Paramedic should not attempt to remove any foreign body in the vagina as it is difficult to determine if internal injury occurred without further testing at the emergency department. These foreign bodies cause a wide range of complaints from mild discomfort to severe pain. Foreign bodies that have been lodged for a period of time are prone to cause infection and may be a source of sepsis in an otherwise young and healthy woman.

18. The amount of vaginal bleeding is often measured by the number of pads the woman uses over a period of time. If the patient describes using one pad every two hours, she is likely having more bleeding than if she used one pad every four hours. Patients who use one pad or more per hour are having severe bleeding and are at risk for developing hemorrhagic shock.

19. Patients with vulvovaginitis or pelvic inflammatory disease may report vaginal itching or pain. The pain of both conditions may increase with urination or sexual intercourse. Vaginal discharge is often described as being thick and having a foul odor.

20. Conditions that can cause vaginal bleeding are spontaneous abortion, threatened abortion, placenta previa, and placental abruption.

Fill in the Blank

21. metromenorrhagia
22. ectopic
23. spotting

24. introitus
25. miscarriage

Chapter 35

Case Study
Chief Concern

1. *What are some of the possible causes of the patient's abdominal pain?*

   Extrauterine causes of abdominal pain include appendicitis, bowel perforation, common gastroenteritis, diabetic ketoacidosis, kidney stones, and urinary tract infections.

2. *How can the pregnancy and the abdominal pain be related?*

   Pregnancy-related causes of abdominal pain include placental abruption, premature labor, and uterine rupture.

History

1. *What are the elements of the history of pregnancy?*

   Using the GPA system, this patient is a gravida 2, para 1, and abortus 0.

2. *What is the probable explanation for the abdominal pain when coughing?*

   The patient is probably experiencing round ligament pain, since the symptom complex matches.

3. *Using Naegle's rule, calculate the patient's last menstrual period.*

   With the expected date of delivery (EDD) of June 30th, the patient's last menstrual period would be September 23rd.

Examination

1. *What are the elements of the physical examination of a patient with suspected tachydysrhythmia?*

   The Paramedic should examine the abdomen of a pregnant woman using a "look, listen, and feel" approach. First, the Paramedic should observe the abdomen for bruising, which can occur because of falls. The Paramedic should then observe for fetal movement. Fetal movement is indicative—but not absolutely indicative—of fetal health. Next, the Paramedic should estimate the fundal height.

2. *Why is a fundal height a critical element in this examination?*

   While the quickening, fetal heart sounds, and detection of fetal movement all suggest a viable neonate (i.e., approximately 20 weeks), they are not dependable. When the fundus is at the umbilicus, the fetus is approximately 20 weeks and therefore potentially viable.

Assessment

1. *What diagnosis did the Paramedic announce to the patient?*

   Differentiation between common discomforts of pregnancy and potential complications of pregnancy is difficult since normal discomforts and physiologic adaptations of pregnancy often mimic more serious issues.

2. *Are there any non-pregnancy-related causes for the abdominal pain?*

   Pregnant women with abdominal pain often experience appendicitis as well as cholecystitis.

Treatment

1. *What is the standard of care of patients with potential pregnancy-related abdominal pain?*

   Supportive care is indicated. To treat the mother is to treat the fetus; therefore, the mother's welfare is most important for the fetus's survival.

2. *How can the Paramedic ascertain if the fetus is in distress and how can it be treated?*

   After 24 weeks it may be possible to appreciate fetal heart tones. If the Paramedic is able to count the heart beat, then the fetus is in distress and the Paramedic should consider fluid resuscitation.

Evaluation

1. *What are some of the predictable complications associated with laying a pregnant woman flat?*

   The symptom pattern (tachycardia, dizziness, cool and clammy skin) matches supine hypotensive syndrome.

2. *What is the treatment for this condition?*

   Place the patient in the left lateral recumbent position or manually displace the uterus off the vena cava if placing her in the left lateral recumbent position is not possible.

Disposition

1. *What is the most appropriate transport decision that will get the patient to definitive care?*

   The decision is premised on one of three factors. If the abdominal pain appears to be pregnancy-related, then the patient should probably be sent to a birthing unit equipped to handle obstetric emergencies.

   If the problem appears to be extrauterine, then the emergency department can be used to stabilize the patient, though birthing center nurses are often called down to help monitor the patient using fetal monitors.

2. *Would the destination change if the patient were to become unconscious?*

If the problem appears to be immediately life-threatening, as evidenced by hypotension, loss of consciousness, and so on, then the patient should be brought to a facility capable of emergency surgery (i.e., cesarean section). Most emergency departments are capable of performing an emergency cesarean section.

Practice Questions
Multiple Choice

1. a	9. b
2. d	10. b
3. b	11. a
4. d	12. d
5. c	13. a
6. d	14. d
7. b	15. b
8. d	

Short Answer

16. Supine hypotensive syndrome, also known as inferior vena cava syndrome, becomes more common in the third trimester. This condition commonly occurs when a pregnant woman lies in the supine position. The weight of the uterus and its contents compresses the inferior vena cava and aorta, decreasing venous return to the heart, which in turn causes arterial hypotension.

17. Extrauterine causes of abdominal pain include appendicitis, bowel perforation, common gastroenteritis, diabetic ketoacidosis, kidney stones, and urinary tract infections, to name a few.

18. Round ligament pain is a type of short, jagging, pelvic pain that occurs with change in position and is caused by the stretching of the round ligament (this is more common on the right side). The round ligament helps to support the uterus and is stretched by the expanding uterus. Round ligament pain can also occur with coughing, or even when the patient is rolling over in bed.

19. A shorthand system for documenting the obstetric and gynecologic history is GPA, which stands for gravid, para, and abortus.

20. TPAL is a system sometimes used for the obstetric history. In TPAL the T stands for number of term deliveries the mother has had, the P stands for the number of preterm births, the A stands for the number of abortions (both spontaneous and therapeutic), and the L stands for living infants.

Fill in the Blank

21. quickening	24. hyperemesis gravidarum
22. appendicitis	25. Naegle's rule
23. tocolysis	

Chapter 36
Case Study
Chief Concern

1. *How might a pregnant woman experience shock trauma differently from others?*

A pregnant woman can experience the same injuries as any other patient. Pregnant women have an increase in blood volume, about 35% to 40%, but a decrease in hematocrit (percentage of red blood cells in a volume of blood). Thus, these women can hemorrhage 15% to 20% without outward signs of shock. At approximately 25% blood loss, the woman will show the sympathetic-mediated consequences of hemorrhage.

A combination of venodilation and placental arteriovenous shunting lowers the resting blood pressure of healthy pregnant patients, who are at approximately 28 weeks, by about 30%, which is compensated by an increased heart rate of 15 beats per minute. This combination may lead the Paramedic to suspect compensated shock when none exists.

2. *How would the pregnancy affect the patient's breathing?*

The increasing size of the pregnant woman's uterus impinges the diaphragm, leading to an increase in respiratory rate (15%). During trauma, a combination of reduced functional capacity and increased oxygen demand can rapidly lead to hypoxia.

History

1. *What are the important elements of the history that a Paramedic should obtain?*

The Paramedic should try to ascertain the exact location of the pain, if possible (i.e., upper abdomen, mid-abdomen, or lower abdomen). Generalized pain with rebound tenderness and guarding may indicate peritonitis. Midline abdominal pain in the lower third of the abdomen suggests uterine involvement.

Complaints of pain should be either labor-like or not (i.e., waxing and waning similar to severe menstrual cramps and associated with pelvic fullness and/or back pain). The Paramedic should also inquire about fetal movement as well as the estimated date of delivery.

2. *What implication does the pain have along with vaginal discharge in a woman who is 28 weeks' pregnant?*

The vaginal discharge may be the result of placental abruption, urinary bladder disruption, or uterine rupture. The fluid could be the result of a "bloody show" from loss of the cervical plug or frank blood from the uterus.

Examination

1. *What are the elements of the physical examination of a pregnant patient with trauma?*

The abdomen, particularly the lower abdomen, should be inspected for ecchymosis, which is suggestive of seat belt injury. Next, the Paramedic should gently palpate the abdomen for tenderness, guarding, and uterine contractions.

2. *What are the elements of the physical examination of the fetus of a pregnant woman who has experienced trauma?*

Auscultation of fetal heart sounds should be undertaken if the patient is greater than 20 weeks' pregnant if, using Leopold's maneuvers, the lie of the fetus and the fetal spine can be determined. Minimally, the fundal height should be estimated, remembering that a fundus above the umbilicus generally means 20 weeks' gestation and potential fetal viability. Finally, the Paramedic should assess the pelvis for integrity.

Assessment

1. *What are the possible obstetric causes of bleeding in a pregnant woman* involved in a motor vehicle collision *at 28 weeks?*

The possible causes of internal bleeding in a trauma patient who is 28 weeks' pregnant are numerous. Obstetric-related causes include placental abruption and uterine rupture, to name just two.

2. *What are the possible non-obstetric causes of bleeding in a pregnant woman involved in a motor vehicle collision?*

Traditional non-obstetric causes of internal hemorrhage can be due to liver laceration and/or splenic injury, as well as pelvic and long bone fractures.

Treatment

1. *What is supine hypotensive syndrome and how is it treated?*

Past the 20th week the weight of the gravid uterus compresses the inferior vena cava, thereby reducing venous return and cardiac preload. This, in turn, reduces cardiac output and causes hypotension.

The obviously pregnant woman should be rolled into the left lateral recumbent position, the backboard should be tilted 15 degrees, or the uterus should be manually displaced. Vena cava syndrome can reduce cardiac output by over one-fourth.

2. *What is the standard of care for patients with bleeding during pregnancy?*

Beyond positioning on the backboard, standard trauma resuscitation is in order, including supplemental oxygen, assisted ventilation, and fluid resuscitation.

Evaluation

1. *Why is treating the mother important to fetal survival?*

   It has been estimated that the most common cause of fetal death, in over 75% of cases, is maternal shock.

2. *What safeguards does the fetus have against trauma?*

   The soft tissues of the uterus, coupled with amniotic fluid, absorb a considerable amount of energy in blunt trauma and save the fetus from injury in the process.

Disposition

1. *What is the most appropriate transport decision that will get the patient to definitive care?*

   In most cases, because of its low survival rate, a trauma arrest would be transported to the closest hospital.

2. *What special procedures are going to be carried out in the case of a pregnant woman who is in trauma arrest?*

   Most emergency physicians are capable of performing an emergency cesarean section. A perimortem cesarean section is considered if the mother has severe brain injury or a "nonresuscitable condition" such as trauma arrest. It is imperative that the CPR be continuous and that the cesarean section be performed within the traditional 5- to 10-minute window of brain death.

Practice Questions
Multiple Choice

1. d		9. a
2. a		10. a
3. c		11. c
4. a		12. c
5. b		13. a
6. a		14. d
7. a		15. d
8. b		

Short Answer

16. The adage goes, "Any female, of childbearing age, who presents with lower abdominal pain is pregnant until proven otherwise."

17. Not all cases of placental abruption present with vaginal bleeding. In fact, up to one-third of the cases of placental abruption do not present with vaginal bleeding. In those cases, the bleeding is sequestered behind the placenta as "hidden bleeding."

18. Diabetes complicates the pregnancy. Diabetes contributes to increased risk of developing pregnancy-induced hypertension, polyhydramnios (excessive amniotic fluid), a large-for-gestational-age baby with associated risks for delivery complications, postpartum hemorrhage, infection, and first trimester spontaneous abortion. There is also an increased risk for the need for cesarean section delivery.

19. Tocolytic agents include fluid bolus, magnesium sulfate, and specific beta/adrenergic agonists. Treatment with tocolytic drugs has not been shown to reduce preterm delivery; however, it can delay delivery for at least 48 hours.

20. The first therapy, a fluid bolus, is premised on the connection between antidiuretic hormone, oxytocin (the labor-inducing hormone), and the posterior pituitary gland. The posterior pituitary gland produces both but has limited production capabilities. Therefore, a fluid bolus challenges the posterior pituitary gland to produce antidiuretic hormone instead of oxytocin. The other agents—magnesium sulfate and beta/adrenergic agonists—work to cause smooth muscle relaxation. As the uterus is made of smooth muscle, these agents suppress the contraction of the uterus and slow delivery.

Fill in the Blank

21. incompetent

22. hydatidiform mole

23. scotomata

24. hemolytic anemia, elevated liver enzymes, low platelet count

25. tocolysis

Chapter 37

Case Study

Chief Concern

1. *How would a Paramedic assess a pregnant woman to see if she is ready to deliver?*

   Traditionally, the expected date of delivery is used. Additional information includes the frequency and duration of contractions as well as the "bloody show."

2. *How would the Paramedic ask about the woman's labor?*

   The woman's chief concern is usually the labor, so the Paramedic's first question should regard when the labor started. Some women may be uncertain of when labor started, as the early symptoms can be nondescriptive flu-like symptoms instead of classic labor. The woman's degree of discomfort is highly variable, depending on cultural and psychological factors. The Paramedic should be accepting of the pain regardless of the pain level the woman describes.

History

1. *What are the important elements of the history that a Paramedic should obtain?*

   With a minor adaptation, the Paramedic can use the SAMPLE method of history gathering to obtain the history of the pregnancy. Using the OPQRST/AMPLE format, the Paramedic should take a history of the labor pain.

2. *How would a Paramedic obtain an obstetric history?*

   Using either the TPAL or GPA system, the Paramedic should inquire about the history of the present pregnancy. Next, the Paramedic should inquire about medications, co-existing medical conditions, and so on, which are all questions that are part of AMPLE.

Examination

1. *What are the elements of the predelivery physical examination of a pregnant patient?*

   With proper draping in place, the Paramedic should check for crowning. Observing the introitus, the Paramedic should observe for blood, perhaps from placenta previa, prolapsed cord, and crowning (the appearance of the newborn's head during contraction).

2. *What are the elements of the predelivery physical examination of the fetus?*

   The Paramedic should try to auscultate heart sounds. Heart sounds above the umbilicus suggest it may be a breech delivery. Heart rates that are too fast to count indicate a healthy baby, whereas those less than 120 bpm may mean fetal distress and possible meconium aspiration. Next, the Paramedic should gently palpate the abdomen for signs of fetal movement.

Assessment

1. *What is the significance of the crowning and urge to move the bowels?*

   A pregnant patient's urge to push, or to move her bowels, coupled with crowning is indicative of imminent delivery. First-time mothers may take up to three hours of pushing to give birth in what is considered a normal labor. Imminent birth is suspected when rectal bulging, perineal bulging, defecation, and/or progressive visibility of the fetal head are observed.

2. *Why did the Paramedic ask the mother what position she would prefer to be in for the delivery?*

   She should be encouraged to assume a position that she finds most acceptable, while avoiding being flat on her back. Although lying supine in the lithotomy position may be convenient to the Paramedic, it is not—physiologically speaking—the best position for the patient. A good position for the mother to be in is the lateral recumbent position (Sim's position). Alternatively, the patient may prefer to squat or sit on the edge of a chair. This position takes advantage of gravity and helps the pelvis widen.

Treatment

1. *What equipment will be needed to deliver a baby?*

   The equipment needed—which should be set up on a sterile field, if possible—includes clamps (at least two are ideal), scissors for cutting the umbilical cord, a bulb syringe, oxygen and suction (if available), equipment for neonatal resuscitation, extra towels or pads, and personal protective equipment as well as adequate lighting.

2. *Explain the process of assisting with delivery.*

   As the head starts to emerge (crowning), the Paramedic should place a gauze pad against the perineum and apply gentle counterpressure with the pads of the fingers. As the newborn begins to crown in a normal head first, or vertex, delivery, the Paramedic should provide gentle pressure on the occiput or top of the baby's head to slow flexion. However, she should avoid applying any pressure to the infant's fontanels. If an umbilical cord is present around the neck, called a nuchal cord, the Paramedic has to judge whether the cord is tightly or loosely wrapped around the neck. If the cord is loose, it should be slipped over the baby's head. If the cord is too tight to slip over the baby's head, but loose enough to move (not tight around the neck), the umbilical cord should be slipped over the shoulders as the baby's body is born. At this point, the baby will change position to permit delivery of the shoulder and will externally rotate. The Paramedic supports the baby's head by placing a hand underneath it, without directing the head in any direction. The Paramedic will slide the posterior hand down the baby's body as the body delivers, keeping the head supported by the other hand or the forearm. She then places the baby immediately on the mother's abdomen, skin-to-skin, and dries the baby with a clean towel.

Evaluation

1. *What are the initial steps in neonatal resuscitation/newborn care?*

   With the newborn on the mother's abdomen, the Paramedic should vigorously dry the newborn with a towel. This serves the two-fold purpose of drying the infant (and thereby preventing hypothermia) as well as stimulating the newborn. If the newborn needs more stimulation to encourage it to breathe, then the Paramedic may elect to rub the newborn's back or smartly flick the soles of the newborn's feet.

2. *What is the APGAR score?*

   In the 1920s, Dr. Virginia Apgar developed a simple scoring method for purposes of trending a newborn's progress. This scale, called the APGAR score, takes into account the newborn's appearance, the newborn's pulse, reactivity via facial grimace, activity as a function of muscle tone, and respirations. These elements are rated on a 0 to 2 scale at one minute following birth and at five minutes of life.

Disposition

1. *What is the last stage of labor?*

   The last stage of labor is the delivery of the placenta. The placenta usually separates from the uterine wall within 5 to 10 minutes after the baby is born; however, up to 30 minutes is considered to be within normal limits. Signs of placental separation include a small trickle or sudden gush of blood and/or lengthening of the umbilical cord as it extrudes from the vagina. The Paramedic may note a change in the shape or contour of the fundus, and the woman may report a sense of fullness or urge to bear down again as well.

2. *What should the Paramedic observe on the placenta?*

   The Paramedic should examine the margins of the placenta. The margins should be relatively smooth and make a complete oval or circular shape. An incomplete placental detachment leaves partial products of conception in the uterus.

Practice Questions

Multiple Choice

1.	d	9.	a
2.	a	10.	a
3.	a	11.	c
4.	b	12.	a
5.	d	13.	a
6.	b	14.	a
7.	c	15.	c
8.	a		

Short Answer

16. It is essential that the Paramedic, before anything else, protect the patient's modesty, maintain a degree of privacy, and be empathetic. Childbirth, especially for a first-time mother, is a time of great anticipation and excitement. A misspoken word can be devastating to the patient–Paramedic relationship.

17. The needed equipment—which should be set up on a sterile field, if possible—includes clamps (at least two are ideal), scissors for cutting the umbilical cord, a bulb syringe, oxygen and suction (if available), equipment for neonatal resuscitation, extra towels or pads, and personal protective equipment.

18. As the head starts to emerge (crowning), the Paramedic should place a gauze pad against the perineum and apply gentle counterpressure with the pads of the fingers. This will allow for a slower distention of the perineum, reducing the risk of perineal lacerations. Some Paramedics may place the index finger just inside the birth canal and gently rub back and forth to help thin the perineum and to help prevent tears; this is referred to as *ironing* the perineum.

19. With the newborn on the mother's abdomen, the Paramedic should vigorously dry the newborn with a towel. This serves the two-fold purpose of drying the infant (and thereby preventing hypothermia) as well as stimulating the newborn.

20. After the placenta is delivered, the Paramedic should massage the fundus to decrease the risk of obstetric hemorrhage from uterine atony. Initially, the uterus will be soft or "boggy" and the Paramedic will have to massage the uterus until it is firm. To massage the uterus, the Paramedic "traps" the uterus by placing one hand at the top of the symphysis pubis horizontally and another at the top of the fundus of the uterus. The upper hand should massage the fundus of the uterus until it starts to contract, ultimately contracting to about the size of a softball and the consistency of a grapefruit. The fundus of the uterus should be at about the level of the mother's umbilicus when the uterus is firm.

Fill in the Blank

21. polyhydramnios

22. Braxton–Hicks contractions

23. meconium

24. uterine atony

25. amniotic fluid embolism

Chapter 38

Case Study

Chief Concern

1. *What are the issues that a normal newborn must overcome?*

   The pivotal issue the newborn must overcome to survive is the transition from dependence on the mother to physiologic independence.

2. *What are the newborn's first two challenges?*

   The newborn must achieve thermoregulation, in order to maintain an ideal body temperature. The newborn must also obtain glucose as a source of energy.

History

1. *What are the important elements of the history that a Paramedic should obtain?*

   The question of prenatal care is important. A nurse–midwife or physician might be aware of any congenital anomalies. The Paramedic should also inquire about the mother's health (i.e., gestational diabetes, pregnancy-induced hypertension, etc.), remembering she has two patients now.

2. *What are the risks associated with prematurity?*

   The complications of prematurity include retinopathy of prematurity, patent ductus arteriosus, hypoglycemia, sepsis, and respiratory distress syndrome secondary to hyaline membrane disease.

Examination

1. *What are the elements of the physical examination of a newborn?*

   The three H's of a newborn assessment are hypothermia, hypoxia, and hypoglycemia. With these three conditions assessed and corrected as needed, the Paramedic should proceed with a head-to-toe examination.

2. *Why is a head-to-toe examination a critical element in this evaluation?*

   Starting at the head, the Paramedic should look for signs of birth trauma to the skull, such as caput succedaneum and cephalhematoma. Moving to the face, the Paramedic should examine the child for dysmorphic features that may suggest Down syndrome or fetal alcohol syndrome as well as a cleft palate.

   Turning to the torso, the Paramedic should examine the chest for equal expansion (to rule out diaphragmatic herniation) and abdominal wall defects such as omphalocele and gastroschisis.

   Turning the newborn over, the Paramedic should examine for neural tube defects, such as meningocele. Finally, the Paramedic should examine the extremities for polydactyly and syndactyly.

Assessment

1. *What is the significance of "bonding"?*

   Maternal–child bonding is the first step in a life-long relationship. It is critical for a mother to accept and want to nurture a newborn. Failure to thrive is the diagnosis given to infants whose mothers did not bond with them.

2. *What is the importance of mother's first milk?*

   Mother's first milk, or colostrum, contains easily digestible nutrients as well as antibodies to protect the newborn during this transient period.

Treatment

1. *What is the APGAR score?*

   The APGAR is a score of newborn health and vitality that serves, initially, as a baseline, then as a trend of newborn progress with transition. Assignment of a "score" is based on five elements: appearance (color), pulse (heart rate), grimace (reflex irritability), activity (muscle tone), and respiratory effort. All five elements are evaluated at one minute of age and again every five minutes until a score of greater than or equal to seven is reached, or neonatal death has been declared.

2. *What is the treatment priority?*

   The treatment priority is to maintain the newborn's warmth.

Evaluation

1. *Why is a blood glucose reading important for a newborn?*

   Hypoglycemia is a common problem for the neonate, one the Paramedic must immediately address. Failure to address hypoglycemia can lead to developmental delays and even permanent neurological impairment.

2. *What is the treatment for hypoglycemia in a newborn?*

   A blood glucose of less than 40 mg/dL should be treated with a gentle infusion of either 2 to 3 mL/kg of $D_{10}W$ or, preferably, 5 mL/kg of D_5W. The Paramedic should perform repeat blood glucose measurements to monitor for rebound hypoglycemia.

Disposition

1. *What is the most appropriate transport decision that will get the patient to definitive care?*

   If the newborn had any of the aforementioned congenital anomalies, then the newborn should be transported to a hospital, one with a neonatal intensive care unit.

2. *Do all newborns need to be transported to the hospital?*

   If resuscitation has been used for more than the provision of supportive care, then the newborn should be transported to a hospital.

Practice Questions
Multiple Choice

1. c		9. b	
2. b		10. b	
3. c		11. d	
4. a		12. d	
5. c		13. d	
6. d		14. c	
7. d		15. d	
8. d			

Short Answer

16. The premature infant's lungs have not developed sufficient surfactant, a complex lipid–protein compound that reduces the surface tension of the fluid that covers the intra-alveolar space, so as to inflate the lungs at birth. The resulting atelectasis causes hypoxia.

17. The gastroschisis defect is typically lateral to the umbilicus, on the right side of the abdominal wall, and the bowel is external to the body without the covering membrane. The newborn should be kept as warm as possible. The Paramedic should apply a sterile, warmed, saline-soaked gauze pad to the abdomen, after which the abdomen is wrapped in sterile gauze to keep the sterile saline-soaked gauze in place.

18. To help prevent meningitis, and to protect the cyst, a sterile, warm saline dressing is applied to the area, which is then wrapped in additional sterile gauze. The newborn is then transported in the prone position (or any position that will keep pressure off the defect).

19. The newborn is placed on the maternal abdomen, skin-to-skin with the mother, to increase heat gain from the mother's abdomen. This also helps the infant avoid heat loss due to contact with cold surfaces. After the newborn has been placed on the mother's abdomen, the newborn is dried with a towel or blanket (preferably prewarmed), after which this wet cloth is set aside. A clean, dry cloth is then placed over the newborn. Paramedics use a swaddling technique to keep the newborn warm.

20. The complications of prematurity include retinopathy of prematurity, patent ductus arteriosus, hypoglycemia, sepsis, and respiratory distress syndrome secondary to hyaline membrane disease.

Fill in the Blank

21. congenital anomalies

22. macrosomia

23. cephalopelvic disproportion

24. spina bifida occulta

25. noncephalic

Chapter 39

Case Study

Chief Concern

1. *What are some of the possible problems of prematurity?*

   Problems of prematurity include neonatal respiratory insufficiency, neonatal hypothermia, and hypoglycemia.

2. *What is the implication of the patient's statement that the baby is blue?*

   Using a "hope for the best and treat for the worst" mentality, the Paramedic should be prepared to treat for neonatal respiratory insufficiency, hoping that the neonate has acrocyanosis.

History

1. *What are the important elements of the history of the delivery that a Paramedic should obtain?*

   The history of pregnancy should include the EDD, prenatal care, possibility of multiple births, and a determination if this premature birth was anticipated.

2. *What are the important elements of the maternal history that a Paramedic should obtain?*

   The maternal history should include gestational diabetes (suggestive of a macrosomic neonate with possible shoulder dystocia, among other issues) and pregnancy-induced hypertension, leading to preeclampsia and risk of seizures.

Examination

1. *What are the initial problems of transition that a newborn must overcome?*

   The premature neonate is at risk for apnea. The Paramedic must be prepared to stimulate the neonate, including the use of blow-by oxygen, and be prepared for secondary apnea, including assisted ventilation.

2. *Why is wrapping the preterm newborn in plastic wrap important?*

   The premature neonate has immature skin and is at extreme risk for hypothermia. The Paramedic should protect the skin with plastic wrap and then swaddle the neonate to preserve heat, plus add an additional heat source.

Assessment

1. *What is the most common "pathway" for newborn care?*

   Similar to pediatric care, neonatal resuscitation includes a sick vs. not sick aspect. If the neonate is sick, then the primary assessment (i.e., ABC) is in order, with the same "assess, then treat" approach at each level. Not sick neonates need warmth and time with the mother for bonding.

2. *What is the current thinking about meconium?*

   Current practice suggests that the newborn's condition—not the presence of meconium—should be the indication for emergent intubation and use of a meconium aspirator.

Treatment

1. *What is the standard of care for neonatal resuscitation?*

   The American Heart Association's neonatal resuscitation program has become the standard for neonatal resuscitation.

2. *What are some of the patient-specific concerns of a Paramedic during a neonatal resuscitation?*

   Patient-specific concerns include obtaining and maintaining an airway, ensuring adequate ventilation with prevention of apnea, and preventing hypoxia, hypothermia, and hypoglycemia.

Evaluation

1. *What are some of the predictable complications associated with neonatal resuscitation?*

   As maintenance of an airway and adequate ventilation, including exhalation of carbon dioxide to prevent acidosis, are critical, the Paramedic may elect to intubate. However, ventilation of the neonate is a delicate matter with predictable complications.

2. *What is a simple mnemonic to remember the complications of newborn intubation?*

Complications of newborn intubation can be remembered by the mnemonic DOPE: displaced endotracheal tube, obstruction, pneumothorax, and equipment failure.

Disposition

1. *What is the most appropriate transport decision that will get the patient to definitive care?*

Premature neonates need immediate transportation to a hospital with a neonatal intensive care unit, neonatologists, and neonatal nurses.

2. *Why must the heat pack be wrapped?*

The preterm newborn has fragile skin that may be easily burnt.

Practice Questions
Multiple Choice

1. a
2. b
3. b
4. a
5. a
6. d
7. d
8. d
9. a
10. c
11. b
12. b
13. c
14. d
15. b

Short Answer

16. Unlike adults, newborns do not shiver to produce heat. Instead, they rely on metabolism of brown adipose tissue for heat production.

17. Meconium aspiration syndrome causes respiratory distress in the neonate by creating an airway obstruction, causing surfactant dysfunction, and eventually leading to chemical pneumonitis.

18. To place an orogastric tube (OGT), the Paramedic typically selects an 8 French OGT and measures it from the bridge of the nose to the earlobe and then to the xiphoid process. This measurement can be done without interrupting ventilation. The OGT is then inserted through the mouth and placed into the stomach by advancing the OGT along the posterior pharyngeal wall (the esophagus is posterior to the trachea).

19. Directly after birth and resuscitation, the neonate should be swaddled in a clear plastic wrap, followed by warm dry blankets, to decrease insensible water loss through the skin and to help with thermoregulation.

20. Kangaroo care (i.e., placing the newborn to the mother's chest and swaddling mother and child) encourages skin-to-skin contact between mother and child and fosters maternal bonding. Kangaroo care has also been shown to help stabilize the newborn's temperature, breathing, and heart rate.

Fill in the Blank

21. neutral thermal
22. primary apnea
23. choanal atresia
24. fontanels
25. periventricular hemorrhage, intraventricular hemorrhage

Chapter 40

Case Study

Chief Concern

1. *What are the elements of the Pediatric Assessment Triangle?*

   The Pediatric Assessment Triangle consists of appearance (mental status), work of breathing (respiratory effort), and circulation (color).

2. *What is the utility of the Pediatric Assessment Triangle?*

   The Pediatric Assessment Triangle is most useful for younger pediatric patients and will allow the Paramedic to differentiate between those patients that require an immediate hands-on assessment and intervention and those that are stable enough so that more time can be taken in gaining the child's trust.

History

1. *What are the important elements of the history that a Paramedic should obtain?*

   The history obtained for a well/stable child is no different than that of an adult. However, the Paramedic must take into account the developmental differences and custom tailor the approach to the child and the circumstances.

2. *How is obtaining a history different with children of different ages?*

   For the toddler, the Paramedic should kneel down to talk with the child and the parent, looking the child in the eyes during the introduction. Speaking to the child before making physical contact will allow the toddler time to get comfortable with the Paramedic's presence and allow a more reliable physical examination.

   For the school-age child, the Paramedic should kneel down to the child's level to allow better eye contact and gain the child's trust. He should speak softly, calmly, and clearly while looking at the child, and use age-appropriate language, providing examples the child may understand. The Paramedic should be honest with the child and answer her questions to the best of his ability.

   For the teenager, the Paramedic should introduce himself to the patient first and then her caregivers. At this point, the Paramedic should be able to obtain most of the history directly from the patient.

Examination

1. *What are the elements of the physical examination of a pediatric patient?*

   The elements of the physical examination of a pediatric patient are the same as the elements of the physical examination of an adult.

2. *Is the pediatric patient's physical examination performed differently than an adult's?*

   One potential difference between the pediatric patient's examination and that of an adult is the order of the assessment. In an adult, the examination is usually head-to-toe, whereas in toddlers, preschoolers, and school-age children, the order may be toe-to-head.

Assessment

1. *What is used to decide sick versus not sick?*

   The Pediatric Assessment Triangle assists the Paramedic in rapidly differentiating between pediatric patients who are critically ill and those who are not critically ill.

2. *What creates the urgency in this case?*

   The child experienced an unexplained syncope. The syncope could be the result of a seizure, which has many ominous implications.

Treatment

1. *How is the treatment of pediatric patients different from treating other patients?*

   The use of appropriately sized pediatric equipment is essential to properly care for pediatric patients. The physical proportions of pediatric patients are different than those of adult patients.

2. *How is the treatment of pediatric patients similar to treating other patients?*

The primary assessment and treatment (i.e., airway, breathing, and circulation) remain the same for both pediatric and adult patients, as do the advanced life support priorities.

Evaluation

1. *What are some of the predictable complications associated with pediatric care?*

In adults, the transition from normal perfusion to compensated shock and then to decompensated shock occurs fairly smoothly and rapidly. In contrast, the pediatric patient will compensate for a longer period of time and then suddenly decompensate, sometimes progressing rapidly to cardiopulmonary arrest in a matter of minutes.

2. *What is the primary cause of decompensation in children?*

The primary cause of pediatric decompensation is respiratory failure. For this reason, the Paramedic should remain vigilant for signs of respiratory distress.

Disposition

1. *What is the most appropriate transport decision that will get the patient to definitive care?*

The disposition of pediatric patients often varies from community to community. Some communities have a dedicated pediatric emergency department, either as part of a small number of freestanding pediatric hospitals or as part of a larger general hospital. However, some communities do not have a separate pediatric emergency department.

2. *Does the destination decision change if the child has special needs?*

Special care needs of the patient (e.g., multisystem trauma or conditions requiring subspecialty care) may dictate transport directly to a tertiary care center. In some areas, emergency departments may be categorized by pediatric capability where not all emergency departments are credentialed for pediatric patients.

Practice Questions
Multiple Choice

1. a
2. d
3. b
4. c
5. a
6. c
7. d
8. a

9. c
10. b
11. a
12. d
13. b
14. b
15. b

Short Answer

16. The Pediatric Assessment Triangle is most useful for younger pediatric patients and will allow the Paramedic to differentiate between those patients that require an immediate hands-on assessment and intervention and those that are stable enough so that more time can be taken in gaining the child's trust.

17. TICLS stands for tone, interactivity, consolability, look/gaze, and speech/cry.

18. In the mnemonic FLACC, the F stands for face. Is the infant grimacing or calm appearing? The L and A stand for legs and arms. Are they thrashing, drawn up tightly, or generally relaxed? The first C stands for crying and the second for consolability.

19. Some parents choose not to have their children immunized due to religious beliefs or due to fears the vaccines are linked with autism and neurological diseases.

20. Delivery complications may include presence of Group B strep or active herpes, the need for an emergency cesarean section, poor APGAR scores, or other complications during the delivery process.

Fill in the Blank

21. developmental milestones

22. length-based tape

23. quick

24. dehydration

25. increased intracranial pressure

Chapter 41
Case Study
Chief Concern

1. *What are some of the possible causes of pediatric cardiac arrest?*

   Pediatric causes of cardiac arrest are varied but are closely linked with trauma, sudden infant death syndrome (SIDS), drowning, poisoning, choking, asthma or other lung diseases, foreign body aspiration, and pneumonia.

2. *What is the most common cause of pediatric cardiac arrest?*

   The most common cause of pediatric cardiac arrest is respiratory arrest.

History

1. *What are the important elements of the history that a Paramedic should obtain?*

   A detailed history of the present illness will provide the Paramedic with the clues necessary to direct the treatment. However, this is not always possible in the case of cardiac arrest. The Paramedic will often have to rely on caregivers, such as parents and coaches, or teammates and even bystanders to provide a history as most critically ill children will not be able to provide a sufficient history themselves.

2. *What may be the significance of being hit in the chest by a line drive?*

   Abnormal heart rhythms or arrest caused by blunt trauma, such as a line drive to the chest with a baseball or by a hockey puck, is called cordis commotio.

Examination

1. *What are the elements of the physical examination of a child in cardiac arrest?*

   The physical examination of the child in cardiac arrest relies on the primary assessment.

2. *If time permits, what other physical examination should be performed?*

   If there is time following the primary assessment, the Paramedic should perform a rapid head-to-toe examination.

Assessment

1. *What diagnosis did the Paramedic announce to the patient's mother?*

   In the case of cardiac arrest, the diagnosis is rather obvious. What is more difficult to answer is the child's chance for return of spontaneous circulation or complete neurological recovery.

2. *Should the mother be allowed to accompany her son?*

   In most cases, it may be appropriate for the mother to accompany her son. However, if there are any concerns about crew safety, or the mother's interference with patient care, then alternative transportation (e.g., with law enforcement) should be considered.

Treatment

1. *What is the standard of care for tachydysrhythmia in pediatric patients?*

   After ensuring a patent airway, and initiating rescue breathing, the Paramedic should begin cardiac compression at a rate of 100 compressions per minute, depressing the sternum one-third to one-half of the depth of the chest with the heel of one hand. Interruptions of compressions should be minimal.

2. *Should the child be cardioverted?*

   Based on the American Heart Association's standard treatment algorithm for pediatric pulseless cardiopulmonary arrest, the child should be cardioverted with 2 joules per kilogram. This should be followed with epinephrine and, in this case, magnesium sulfate.

Evaluation

1. *What is the treatment for return of spontaneous circulation?*

   In the setting of successful return of spontaneous circulation at any time during the resuscitation, the Paramedic should reassess the child's airway, breathing, and circulatory status. If the airway is not patent, the Paramedic should place an advanced airway to maintain patency. If the patient has inadequate spontaneous respirations, the Paramedic should continue to ventilate the patient to ensure appropriate oxygenation and ventilation. If signs of poor perfusion are present, the Paramedic administers a fluid bolus and reassesses the response.

2. *What is therapeutic hypothermia?*

   Therapeutic hypothermia is the deliberate cooling of the body to slow metabolic processes and allow the body time to recover from the shock.

Disposition

1. *What is the most appropriate transport decision that will get the patient to definitive care?*

   Critically ill children should be taken to the closest appropriate pediatric-equipped emergency department. If a specialized pediatric emergency department is within a reasonable transport distance, it may be appropriate to transport the patient directly to the pediatric emergency department rather than the closest facility.

2. *Are there any special considerations needed as a result of the use of therapeutic hypothermia?*

   Once therapeutic hypothermia has been introduced, the receiving facility must be capable of continuing it for a minimum of 24 hours.

Practice Questions
Multiple Choice

1. c
2. a
3. c
4. a
5. c
6. d
7. b
8. c
9. d
10. d
11. c
12. a
13. d
14. c
15. b

Short Answer

16. A fever is defined as a body temperature above 38°C or 100.4°F in an infant younger than 30 to 60 days old.

17. The three additional elements of the history of present illness for a child are birth history, developmental history, and immunizations.

18. To calculate the normal low systolic blood pressure of a child, double the child's age in years and add 70.

19. All children, regardless of age, should look toward or make eye contact with the Paramedic as she approaches and makes physical contact. The Paramedic may assume a child without a history of cognitive and developmental delay who does not make eye contact or acknowledge the Paramedic has altered mental status until proven otherwise.

20. The Paramedic may use an anterior–posterior approach when using adult paddles in a pediatric arrest. The Paramedic should place one electrode posterior on the patient's back and the second anterior, just left of the sternum.

Fill in the Blank

21. respiratory failure
22. cordis commotio
23. acrocyanosis
24. sudden infant death syndrome
25. long QT syndrome

Chapter 42

Case Study

Chief Concern

1. *What are some of the possible causes of the child's fever?*

   Fever is one of the most common medical concerns for children. Causes of fever range from the common ear infection (otitis media) to meningitis. The usual sources of fever are upper respiratory infections, gastrointestinal infections, and urinary tract infections.

2. *How can the fever and the seizure be related?*

   Fever can induce seizure, particularly in children. The etiology of the seizure can be directly related to the fever (i.e., primary causation), or the fever (and subsequent seizure) can be secondary to an underlying infection, such as meningitis.

History

1. *What are the important elements of the history that a Paramedic should obtain?*

   The standard OPQRST mnemonic, modified for fever, is sufficient: when did the fever start, what other symptoms did the child have (i.e., URI or UTI), have there been changes in the fever's quality, is the child taking any antipyretics for relief, how high was the temperature (what was its severity), and when was the temperature taken? There are three additional elements in the history of an infant: birth history, immunization history, and mother's smoking history. As a potential etiology of a febrile seizure is meningitis, the Paramedic should first examine the child for signs of meningitis, a potentially life-threatening condition. As viral illness is the predominant cause of febrile seizures, the Paramedic should assess the child for symptoms such as myalgia, headache, and so on.

2. *Why are immunizations an important part of the fever history?*

   Although it is unlikely, as most school-age children are required to have certain immunizations, young children and children of immigrants may not have had the required immunizations. Therefore, classic childhood infections, such as mumps, measles, rubella, pertussis, and so on, may be the source of the infection.

Examination

1. *What are the elements of the physical examination of a patient with suspected febrile seizure?*

   As a potential etiology of a febrile seizure is meningitis, the Paramedic should first examine the child for signs of meningitis, a potentially life-threatening condition. However, as upper respiratory infections and ear infections (otitis media) are the more common etiologies of pediatric fever, the Paramedic should assess for catarrhal signs and signs of an ear infection.

2. *Why is a blood glucose a critical element in this examination?*

   While hypoglycemia may be the etiology of a seizure, the fever may simply be a distracter (red herring). The seizure itself may have induced hypoglycemia and the "post-ictal" period may actually be attributed to hypoglycemia.

Assessment

1. *What diagnosis did the Paramedic announce to the patient's mother?*

   The Paramedic should advise the mother that the child has had a febrile seizure and that febrile seizures are not uncommon, as some 5% of children have a febrile seizure before their fifth birthday.

   However, the Paramedic should be aware that febrile seizures in those children who are less than 1 year of age and triggered by a temperature less than 39°C have an increased mortality.

2. *How does the Paramedic answer the mother's question about epilepsy?*

   Although the child with a febrile seizure is at risk, the risk is very low unless there is a family history of seizure or the child has a developmental delay.

Treatment

1. *What is the standard of care of patients with suspected febrile seizure?*

   Generally, care is supportive. If the child is overheated, then the patient's clothing should be removed. Antipyretics are generally not administered in the field.

2. *What is the danger of cooling the child too quickly?*

Caution is advised to not chill the child and induce shivering. Shivering actually increases the child's temperature.

Evaluation

1. *What are some of the predictable complications associated with febrile seizures?*

The saying goes that "seizure begets seizure." In other words, the Paramedic must be prepared for repeated seizure activity. Approximately one-third of children with a febrile seizure will have a reoccurrence, particularly if the child is young, had a relatively low temperature at the time of the seizure, or experienced a brief time between onset of fever and seizure.

Disposition

1. *What is the most appropriate transport decision that will get the patient to definitive care?*

While most febrile seizures can be managed at any emergency department, pediatric patients with repeated febrile seizures may need to be hospitalized, preferably in a children's hospital with pediatricians and pediatric nurses.

2. *What are some medication administration routes for benzodiazepines in children?*

Diazepam and midazolam, two commonly used benzodiazepines, can be administered to children intravenously, via interosseous routes, or per rectum. Midazolam can be administered intranasally as well.

Practice Questions
Multiple Choice

1. b
2. a
3. a
4. c
5. a
6. b
7. d
8. b
9. a
10. d
11. a
12. b
13. d
14. a
15. c

Short Answer

16. In fetal circulation, oxygenated blood starts at the placenta, travels along the umbilical vein, and follows the ductus venosus around the liver and into the inferior vena cava. This oxygenated blood flows through the foramen ovale into the left side of the heart and is pumped out the aorta into the fetal circulation. Deoxygenated blood returns to the right atrium and flows into the right ventricle. Rather than circulating through the lungs, the majority of the deoxygenated blood flows from the pulmonary artery through the ductus arteriosus and into the aorta. This deoxygenated blood flows back to the placenta via the two umbilical arteries.

17. Cystic fibrosis is a genetic condition in which the patient has increased viscosity of mucosal secretions among other enzymatic and autonomic nervous system dysfunctions. Specific respiratory system issues of patients who have cystic fibrosis include chronic respiratory infections due to the inability to clear the secretions as effectively as a person without cystic fibrosis.

18. Status asthmaticus is a severe prolonged asthma attack with significant air trapping and respiratory distress that does not respond to usual treatment aimed at bronchodilation and decreasing inflammation.

19. Croup is most commonly seen in children 3 months to 3 years of age, although it can be seen in older children as well.

20. Status epilepticus traditionally has been defined as seizure activity which lasts for 30 minutes with or without treatment or two seizure episodes without a return to normal mental status in-between seizures.

Fill in the Blank

21. TET spells
22. acyanotic heart disease
23. croup
24. failure to thrive
25. hyaline membrane disease

Chapter 43

Case Study

Chief Concern

1. *What is the implication of domestic violence and child abuse?*

   Violence often begets violence. If domestic violence is seen as acceptable, then child abuse may also be seen as acceptable.

2. *What connection does domestic violence have to a child with a fever of unknown origin?*

   There may be no connection; however, if the infant is lethargic the parents may be trying to convince the Paramedic the lethargy is from the fever as opposed to shaken baby syndrome.

History

1. *What are the important elements of the history that a Paramedic should obtain?*

   While preparing the infant for transport, the Paramedics in this case should obtain a standard SAMPLE history including a search for chronic medical conditions that might explain his size, such as an inborn error of metabolism.

2. *What is the implication assumed when the mother changes her mind about EMS as soon as the police arrive?*

   It might be assumed that the mother does not want EMS to uncover any child abuse that could be reported to the police.

Examination

1. *What are the elements of the physical examination of a patient with suspected failure to thrive?*

   While performing a head-to-toe secondary assessment, the Paramedic should look for signs of dehydration (such as poor turgor and sunken fontanels) and malnutrition (such as muscle wasting).

2. *What is a good indicator of good nutrition?*

   The hair is an excellent indicator of overall health. Sparse or coarse hair may mean malnutrition as well. The use of the age-based pediatric tapes may help to establish normal growth.

Assessment

1. *What diagnosis did the Paramedic announce to the patient's mother?*

   While the Paramedic has an order for transport, the Paramedic should emphasize that the child may be ill and must be seen in the emergency department.

2. *Should the Paramedic address the question of malnutrition on-scene?*

   The Paramedic's first priority should be the immediate care of the child. Therefore, the problem of malnutrition should be reported to the emergency department staff to be addressed in a timely manner.

Treatment

1. *What is the standard of care of patients with suspected failure to thrive/neglect?*

   Treatment in the case of suspected child abuse should proceed as normal, focusing on the chief concern and transporting the patient to the hospital for further treatment.

2. *Should the Paramedic approach the mother with an accusation of child abuse?*

   It is not the Paramedic's place—nor does a Paramedic have the education and preparation—to therapeutically intervene when child abuse is suspected.

Evaluation

1. *Does the mother's second refusal raise the level of concern that the police need to be involved?*

   For the refusal of health care to rise to the level of physical neglect, the parent(s) must fail to provide (or allow) needed medical care in accordance with physician recommendations.

2. *Could the Paramedic assume custody of the child?*

   Paramedics should enlist the assistance of law enforcement officers or child protective services to convince the parent(s) that medical care is necessary.

Disposition

1. *Jamila has never reported child abuse and she is concerned about liability. What facts should the supervisor provide to Jamila?*

   In many states, the failure to report suspected child abuse can expose the Paramedic to both criminal and civil penalties including imprisonment and fines. However, to encourage reporting, Paramedics who report suspected child abuse in good faith are granted immunity from liability.

2. *Why is it important to get both the parent's report as well as the Paramedic's report?*

   Paramedics are often the first "reporters" of child abuse, reporting the explanations offered to them. An abusive parent may collaborate with others or with the child to fabricate a story to explain the injuries. This deceit is often discovered when the physician compares the Paramedic's report to the parent's report.

Practice Questions
Multiple Choice

1. d		9. b	
2. c		10. d	
3. d		11. b	
4. d		12. c	
5. b		13. a	
6. a		14. d	
7. a		15. b	
8. c			

Short Answer

16. Every child in the United States has a right to nourishing food, proper clothing, and a safe shelter to rest in at night as well as an education which helps in preparation for the future. Perhaps more importantly, a child should grow up in an environment without fear, especially fear of harm at the hands of loved ones and caregivers.

17. Federal law defines child abuse as any act, or failure to act, on the part of responsible adults which results in death, serious physical or emotional harm, sexual abuse or exploitation, or an act or failure to act which presents an imminent risk of serious harm.

18. These acts permit the parent, or legal guardian, to relinquish care of the newborn to a "safe haven" such as a public safety agency. Typically, the individual is not asked for a name or any other identifying information.

19. In order to gain attention for themselves, a parent may either fabricate or induce an illness in the child so that medical professionals will have to treat it. This is called Munchausen by Proxy.

20. An excited utterance occurs when a person makes a statement while in the excitement of an event. This statement may be allowed into evidence. Not only is the verbal utterance considered a statement but the child's demeanor also has meaning.

Fill in the Blank

21. sexual abuse

22. sexual exploitation

23. enuresis, encopresis

24. failure to thrive

25. sexual assault nurse examiner

Chapter 44
Case Study
Chief Concern

1. *What are some of the serious causes of abdominal pain in the elderly?*

   Serious causes of abdominal pain in the elderly include appendicitis, small bowel obstruction, and peptic ulcer disease.

2. *What are some potentially life-threatening causes of abdominal pain in the elderly?*

   Some potentially life-threatening causes of abdominal pain in the elderly are aortic aneurysms, mesenteric bowel ischemia, and peritonitis.

History

1. *What are the important elements of the history that a Paramedic should obtain?*

   Beyond the normal OPQRST history taken for those with abdominal pain, the Paramedic should take a careful stool history (i.e., history, frequency, color, last movement).

2. *What questions should the Paramedic ask about the medication history?*

   The Paramedic should ask for a complete history of medications, especially use of opiates. Opiates are known to cause constipation.

Examination

1. *How could Mrs. Johnson be in shock?*

   First, bowel obstructions can sequester large volumes of body fluid in the protuberant abdomen, leading to hypovolemia.

2. *What is another danger of bowel obstructions?*

   A bowel perforation can lead to septic shock. The elderly patient's diminished inflammatory response may not produce the typical signs associated with septic shock.

Assessment

1. *What are some explanations for Mrs. Johnson's shock?*

   An elderly patient with signs of shock and no obvious reason for hypovolemia must be evaluated for occult bleeding, dehydration, vasogenic (septic) shock, hypoxia, and cardiogenic shock.

2. *What are complicating factors that make ascertaining the source of the shock more difficult in the elderly?*

   Many elderly patients have a decreased sense of pain, as well as an altered physiologic response to infection, including absence of fever.

Treatment

1. *What are the concerns about using "standard care" for elderly patients?*

   Elderly patients are more fragile. For example, a simple fluid bolus may be too much for their cardiovascular system, putting them at risk for congestive heart failure. Every treatment should be considered carefully with an understanding of the unique physiology of the elderly.

2. *How might treating the elderly be different from treating others?*

   In many cases, "standard" doses of medications are hazardous to the health of the elderly patient. These medications may need to be re-dosed to be weight-related or age-related.

Evaluation

1. *Why would the elderly be prone to an AMI?*

   By age 70, approximately 70% of individuals will have significant atherosclerosis, including asymptomatic disease.

2. *Why would elderly female patients be prone to an acute myocardial infarction?*

   Elderly, post-menopausal females, without the protection of hormones, can develop atherosclerosis. These elderly women tend to not have the typical signs of an AMI but rather are particularly prone to "silent MI."

Disposition

1. *What is the most appropriate transport decision that will get the patient to definitive care?*

   If specialty care is not required, then the patient should be transported to the hospital her physician is affiliated with to ensure continuity of care, especially when the patient has a complex medical history and conditions.

2. *What happens if the patient is unstable?*

   A patient who has critical airway, breathing, or circulation issues must be taken to the closest appropriate facility unless the patient can be stabilized and taken to her usual facility.

Practice Questions
Multiple Choice

1. c		9. d	
2. d		10. d	
3. c		11. b	
4. d		12. d	
5. a		13. a	
6. c		14. d	
7. b		15. d	
8. d			

Short Answer

16. Geriatrics is the study of all aspects of aging, including the psychological, pathological, economic, and sociological problems connected with aging.

17. Dementia is a gradual cognitive decline as a patient's medical condition progresses. In contrast, delirium occurs as an acute and typically reversible change in mental status from the patient's baseline mental status.

18. Kyphosis, an increase of the normal forward curve of the thoracic spine, can result from a number of processes, including normal loss of muscle tone, osteoporosis, arthritis, ankylosing spondylitis, and tumors, among other things.

19. Brain atrophy and decreased brain size increase the risk of subdural hematomas due to stretching of the bridging veins that span the space from the dura to the brain tissue.

20. Although the maximum size of the lungs (total lung capacity) does not change with age, functional residual capacity (FRC) and residual volume (RV) both increase so that inspiratory capacity (IC) and vital capacity (VC) both decline.

Fill in the Blank

21. dialysis	24. polypharmacy
22. diverticulitis	25. dysrhythmia
23. presbyopia	

Chapter 45

Case Study

Chief Concern

1. *What are some potential causes of shortness of breath for the ventilator-dependent patient?*

   The most obvious cause of shortness of breath is infection, as iatrogenic ventilator infections are common.

2. *What are some non-ventilator causes of shortness of breath?*

   The shortness of breath may be due to a respiratory disease, such as asthma, or backward heart failure. Fortunately, the care of these conditions is unchanged despite the presence of a ventilator.

History

1. *What are some alarms on a home ventilator?*

   Home ventilators have oxygen alarms, battery alarms, and airway pressure alarms that ensure correct ventilation.

2. *What should the Paramedic do when the ventilator alarm sounds?*

   Whenever the alarms sound, the patient should be disconnected from the ventilator and manually ventilated with a bag–mask assembly until the source of the problem can be identified.

Examination

1. *What are the elements of the physical examination of a ventilator-dependent patient?*

   The examination should start with the patient as the Paramedic assesses for signs of respiratory infection and/or backward failure.

2. *What are the Paramedic's first assessment priorities?*

   As always, the patient's airway, breathing, and circulation are assessed first, followed by a secondary assessment for medical conditions that would cause shortness of breath.

Assessment

1. *What diagnosis did the Paramedic announce to the patient?*

   The development of a paramedical differential diagnosis and impression is the same for patients with special challenges as for patients without those challenges.

2. *What is different in the Paramedic's differential diagnosis of a technology-dependent patient?*

   The only difference with technology-dependent patients is the Paramedic must always take into account the operation of those assist devices, considering malfunction and infection as possibilities.

Treatment

1. *What is the standard of care of patients with suspected ventilator/tracheostomy-related difficulty breathing?*

   The Paramedic may apply the mnemonic DOPE—where the D is for displacement, the O is for obstruction, the P is for pneumothorax, and the E is for equipment failure—as a method of determining the problem with ventilation.

2. *Should the Paramedic attempt to correct or reset the ventilator?*

   The Paramedic need not try to fix a ventilator, since BVM ventilation can sustain the patient until an expert is able to fix the ventilator.

Evaluation

1. *What are some of the predictable complications associated with a manual ventilation of the patient with a tracheotomy?*

   A pneumothorax is a constant concern. Overventilation can lead to barotrauma and pneumothorax. In Charlie's case, it appears that his simple pneumothorax might have progressed to a tension pneumothorax.

2. *What would be the treatment for this patient?*

   Treatment for Charlie includes a needle thoracostomy, assuming that assessment bears out the diagnosis of a tension pneumothorax.

Disposition

1. *What is the most appropriate transport decision that will get the patient to definitive care?*

   Ideally, the Paramedic will transport the patient with special challenges to the facility in which the patient receives most of his chronic care.

2. *Does the destination decision change if the patient is unstable?*

   In a situation of critical illness, the Paramedic may decide it is more appropriate to transport the patient to the closest facility for stabilization, especially if the patient's usual hospital is some distance away.

Practice Questions
Multiple Choice

1. a
2. a
3. c
4. d
5. b
6. a
7. b
8. a
9. d
10. a
11. a
12. a
13. b
14. b
15. c

Short Answer

16. The Paramedic may apply the mnemonic DOPE—where the D is for displacement, the O is for obstruction, the P is for pneumothorax, and the E is for equipment failure—as a method of determining the problem with ventilation.

17. Nerve stimulators are implanted devices that provide electrical pulsations to certain nerves in an effort to control epilepsy and other seizure disorders as well as treat chronic pain. Nerve stimulators have also been used to treat depression, urinary incontinence, Alzheimer's disease, and Parkinson's disease. Finally, nerve stimulators have also been used to treat hemiplegia from stroke.

18. Vascular access devices are central lines placed into the larger caliber subclavian vein, internal jugular vein, or femoral vein. These lines are larger caliber and often have several lumens, allowing simultaneous infusion of multiple medications.

19. Analgesia pumps provide continuous low level analgesia directly to the epidural space around the spinal cord. The pump, which may be implanted under the skin in the abdomen or may be external to the patient, is connected to a flexible catheter that is placed into the epidural space surrounding the spinal cord.

20. Insulin pumps are small programmable pumps approximately the size of a cell phone which hold a cartridge of insulin.

Fill in the Blank

21. Americans with Disabilities Act
22. fenestrated
23. Huber needle
24. Foley catheter
25. autism spectrum disorders

Chapter 46
Case Study
Chief Concern

1. *What is the significance of the pre-existing medical condition to the fall?*

   Chronic diseases, particularly those affecting neuromuscular function (such as muscular dystrophies or multiple sclerosis), may lead to a higher tendency toward trauma, particularly from falls.

2. *Why might there be a "no-lift" policy at the facility?*

Many facilities have adopted a "no-lift" policy for many reasons. One is to ensure the client is not injured during the fall. In this way, it recognizes the frailty of the elderly.

History

1. *What are the different elements of the history that a Paramedic should obtain in the medically fragile patient?*

The most important issue regarding a fall by the elderly is not the injuries sustained during the fall, although those are important, but rather why the patient fell in the first place. A simple trip and fall is understandable, but syncope before a fall could be a sign of a potentially life-threatening condition.

2. *What is the advantage of a MOLST?*

The MOLST form includes information about the patient's wishes related to artificial hydration and nutrition, antibiotics, and ventilator use. In the prehospital setting, the portions of the form related to CPR and intubation are the most pertinent in direct care decisions. However, relaying information from other parts of the form may assist the medical control physician in directing the Paramedic about intravenous and medication use or about BLS airway and ventilation measures.

Examination

1. *Why is the comparison between the patient's present condition and baseline important?*

It is important that an EMS provider question whether any abnormalities are consistent with the patient's baseline status. Asking about the patient's usual status and how things are different currently can be very helpful to the Paramedic in determining the severity of the problem at the present time.

2. *Why is it important to ask why EMS was summoned?*

It is helpful to ask a patient who has chronic symptoms why he or she decided to call EMS, since there is almost always some change in the symptoms that prompted the emergency call. This change may lead to a diagnosis.

Assessment

1. *Why is the staff members' input important?*

Staff members in these assisted living centers are most aware of ongoing changes in the patient's status.

2. *What diagnosis will the Paramedic announce to the patient?*

The Paramedic should explain to the patient that recurrent falls may be a symptom of a deeper underlying medical condition.

Treatment

1. *What is the standard of care for fluid resuscitation of an extreme elderly patient?*

Fluid administration needs to be monitored very closely in patients with ongoing cardiac, pulmonary, or renal problems because of the possibility of the patient developing pulmonary edema. Intravenous access should be considered because of the potential for deterioration. It can be difficult to obtain intravenous access on patients with chronic illnesses because of the disease process itself, or because they have needed frequent blood draws or intravenous treatments.

2. *What are some of the patient-specific concerns for spinal immobilization of the extreme elderly?*

Patient treatment can become more complicated in an extreme elderly patient. Spinal immobilization may be difficult in a patient with bony deformities such as kyphosis, or in a patient with a congestive heart disease history who experiences dyspnea when supine.

Evaluation

1. *What are some of the implications of the MOLST form?*

Early in an EMS call, the information on the MOLST form may not seem particularly pertinent because the patient may have a relatively minor injury or illness. However, because patients with chronic medical problems—especially those with significant cardiac, chronic lung, and renal problems—can deteriorate so quickly, it is prudent to transport the document to the hospital with the patient.

2. *What value does the MOLST form have for the Paramedic?*

If the patient's status worsens en route to the hospital, significant information about the patient's desire for resuscitation found on the form can provide direction to the Paramedic about whether to provide CPR if the patient proceeds to cardiac or respiratory arrest. Even if arrest does not occur, information about the patient's desires related to fluid administration or medications for nonlethal cardiac dysrhythmias can be relayed to the medical control physician for appropriate orders.

Disposition

1. *What is the most appropriate transport decision that will get the patient to definitive care?*

Chronically ill patients are more likely to need hospitalization or transport to an emergency department by ambulance. It is usually best to take patients to the hospitals where they have been treated previously so that their medical records—and in some cases, medical personnel who are familiar with their histories—are more readily available.

2. *Why is a good patient report important?*

Hospital admission, observation, and treatment may be more likely in many patients with chronic illnesses. The information that the Paramedic provides may assist in decision making for admission.

Practice Questions
Multiple Choice

1. c	9. c
2. b	10. a
3. a	11. d
4. c	12. c
5. b	13. d
6. c	14. d
7. c	15. a
8. d	

Short Answer

16. A patient is medically fragile if a minor illness or minor trauma adversely affects his health.

17. Hospice is a palliative care facility that provides patients with quality comfort care.

18. Almost all of the states have either an explicit recognition of immunity from civil and criminal liability for withholding resuscitative measures when a valid DNR/DNAR is available, or immunity is implicit in other portions of state health codes.

19. A durable power of attorney is in force even "after death" whereas the typical power of attorney is only in force during a patient's life.

20. Hospital admission, observation, and treatment may be more likely in many patients with chronic illnesses. The information that EMS provides may assist in decision making.

Fill in the Blank

21. medically fragile

22. healthcare proxy

23. assisted living

24. enriched living

25. hospice

Chapter 47

Case Study

Chief Concern

1. *What are some of the reasons that a college co-ed might press the panic alarm?*

   Sexual assault, in the form of nonconsensual sex is an unfortunate reality of college life.

2. *What are the forms of nonconsensual sex?*

   Both date rape and drug-facilitated sex are forms of nonconsensual sex.

History

1. *What are the important elements of the history that a Paramedic should obtain?*

   The assessment should include the patient's feeling of danger and lethality, the patient's safety concerns, the patient's present health status, a review of the patient's medications, a physical assessment for trauma and other signs of illness, an evaluation of level of consciousness (LOC), and the ABC principles.

2. *What resources could the Paramedic request to help on-scene?*

   While the patient's physical health is the first priority, many campuses have rape assistance programs and mental health counselors that may be part of the response to the scene of a sexual assault.

Examination

1. *What additional responsibilities does the Paramedic have during the physical examination of a patient with suspected violence?*

   The Paramedic's main responsibility is assessing for signs of domestic violence and sexual assault (i.e., choking, strangulation, ligature marks, bite marks, or burns).

2. *What responsibility does the Paramedic have in caring for the evidence?*

   The Paramedic must use caution and maintain the integrity of evidence (i.e., maintaining the chain of custody) while treating the patient.

Assessment

1. *What is the common sequela of sexual assault and rape?*

   The psychological sequela of sexual assault (rape) may include isolation, depression, anxiety, suicide attempts, and post-traumatic stress disorder (PTSD).

2. *What psychological symptoms might the patient manifest following a sexual assault and rape?*

   There are four common signs and symptoms: (1) reliving the experience, (2) social withdrawal, (3) avoidance, and (4) increased physiological arousal (somatic complaints).

Treatment

1. *What is the first priority of care of patients with suspected sexual assault?*

   The Paramedic should ensure that the "ABC's" are maintained.

2. *What is the other patient care priority?*

   The other priority is treatment focused on providing psychological "first aid" to the patient.

Evaluation

1. *What do the patient's behaviors represent?*

   Some women are demonstrative (i.e., crying or sobbing), whereas other women attempt to regain control of their emotions by appearing calm and collected. In both cases, the patient is trying to respond to an extreme stress.

2. *What is the Paramedic's responsibility during care and transport of the patient?*

   Since the traumatized patient is fearful, it is the Paramedic's responsibility to try to make the patient feel as safe as possible.

Disposition

1. *What is the most appropriate transport decision that will get the patient to definitive care?*

   If possible, the patient should be transported to a SAFE center. Sexual assault forensic examination (SAFE) centers provide victims of sexual assault with access to trained staff 24 hours per day 7 days per week to assist victims of sexual assault with forensic exams and other needed services. They are offered prophylactic post-exposure treatment for sexually transmitted infections (STI), including the HIV post-exposure prophylaxis (HIV-PEP) kit and hepatitis B virus (HBV) immune globulin. All victims who are considered fertile are offered emergency contraception (EC).

2. *What are the documentation standards for wounds?*

   The BEARS mnemonic is often used to document injuries to victims of sexual assault: B for bruises, tears, lacerations, and so on; E for ecchymosis/bruises; A for abrasions, R for redness, and S for swelling.

Practice Questions
Multiple Choice

1. d	9. a
2. b	10. d
3. c	11. c
4. d	12. d
5. d	13. d
6. d	14. d
7. d	15. c
8. d	

Short Answer

16. Youth violence has been defined as "the intentional use of physical force or power, threatened or actual, exerted by or against children, adolescents or young adults ages 10–19 which results in or has a high likelihood of resulting in injury, death, psychological harm, mal-development or deprivation."

17. The cycle of abuse is tension, crisis, and calm.

18. Rape is a crime of violence that involves the use (or threat) of force that is motivated by power, control, aggression, anger, and rage.

19. Sexual elder abuse has been defined as the coercing or the use of (or threat of) force against an elderly person to cause such person to engage in sexual acts against his or her will.

20. Some of the first steps in providing care to elderly victims of abuse are to accurately assess, treat, and stabilize. The next important steps are to identify signs of abuse and accurately document and report physical findings. Lastly, the prehospital medical personnel must also be astute and preserve evidence.

Fill in the Blank

21. intimate partner violence	24. adult protective services
22. sexual assault nurse examiner	25. elder sexual abuse
23. rape trauma syndrome	